Botulinum Toxin Treatment in Surgery, Dentistry, and Veterinary Medicine

Bahman Jabbari

Editor

Botulinum Toxin Treatment in Surgery, Dentistry, and Veterinary Medicine

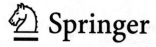 Springer

Editor
Bahman Jabbari MD, FANN
Professor Emeritus of Neurology
Yale University School of Medicine
New Haven, CT, USA

Clinical Professor of Neurology
University of California
Irvine, CA, USA

ISBN 978-3-030-50693-3   ISBN 978-3-030-50691-9   (eBook)
https://doi.org/10.1007/978-3-030-50691-9

This Springer imprint is published by the registered company Springer Nature Switzerland AG
The registered company address is: Gewerbestrasse 11, 6330 Cham, Switzerland

Preface

Over the past 30 years, botulinum toxins A and B have proved efficacious in treatment of the symptoms of a variety of chronic medical disorders. Currently, the FDA-approved indications of Botulinum Neurotoxin (BoNT) therapy include cervical dystonia, blepharospasm, hemifacial spasm, chronic migraine, adult and childhood spasticity, sialorrhea, axillary hyperhidrosis, neurogenic bladder, overactive bladder as well as aesthetic indications (frown lines, wrinkles, glabellar lines). The medical use of botulinum toxins have been discussed in several recently published books including three previous books of this editor.

For the past 15 years, an increasing number of publications have demonstrated the utility of BoNT therapy in post-surgical pain as well as in dentistry and veterinary medicine; hence, it became apparent that a book with information on these novel applications could benefit the medical community. This book, *Botulinum Toxin Treatment in Surgery, Dentistry and Veterinary Medicine*, is designed to provide updated information on the utility of BoNT therapy in these fields. In this book, the history of BoNTs is discussed in Chap. 1, molecular structure and mechanisms of actions in Chap. 2, differences in the variety of available BoNTs in Chap. 3 and the already established medical indications of BoNT therapy in Chap. 4. Chapters 5–15 discuss different surgical indications of BoNTs. Chapter 16 is on dentistry and Chap. 17 discusses indications in veterinary medicine. Chapter 18, Future Perspectives, addresses potential future uses of BoNTs in dentistry.

I am grateful to the authors of different chapters of this book who accepted to write various chapters in their busy schedule. Drs. Fattaneh Tavassoli and Shahroo Etemad-Moghadam furnished valuable editorial help. Tahereh Mousavi, M.D., and Damoun Safarpour, M.D., provided the drawings for this book. Carolyn Spence from Springer was the source of constant guidance and encouragement.

Hopefully, this book will help surgeons, dentists and veterinarian in their practice, ultimately benefitting the patients.

New Port Coast, CA, USA   Bahman Jabbari
February 9, 2020

Contents

Chapter 1
The History of Botulinum Neurotoxins: From 1820 to 2020

Bahman Jabbari

Abstract Nearly 200 years ago (1820), a young German physician Justinus Kerner predicted that the agent responsible for "sausage poisoning "could have therapeutic implications. The agent *Clostridium botulinum* was discovered at the end of the nineteenth century by the Belgian bacteriologist Emile Van Ermengem. Close to end of World War II, the toxin was isolated and purified by Lamanna and Duff and was prepared and produced for clinical use by Schantz. Allen Scott, following a series of studies in monkeys, published the first utility of botulinum neurotoxin (BoNT) in humans for correcting strabismus in 1980. The past 40 years witnessed the development of vast clinical indications of botulinum neurotoxin (BoNT) therapy. This chapter, in addition to the older historical data, also briefly discusses the contribution of some of contemporary basic scientists and clinical neurotoxicologists who are responsible for the therapeutic success of BoNT therapy in medical and surgical fields.

Keywords History of botulinum toxin · Sausage poisoning · Justinus Kerner · Van Ermengem · Allen Scott

Introduction

Nearly 200 years has passed since 1820 when Justinus Kerner published the first comprehensive account of botulinum toxin intoxication, then known as sausage poisoning. The part of southern Germany where Kerner was born and practiced medicine, Swabia (now Bavaria and Baden-Wurttemberg) had been experiencing outbreaks of "sausage poisoning" during the second half of the eighteenth century. These outbreaks increased during the Napoleonic Wars (1796–1813) when the ravished area suffered from poverty and smoking the sausage was performed under poor hygienic conditions. The issue of sausage poisoning was discussed during

B. Jabbari (✉)
Department of Neurology, Yale University School of Medicine, New Haven, CT, USA
e-mail: bahman.jabbari@yale.edu

© Springer Nature Switzerland AG 2020   1
B. Jabbari (ed.), *Botulinum Toxin Treatment in Surgery, Dentistry,*
and Veterinary Medicine, https://doi.org/10.1007/978-3-030-50691-9_1

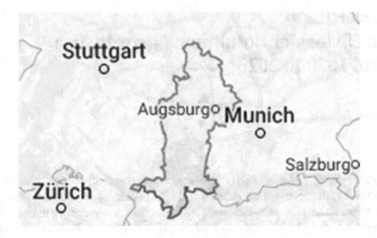

Fig. 1.1 Swabia with its capital Augsburg located between Munich and Stuttgart

these years in the Department of Medical Affairs of Kingdom of Wurttemberg several times seeking opinions from University professors in Tuningen and Stuttgart. A new outbreak in 1815, during which three of seven intoxicated patients died, further put demands on the medical community of the region to find the cause and remedy of sausage poisoning.

Justinus Kerner (Fig. 1.1), as a young physician and a native of the land, took an interest in the issue and first published a brief account of this illness in 1817. His more detailed paper of 1820 was based on observation of 76 patients. In this paper, Kerner described nearly all major symptoms of botulinum toxin intoxication, as we recognize today such as muscle weakness, paralysis of eye muscles, difficulty in swallowing, dry mouth, and some other signs of autonomic dysfunction. He then reported a larger observation on 155 patients in 1922. This was followed by a series of in vivo animal experimentations including a brief experiment on himself where he noticed severe dryness of the mouth after placing a small fragment of a spoiled sausage on his tongue. He concluded from his experiments that the toxin, potentially lethal, develops in the spoiled sausage in anaerobic milieu and exerts its ill effect mainly upon the motor and autonomic systems, sparing the sensory system (Fig. 1.2).

Kerner was the first to suggest that the "fatty toxin" in the spoiled sausage could find medicinal use in the future, especially in the area of hyperactive (hyperkinetic) movement disorders due to its muscle weakening effect; as an example, he mentioned the involuntary movement of chorea. Kerner also believed that, contrary to the common belief of the time that the culprit in the spoiled sausage was a chemical (fatty acid, prussic acid), it was probably a biologic (zoonotic) toxin.

We owe much of the information about Kerner to the German medical historian FJ Erbguth who has researched and described in detail Kerner's medical accomplishments in a series of articles [1–3]. Kerner was also an accomplished poet and avid traveler who was considered by Hermann Hesse – the Nobel Laureate of

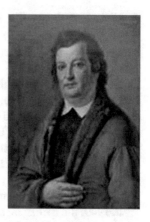

Fig. 1.2 Justinus Kerner 1786–1862. (From Erbguth reproduced with permission from Springer)

a

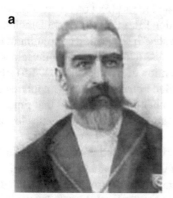

b

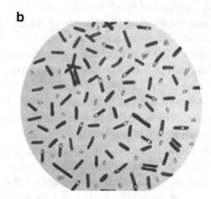

Fig. 1.3 (**a**) Emile Van Ermengem 1851–1932. (**b**) *Clostridium botulinum.* (From FJ Erbguth reproduced with permission from Springer)

Germany (1946) – as one of the three true German poets of his era. Interestingly, poisoning from blood sausage was recognized during the medieval era as well. The Byzantine emperor Leo the IV (750–780 AD) signed an order to stop the making and eating of blood sausage prepared in the pig stomach [4].

The next major event was the discovery of the responsible agent in 1895. On December 14, 1895, a group of 34 musicians who had attended a funeral became very sick and developed signs of botulism after consuming spoiled ham. Three of the 34 musicians died. The ham was sent to Emile Van Ermengem, professor of bacteriology at Ghent University, Belgium (Fig. 1.3a). Ermengem was able to produce similar signs of illness in animals after injecting them with the tissue containing the toxin. His microscopic examination revealed anaerobic Gram-positive, rod-shaped bacteria in the spoiled ham and tissue obtained from the dead musicians; he named the organism *Bacillus botulinus*, believing it to be the source of the culprit toxin in the ham (Fig. 1.3b).

In 1919, A. Burke from Stanford University published a paper on the serological types of botulinum toxins defining type A and type B toxins. In 1924, at the suggestion of Ida Bengtson, a Swedish-American bacteriologist, the name *Bacillus botulinus* was changed to *Clostridium botulinum*. The word clostridium is derived from Greek word "Kloster," meaning spindle. The genus *Clostridium* includes a group of anaerobic bacteria such as *Clostridium tetani* responsible for the production of tetanus toxin.

During World War II, all parties were very interested to purify and develop botulinum toxin both as a weapon and to find measures to protect the soldier in case of exposure. Close to the end of the war, James Lamanna and Richard Duff working at Fort Detrick, Maryland, a US Army facility, discovered a technique to crystalize and concentrate botulinum toxin. In 1946, Edward Schantz, working at the same facility, purified and produced a large amount of the toxin. Schantz then moved to the University of Wisconsin where, in collaboration with Erik Johnson (Fig. 1.4), he further refined the toxin and made it available for clinical research.

In 1949, the British investigator A. Burgen and his colleagues discovered that the paralytic effect of botulinum neurotoxin is related to its effect on the neuromuscular junction via blocking the release of acetylcholine [5]. In 1964, Daniel Drachman at Johns Hopkins using Schantz's toxin demonstrated that injection of botulinum toxin A into the hind limb of chicken's embryo can cause a dose-dependent muscle weakness and atrophy [6]. His work came to the attention of Allen Scott (Fig. 1.5) and his colleague Carter Collins, ophthalmologists in San Francisco, who were interested in improving strabismus in children by methods other than surgery. At that time, their research focused on injection of anesthetic agents into monkey's eye muscles under electromyographic guidance.

For the next decade, Dr. Scott, borrowing botulinum toxin from Edward Schantz laboratory in Wisconsin, conducted a series of experiments in monkeys by injecting the toxin into the extraocular muscles. His seminal publication in 1973 showed that injection of botulinum toxin can weaken the eye muscle of the monkeys, and this selective weakening had the potential of improving strabismus. His subsequent important work published in 1980 on 67 patients under an FDA-approved protocol demonstrated that BoNT injection into selected eye muscles can indeed improve

Fig. 1.4 Edward Schantz and Erik Johnson. (From Dressler and Roggenkaemper, reproduced by permission from Springer)

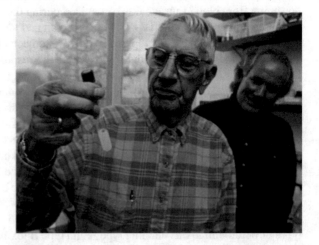

Fig. 1.5 Dr. Alan Scott who pioneered BoNT therapy in humans. (From FJ Erbguth reproduced with permission from Springer)

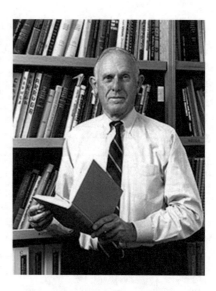

strabismus in human subjects [7]. During the 1980s in a number of small open label studies, Scott and his colleagues showed that injection of BoNTs into the face can improve hyperactive face movements such as blepharospasm and hemifacial spasm. Scott was also first to show that injection of 300 units of onabotulinumtoxinA (then called oculinum) in a single session (for spasticity) is safe, a safety margin that was not known prior to his observation [8].

These observations were of great interest to movement disorder specialists and led to conduction of several small blinded protocols by US (Fahn, Jankovic, Brin, and others) and Canadian (Tsui and others) investigators in the 1980s, ultimately resulting in FDA approval of botulinum toxin A in 1989 for blepharospasm, hemifacial spasm, and strabismus (based on Scott's work) (Table 1.1).

The initial name of oculinum used in earlier studies was changed to Botox, 2 years later, when Allergan Inc. acquired the right of the toxin distribution and marketing.

Along these clinical developments, our knowledge about the molecular structure of the toxin and where and how it works improved significantly through the tireless efforts of biologist and basic scientists; the contributions of some of them are described briefly at the end of this chapter (Fig. 1.6).

What happened next is one of the most amazing developments in clinical pharmacotherapy. A feared and lethal toxin was shown to be effective and relatively safe for treatment of a large number of medical and surgical conditions [9]. More recently, its use has been extended to the field of dentistry and veterinary medicine (Chaps. 16, 17, and 18 of this book). Other botulinum neurotoxins (incobotulinumtoxinA, abobotulinumtoxinA) and BoNT-B (rimabotulinumtoxinB) have found to be effective in several medical and surgical conditions as well. Newly developed botulinum toxins such as Korean toxin Meditox and Chinese toxin (Prosigne) have also shown promise in a number of neuropathic pain conditions [10]. A new form of

Table 1.1 Important timelines of botulinum toxin (BoNT) development for clinical use

Year	Investigator(s)/FDA approvals	Comment
1820–1822	Justinus Kerner	Describes details of botulism; predicted the toxin can be used in the future as medical remedy
1895	Emile Van Ermengem	Discovery of bacteria causing botulism
1944–1946	Lamanna and Duffy	Concentrated and crystalized the toxin
1946	Edward Schantz	Purified and produced the toxin in form suitable for medical research
1949	A. Burgen	Acetylcholine identified as the chemical blocked by BoNT at nerve muscle junction
1953	Daniel Drachman	Intramuscular injection Schantz's toxin can be quantified and causes dose-dependent muscle weakness in chicks
1973	Alan Scott	Injection of type A toxin improves strabismus in monkeys
1980	Alan Scott	Controlled human study showed efficacy in strabismus. Observations on potential use for blepharospasm, hemifacial spasm, spasticity
1985–1988	Fahn, Jankovic,Brin, Tsui	Controlled and blinded studies show efficacy in blepharospasm and cervical dystonia
1989	FDA approval of type A toxin (oculinum – name later changed to Botox)	Blepharospasm, hemifacial spasm, and strabismus
1989–present	FDA approved several other indications	Facial wrinkles, frown lines, cervical dystonia, chronic migraine, bladder dysfunction, upper and lower limb spasticity, axillary sweating

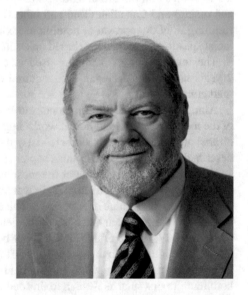

Fig. 1.6 Dr. James Rothman, Yale cell biologist who won the Nobel Prize in 2013 for his work on synapse physiology. His laboratory purified the SNARE complex

botulinum toxin A (prabotulinumtoxinA, Jeuveau) recently received approval for treatment of frown lines in the USA. Chapter 3 of this book describes the characteristics of available and marketed botulinum toxins as well as their similarities and differences. The list of US marketed botulinum neurotoxins, their clinical indication, and the year of FDA approval for each indication is presented in Table 1.2.

This brief account of botulinum toxin history will not do justice to the subject if it did not include significant contribution of recent contemporary basic scientists and clinical neurotoxicologists who have been instrumental for the current status of

Table 1.2 Clinical indications approved by FDA for botulinum toxins marketed in the USA

Generic and trade names	Abbreviation	Manufacturer	Approved indication (FDA)	Year of FDA approval
OnabotulinumtoxinA; Botox	OnaBoNT-A	Allergan Inc.; Dublin, Ireland	Blepharospasm	1989
			Hemifacial spasm	1989
			Strabismus	1989
			Cervical dystonia	2000
			Glabellar lines	2002
			Axillary hyperhidrosis	2004
			Chronic migraine	2010
			Upper limb spasticity	2010
			Neurogenic bladder	2011
			Lateral canthal lines	2013
			Overactive bladder	2013
			Adult lower limb spasticity	2016
			Forehead lines	2017
			Pediatric lower and upper limb Spasticity	2019
IncobotulinumtoxinA; Xeomin	IncoBoNT-A	Merz Pharma GmbH & Co; Frankfurt, Germany	Cervical dystonia	2010
			Blepharospasm	2010
			Glabellar lines	2011
			Adult upper limb Spasticity	2015
			Sialorrhea	2018
AbobotulinumtoxinA; Dysport	AboBoNT-A	Ipsen Pharmaceutical; UK	Cervical dystonia	2009
			Glabellar lines	2009
			Adult upper limb spasticity)	2015
			Pediatric lower limb spasticity	2016
			Adult lower limb spasticity	2017
			Wrinkles	2019?
RimabotulinumtoxinB; Myobloc/Neurobloc	RimaBoNT-B	US World Med-Solstice	Cervical dystonia	2009
			Sialorrhea	2010
PrabotulinumtoxinA Jeuveau	PraboBoNT-A	Evolus Inc.; Santa Barbara, CA	Frown lines	2019

BoNT therapy in 2020. Some of the most influential individuals in this field are discussed below. The list is by no means complete.

Biology and Basic Science

James E. Rothman, PhD, chairman of the department of cell biology at Yale University, revolutionized the field of cell biology by studying the molecular processes in a cell-free system. His work discovered many genetic and functional aspects of synapse physiology including vesicular trafficking, vesicular fusion, and proteins involved in this function. He identified genes and enzymes responsible for the budding of vesicles and their fusion with membranes. Dr. Rothman's laboratory succeeded in purification of the SNARE complex and provided pivotal evidence for establishing the central role of the SNARE complex (proteins targeted by botulinum toxins) in mediating membrane fusion. In 2013, Dr. Rottman was awarded the Nobel Prize in Medicine and Physiology.

Cesare Montecucco's first seminal work on BoNTs was the proposal of the double-receptor model in 1986 that is now well established for the majority of BoNTs. In 1992, he demonstrated that the common belief that the opposite symptoms of botulinum and tetanus toxins (flaccid versus spastic paralysis, respectively) are induced by different molecular actions is incorrect. In fact, the cleavage of a single protein is essential for the function of both toxins. The opposite symptoms are simply due to the different neurons targeted by tetanus and botulinum neurotoxins: the inhibitory interneurons of the spinal cord and the peripheral cholinergic neurons, respectively [11]. This was a major breakthrough in the understanding of the molecular pathogenesis of these diseases.

Gianmpietro Schiavo with a series of pioneering experiments, together with Cesare Montecucco, demonstrated that the inhibition of synaptic activity caused by tetanus and botulinum neurotoxins is due to a specific protease activity [12]. He showed that these neurotoxins cleave three synaptic proteins that play fundamental roles in neurotransmitter release. This discovery was instrumental for the field of SNARE biology and generated great interest worldwide. The seminal discovery of SNARE proteins as the substrates for BoNTs and TeNT in the early 1990s, led by Giampietro Schiavo and Cesare Montecucco, along with the groundbreaking work from James Rothman's laboratory on the purification of the SNARE complex, provided pivotal evidence for establishing the central role of the SNARE complex in mediating membrane fusion.

Matteo Caleo research on botulinum neurotoxins was devoted to their central effects. In collaboration with Cesare Montecucco in Padua and Gipi Schiavo in London, he demonstrated that BoNTs are retrogradely transported from the injected muscle along the axons of motoneurons and directly affect neurotransmission in central areas [13].

Ornella Rossetto's collaboration with Prof. Montecucco and Prof. Giampietro Schiavo led to the discovery of the zinc-endopeptidase activity of tetanus and botulinum neurotoxins and provided initial experimental evidence that the molecular basis of their exceptional specificity is based on a double recognition of the substrate, i.e., of the cleavage site and of other regions outside the cleavage site termed SNARE motif.

Zdravko Lackovic, chairman of department of pharmacology in Zagreb, Croatia, along with his colleagues **Ivica Matak, Lidjia Back-Rojecky, and Boris Filipovic** through a series of elegant experiments, provided strong evidence for the central action of botulinum toxins in the pain pathways [14, 15]. Their findings have improved our knowledge about the central analgesic mechanisms of botulinum neurotoxins in pain. Their contributions to this field have opened the path and encouraged many clinical neurotoxicologist to conduct controlled clinical trials in different pain disorders.

Oliver Dolley, research professor and director of the International Center for Neurotherapeutics (ICNT) in Dublin, has done multidisciplinary investigations on the molecular basis of communications in the nervous system searching for proteins responsible for the fundamental process of transmitter release and its indirect regulation of voltage-sensitive K+ channels. His investigations have provided important information on endocytosis of botulinum neurotoxins by glutamatergic and peptidergic neurons. His most recent work has focused on selective targeting of sensory spinal cord by different agents to achieve analgesia. He has been successful in producing analgesia in rats by using a novel A/E toxin chimera [16].

Pietro De Camilli, MD, PhD

Dr. De Camilli is professor of neuroscience and cell biology at Yale University and founding director of the Yale Program in Cellular Neuroscience, Neurodegeneration, and Repair. His research has provided insight into mechanisms of membrane fission and has revealed ways through which membrane-associated proteins can generate, sense, and stabilize lipid bilayer curvature. His discovery and characterization of the role of phosphoinositide metabolism in the control of endocytosis have broad implications in the fields of phospholipid signaling and of membrane traffic. Dr. De Camilli and his collaborators were to first to discover that the synapse protein targeted by BoNT-A is SNAP-25 [17].

Neurologists: Clinical Neurotoxicologists in the USA

Joseph Jankovic, MD

Joseph Jankovic MD, professor of neurology at Baylor College of Medicine, is probably the most influential clinician/neuroscientist in discovering and promoting different clinical indications for the use of botulinum neurotoxins in medicine. He has contributed, often as a leader, in many well-designed clinical trials with botulinum toxins for different indications. His rating scale for blepharospasm is widely used specially in clinical trials of botulinum toxins. He is an outstanding teacher, who over the years has trained many fellows and young physicians for proficiency in botulinum toxin treatment. As a prolific writer, his list of publication in Medline as of February 1, 2020, includes 177 articles on the subject of botulinum neurotoxins. Dr. Jankovic has held many important positions in national and international toxin-related forums. He is the recipient of lifetime achievement award at the international Toxin conference in 2019.

Mark Hallett, MD
Dr. Mark Hallett is Chief human motor control section in NINDS, National Institutes of Health at Bethesda, Maryland. As an internationally renowned figure in the field of movement disorders and clinical neurophysiology, Dr. Hallett has provided evidence that intramuscular injection of botulinum toxins changes the electrophysiology of muscle, peripheral nerves, and central nervous system. Under his watch, botulinum toxin treatment of movement disorders developed in NIH. Young and brilliant faculties such as Leonard Cohen, Barbara Illowsky Karp, Cordin Lungu, and Kathrine Alter developed expertise in different areas of their interest and rose to level of international experts in this field. His group conducted the most comprehensive studies of BoNT therapy in task-specific dystonias (Medline articles related to BoNTs: 60). He is the recipient of life time achievement award in international Toxin conference in 2017.

Michell Brin, MD
Dr. Brin was trained under Stanley Fahn, MD, at Columbia University, NY, and conducted some of the earliest studies of onabotulinumtoxinA efficacy in movement disorders (mostly tremor and dystonia). Over the past 30 years, he has been a key investigator in a large number of clinical trials. As an executive at Allergan Inc., he has been a key player in FDA approval of onabotulinumtoxinA for several clinical conditions (migraine, spasticity, cervical dystonia, axillary hyperhidrosis) (Medline articles related to BoNTs: 98).

Cynthia Comella, MD
Professor of neurosurgery and neurological sciences at Rush Medical School, Chicago, Ill, Dr. Comella has been a major contributor and investigator in several multicenter studies conducted on botulinum toxin therapy in the USA. Her major area of work has been on investigating the effect of botulinum toxins in cervical dystonia. Through her efforts and those of her collaborators, all four marketed BoNTs in the USA received approval by FDA for US use in cervical dystonia. As an expert electromyographer, Dr. Comella defined precise injecting methods to target difficult neck muscles in cervical dystonia. Her educational workshops in the annual meetings of the American Academy of Neurology are popular and well received (Medline articles related to BoNTs: 55).

David M. Simpson, MD
David M. Simpson, MD, FAAN, is professor of neurology at the Icahn School of Medicine at Mount Sinai, Department of Neurology. He is director of the Neuromuscular Diseases Division and the Clinical Neurophysiology Laboratories. His main area of toxin work focuses on the study of BoNTs in spasticity. He and his colleagues have shown, in an important study, that up to 800 units of

incobotulinumtoxinA in one session can be used for treatment of poststroke spastic-ity without serious side effects [18]. He is the chair of the Guidelines and Assessment Subcommittee of AAN that periodically assesses the efficacy of BoNTs for different neurological disorders (Medline articles related to BoNTs: 36).

Daniel Troung, MD
Dr. Truong has been a major contributor to multicenter studies in cervical dystonia and blepharospasm. His book *Manual of Botulinum Toxin Therapy* has been received with enthusiasm worldwide due to its practical points delivered with remarkable anatomical drawings. The book has been translated in many languages (Medline articles related to BoNTs: 40).

Bahman Jabbari, MD
Bahman Jabbari, emeritus professor of neurology at Yale University, started his practice and research on BoNT therapy in 1990 by establishing a comprehensive BoNT therapy clinic at Walter Reed Army Medical Center, Washington, DC, and 15 years later at Yale University School of Medicine in New Haven, CT. He and his colleagues were first to show the efficacy of BoNT therapy in plantar fasciitis and in nonsurgical low back pain. His most recent contribution is designing a special EMG-guided method that can significantly reduce the incidence of hand and finger weakness after BoNT injection into the forearm muscles of patients with Parkinson tremor and ET. Dr. Jabbari is the author of two books on botulinum toxin therapy and editor of two books on the same subject (Medline articles related to BoNTs: 45).

PREEMPT Group (Drs. Silberstien, Dodick, Aurora, Lipton, Blumenfeld, and Others)

A group of investigators, expert in treatment of headache, through two well-designed multicenter, blinded clinical trials (PEEMPT I and II), demonstrated the efficacy of onabotulinumtoxinA injections in chronic migraine [19] that led to its FDA approval in 2010. Subsequently, in a series of articles using the large PREEMPT cohort, they have shown that BoNT therapy in chronic migraine also improves the patients' quality of life and is effective in migraineurs with medication overuse. BoNT ther-apy is now an established treatment for chronic migraine worldwide.

Germany

Dirk Dressler, MD
Dr. Dressler, director of division of movement disorders in the University of Hanover, Germany, is probably the most influential clinical neurotoxicologist and clinical toxin researcher in Europe. He developed an interest in BoNT therapy

during his training with late David Marsden in National Hospital of London (the 1980s). He was the first person who organized BoNT therapy in Europe and is the individual with most clinical toxin-related publications in the European continent [20]. Dr. Dressler is the author of two books on botulinum toxin therapy, the first one in German and the second in English.

Reiner Benecke, MD
Dr. Benecke, like Dr. Dressler, developed his interest in clinical use of botulinum neurotoxins while working with Marsden's group in London. Dr. Beneke and Dr. Dressler participated in the development of incobotulinumtoxinA (Xeomin), then called NT201 (in research protocols), during their several years of partnership in Rostock, Germany. Their publications on merits of incobotulinumtoxinA as a BoNT free of neutralizing proteins and on immunology of botulinum neurotoxins paved the way for extensive use of this form of BoNT-A in Europe and the USA. The list of other German physicians with expertise in botulinum toxin therapy and significant contributions to this field include (but not limited to) Wolfgang Jost, Gerhard Reichel, Markus Naumann, Jorg Wissel, and Fereshteh Adib Saberi.

Austria

Werner Poewe, MD
Professor Poewe is the chairman of the Department of Neurology in Medical University of Innsbruck, Austria. He conducted several clinical trials assessing the efficacy of BoNTs in different movement disorders and spasticity. In an early study, he has shown that in children and young adults, 200 units of onabotulinum injected per leg is relatively safe and is more effective than a lower dose of 100 units. He served as president of the International Movement Disorder Society from 2000 to 2002 and as president of the Austrian Society of Neurology from 2002 to 2004. He is the author of a book entitled *Botulinum Toxin in the Treatment of Cerebral Palsy* (Medline articles related to BoNTs: 38).

References

1. Erbguth FJ. Botulinum toxin, a historical note. Lancet. 1998;351(9118):1820. https://doi.org/10.1016/S0140-6736(05)78793-6.
2. Erbguth FJ. Historical notes on botulism, Clostridium botulinum, botulinum toxin, and the idea of the therapeutic use of the toxin. Mov Disord. 2004;19(Suppl 8):S2–6. https://doi.org/10.1002/mds.20003.
3. Erbguth FJ. From poison to remedy: the chequered history of botulinum toxin. J Neural Transm (Vienna). 2008;115(4):559–65. https://doi.org/10.1007/s00702-007-0728-2.
4. Whitcup SM. The history of botulinum toxins in medicine: a thousand year journey [published online ahead of print, 2019 Aug 27]. Handb Exp Pharmacol. 2019; https://doi.org/10.1007/164_2019_271.

5. Burgen AS, Dickens F, Zatman LJ. The action of botulinum toxin on the neuro-muscular junction. J Physiol. 1949;109(1–2):10–24. https://doi.org/10.1113/jphysiol.1949.sp004364.
6. Drachman DB. Atrophy of skeletal muscles in chicks embryo treated with botulinum toxin. Science. 1964;145(3633):719–21. https://doi.org/10.1126/science.145.3633.719.
7. Scott AB. Botulinum toxin injection into extraocular muscles as an alternative to strabismus surgery. J Pediatr Ophthalmol Strabismus. 1980;17(1):21–5.
8. Scott AB. Development of botulinum toxin therapy. Dermatol Clin. 2004;22(2):131–v. https://doi.org/10.1016/s0733-8635(03)00019-6.
9. Jankovic J. Botulinum toxin: state of the art. Mov Disord. 2017;32(8):1131–8. https://doi.org/10.1002/mds.27072.
10. Jabbari B. Botulinum toxins in pain disorders: Springer Nature; New York 2015.
11. Schiavo G, Benfenati F, Poulain B, et al. Tetanus and botulinum-B neurotoxins block neurotransmitter release by proteolytic cleavage of synaptobrevin. Nature. 1992;359(6398):832–5. https://doi.org/10.1038/359832a0.
12. Schiavo G, Rossetto O, Santucci A, DasGupta BR, Montecucco C. Botulinum neurotoxins are zinc proteins. J Biol Chem. 1992;267(33):23479–83.
13. Caleo M, Spinelli M, Colosimo F, et al. Transynaptic action of botulinum neurotoxin type a at Central Cholinergic Boutons. J Neurosci. 2018;38(48):10329–37. https://doi.org/10.1523/JNEUROSCI.0294-18.2018.
14. Filipović B, Matak I, Bach-Rojecky L, Lacković Z. Central action of peripherally applied botulinum toxin type A on pain and dural protein extravasation in rat model of trigeminal neuropathy. PLoS One. 2012;7(1):e29803. https://doi.org/10.1371/journal.pone.0029803.
15. Matak I. Evidence for central antispastic effect of botulinum toxin type A. Br J Pharmacol. 2020;177(1):65–76. https://doi.org/10.1111/bph.14846.
16. Wang J, Casals-Diaz L, Zurawski T, et al. A novel therapeutic with two SNAP-25 inactivating proteases shows long-lasting anti-hyperalgesic activity in a rat model of neuropathic pain. Neuropharmacology. 2017;118:223–32. https://doi.org/10.1016/j.neuropharm.2017.03.026.
17. Blasi J, Chapman ER, Link E, et al. Botulinum neurotoxin A selectively cleaves the synaptic protein SNAP-25. Nature. 1993;365(6442):160–3. https://doi.org/10.1038/365160a0.
18. Dodick DW, Turkel CC, DeGryse RE, et al. OnabotulinumtoxinA for treatment of chronic migraine: pooled results from the double-blind, randomized, placebo-controlled phases of the PREEMPT clinical program. Headache. 2010;50(6):921–36. https://doi.org/10.1111/j.1526-4610.2010.01678.x.
19. Wissel J, Bensmail D, Ferreira JJ, et al. Safety and efficacy of incobotulinumtoxinA doses up to 800 U in limb spasticity: the TOWER study. Neurology. 2017;88(14):1321–8. https://doi.org/10.1212/WNL.0000000000003789.
20. Dressler D, Roggenkaemper P. A brief history of neurological botulinum toxin therapy in Germany. J Neural Transm (Vienna). 2017;124(10):1217–21. https://doi.org/10.1007/s00702-017-1762-3.

Chapter 2
Molecular Structure and Mechanisms of Action of Botulinum Neurotoxins

Ornella Rossetto and Marco Pirazzini

Abstract Botulinum neurotoxins (BoNTs) are a growing family of bacterial protein toxins that cause a generalized flaccid paralysis of botulism by inactivating neurotransmitter release at peripheral nerve terminals. They are the most potent toxins known thanks to the marvel of their protein design, which underlines their mechanism of action. Their unique biological properties have led them to become also highly effective and successful therapeutic agents for the treatment of a variety of human syndromes. This chapter reports the progress on our understanding of BoNTs, highlighting the different steps of their molecular mechanism of action as key aspects to explain their extreme toxicity but also their unique pharmacological properties.

Keywords Botulinum neurotoxins · Mechanism of action · SNAREs · Peripheral nerve terminal · Duration of paralysis

Introduction

Botulinum neurotoxins (BoNTs) are a large family of bacterial protein toxins responsible for the animal and human neuroparalytic disease botulism. They are produced by bacteria of the genus Clostridia, but other bacteria of different classes may have the gene coding for BoNT or BoNT-like toxins and more than 40 different BoNT protein sequences have been described to date [1]. BoNT-producing Clostridia are widely distributed in the environment, including food particularly for *Clostridium botulinum*, where they can survive for a long time as spores. They are classified in eight different serotypes (BoNT/A, /B, /C, /D, /E, /F, /G and /X) on the basis of their immunological properties [2]. Among the BoNT serotypes, types A, B, E, and F are associated with botulism in both humans and animals, whereas BoNT/C and /D primarily cause disease in domestic animals. Many subtypes of serotypes are known

O. Rossetto (✉) · M. Pirazzini
Dipartimento di Scienze Biomediche, Università di Padova, Padova, Italy
e-mail: ornella.rossetto@unipd.it

© Springer Nature Switzerland AG 2020
B. Jabbari (ed.), *Botulinum Toxin Treatment in Surgery, Dentistry, and Veterinary Medicine*, https://doi.org/10.1007/978-3-030-50691-9_2

and designated with an arabic number (e.g., BoNT/A1-A8) in addition to chimeric neurotoxins (BoNT/CD, BoNT/DC, BoNT/FA), and this figure is bound to increase with expanding DNA sequencing of strains and novel isolates [3–6].

BoNTs are the most lethal toxins and their high toxicity is due to a multi-step molecular mechanism: they target peripheral nerve terminals by a unique mode of binding and enter into their cytosol where they cleave SNARE proteins, thus inhibiting the neurotransmitter release. The specificity and rapidity of binding and its reversible action make BoNT a valuable pharmaceutical to treat neurological and non-neurological diseases characterized by hyperactivity of cholinergic nerve terminals. Several BoNT preparations based on serotype A1 are licensed for clinical use, whereas only one is based on serotype B1 [7]. This chapter reports the progress on our understanding of botulinum neurotoxins, highlighting the structure–activity relationship of the BoNT domains and their multi-step molecular mechanism of action as key aspects to explain the extreme toxicity but also their unique pharmacological properties.

Structural Organization of Botulinum Neurotoxins

BoNTs are produced by bacteria together with nontoxic accessory proteins to form high-molecular-weight progenitor toxin complexes (PTC) of various sizes. The toxin molecule interacts directly with a homologous non-toxic non-hemagglutinin component (NTNHA), with whom it forms a hand-in-hand shaped heterodimer named M-PTC (Fig. 2.1a). This is much more stable than BoNT alone to the acidic and proteolytic conditions found in the gastrointestinal tract [8] and in decaying biological materials where BoNT is produced. This heterodimer assembles with hemagglutinin components (HAs) or OrfX proteins to form higher molecular weight PTCs (L-PTCs/A1 ≈ 500–900 kDa) (Fig. 2.1b), which rapidly dissociate under slightly alkaline physiologic solutions. HA proteins of PTCs present multiple carbohydrate-binding sites and are believed to mediate the binding of the complex to the intestinal mucus layer and the polarized intestinal epithelial cells of the intestinal wall through which BoNTs enter into the lymphatic circulation and then in the blood circulation [9–11]. Among the major brands of BoNT/A for clinical use, onabotulinumtoxinA and abobotulinumtoxinA are purified PTCs, whereas incobotulinumtoxinA contains only the purified BoNT/A1 neurotoxin [7].

Despite the existence of a high number of isoforms, all the BoNT 150 kDa neurotoxins are structurally similar and consist of two chains: a light chain (L, 50 kDa) and a heavy chain (H, 100 kDa) linked by an essential interchain disulfide bridge (Fig. 2.1a). The full-length crystal structures of BoNT/A1, BoNT/B1, BoNT/E1 have been determined and reveal a three-domain architecture, composed of the L, HN (the N-terminal part of the H), and HC (the C-terminal part of H) (Fig. 2.1a) [12–14]. BoNT/A1 and BoNT/B1 have a linear domain arrangement, with the HC isolated from the L, while BoNT/E has a more-compact globular shape with the L and HC located on the same side of HN, with interactions between all three domains [15].

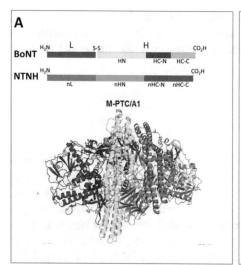
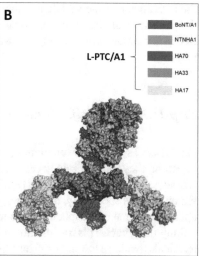

Fig. 2.1 Molecular structure of BoNT/A1 neurotoxin and its progenitor protein complexes (PTCs). (**a**) Schematic organization and crystal structure of BoNT/A1 in complex with NTNH/A1 protein (M-PTC/A1) (PDB accession: 3VOC). (**b**) Structure of the precursor toxin complex of BoNT/A1, which consists of the NTNH/A1-BoNT/A1 heterodimer and the hemagglutinin proteins (HA) forming the so-called L-PTC/A1. There are 6 HA33 proteins, 3 HA17 proteins, 1 HA70 per 1 NTNHA1-BoNT/A1 complex. L-PTC/A1 displays three spider-like legs that are suggested to have a role in binding to the intestinal epithelium to facilitate absorption of the toxin. (Adapted from [1])

The overall similar architecture of BoNTs is strictly linked to their common multi-steps mechanism of intoxication of nerve terminals. The L chain is a zinc-metalloprotease that specifically cleaves the three SNARE proteins necessary for neurotransmitter exocytosis; the HN domain assists the translocation of the L chain across the membrane of intraneuronal acidic vesicles into the cytosol; the HC domain is responsible for presynaptic binding and endocytosis and consists of two sub-domains (HC-N and HC-C) with different folding and membrane binding properties. Therefore BoNT is a modular nanomachine, which exploits its sophisticate design at each step of the intoxication process, thereby achieving an exquisite toxicity.

The Conserved Mechanism of Nerve Terminal Intoxication

The modular structure of BoNTs has been shaped by the evolution to deliver the catalytic L chain into the nerve terminal. This remarkable result is attained by exploiting different physiological functions of the host nerve terminals; and it can be conveniently divided into five major steps: (1) binding to nerve terminals, (2) internalisation within an endocytic compartment, (3) low pH-driven translocation of the L chain across the vesicle membrane, (4) release of the L chain in the cytosol by the reduction of the interchain disulphide bond, and (5) proteolytic cleavage of SNARE proteins with ensuing blockade of neurotransmitter release and neuroparalysis [16].

Step 1: Neurospecific Binding

Once BoNTs enter the circulation, following intestinal absorption, inhalation or injection, they rapidly gain access to the peri-neuronal fluid compartment, without crossing the blood–brain barrier [9]. BoNTs have evolved a unique binding mode, which ensures specificity, high affinity, and rapidity of interaction with the presynaptic membrane of peripheral nerve terminals. Indeed, the BoNTs bind with high-affinity presynaptic plasma membrane of skeletal and autonomic cholinergic nerve terminals thanks to the carboxyl terminal domain (HC-C, 25 kDa, green in Fig. 2.1a). This C-terminal sub-domain contains one conserved binding site for a polysialoganglioside receptor, which is highly enriched in the nerve presynaptic membrane, and a second binding site for a protein receptor that is present on the lumenal side of the membrane of synaptic vesicles (SV) [2, 7, 17, 18]. The glycan part of ganglioside receptors provides abundance and specificity and accumulates the toxins onto unmyelinated areas of nerve endings, thus facilitating the interaction with a second receptor [19, 20]. The SV calcium sensors Synaptotagmin I/II (Syt-I and Syt-II) were identified as specific receptors for BoNT/B1, /G, and the mosaic serotype /DC whereas BoNT/A1 and BoNT/E1 bind specifically to two different segments of the fourth luminal loop of the synaptic vesicle glycoprotein SV2A/B/C (for a complete list of references, see [2, 7, 17, 18]). The neurospecific binding of the other BoNTs has not been well characterized and conflicting results have been reported, calling for further investigations. In vitro binding experiments have shown that the affinity of BoNT/B and BoNT/G to the luminal domain of Syt-I and Syt-II decreases in the order B-Syt-II>>G-Syt-I>G-Syt-II>>B-Syt-I [21]. Remarkably, it has been recently shown that human Syt-II is not a high-affinity receptor for BoNT/B and G due to the F54L mutation in its luminal domain, which eliminates one of the three major interactions between Syt-II and BoNT/B [22, 23]. This mutation is present only in humans and chimpanzees and might explain the observed disparity of BoNT/B potency in human and mice [24]. Noteworthy Syt-II is present in every endplate in diaphragm muscle whereas only a subpopulation of neuromuscular junctions (NMJs) additionally expresses Syt-I [25]. The F54L mutation in human Syt-II, together with the low expression at the NMJ of Syt-I, explains why high doses of BoNT/B are required to achieve therapeutic effects in neuromuscular disorders. In contrast, the predominant presence of Syt-I in autonomic and sensory neurons [26] might explain the observed autonomic effects of BoNT/B and the lower BoNT/A:BoNT/B dose ratio for autonomic indications [27].

N-glycosylation plays a critical role for the high-affinity binding of BoNT/A1 to SV2C and of BoNT/E to SV2A/B [28, 29] and the potential clinical relevance of this finding calls for appropriate investigations. In fact, a different pattern of glycosylation among individuals would provide a simple explanation for the variable sensitivity of different patients to BoNT/A1 injection, which is commonly observed in the clinical use of this toxin. Clearly, this consideration might also be applicable to different vertebrate species.

The dual binding interaction with polysialogangliosides and SV receptors increases the strength of BoNT interactions with the membrane as it is the product of the two binding affinities [17]. Besides high-affinity binding to gangliosides and to the protein receptor, hydrophobic loops in the HC-C [30] and the HC-N binding domain could contribute with low affinity, but selective interactions to the overall affinity of the toxins for cell surfaces [31, 32].

The double receptor binding accounts for the extreme potency of BoNTs but does not explain their apparent selectivity for cholinergic nerve terminals, which may be provided by additional receptor(s) still to be identified [33].

Step 2: Toxin Internalization

After binding to the presynaptic receptors, BoNTs enter into the nerve terminal. BoNT/A1, at mouse neuromuscular junction was predominantly visualized within synaptic vesicles and the number of toxin molecules (either 1 or 2) correlates with the number of SV2 molecules in the SV membrane [34, 35]. SV exocytosis is strictly coupled to endocytosis, and this explains the fact that BoNT/A1 paralyses is faster in a synaptic terminal, which is stimulated electrically or by exercise, whilst the lowering of synaptic activity prolongs the time of paralysis development [36]. Recent findings indicate that high activity levels of SV neurotransmitter release leads to full-collapse SV fusion with the incorporation of the SV membrane into the presynaptic membrane [37]. In turn, this would result in an increased extent of exposure of the BoNT luminal SV receptor with a consequent increase of the internalized BoNT. This BoNT would end in the lumen of a bulk endosome, rather than in the SV lumen. However, SV will form rapidly by clathrin-mediated budding of SV from endosomes. Clearly, the recent novel findings on endocytosis at nerve terminals call for further studies to clarify the different forms of vesicular/endosomal trafficking of the various BoNTs into the nerve terminal. Such studies could lead to improved modes of delivery of BoNT to patients.

Step 3: Toxin Translocation

In order to reach the intracellular targets in the cytosol of nerve cells, the catalytically active L domain must be translocated from the SV lumen into the cytosol. To accomplish this, BoNTs have to exploit another physiological function of the synapse; i.e., they parasitize the refilling of neurotransmitter inside empty vesicles. This is powered by the action of an ATPase proton pump present on the SV membrane which injects protons inside to create a transmembrane pH gradient that drives the uptake of neurotransmitter from the cytosol into the lumen. The low pH inside the SV lumen induces a structural change of the HN domain, leading to its insertion into the membrane, and thus an ion translocation channel is formed that assists the passage of the partially unfolded L from the lumenal to the cytosolic side of the SV membrane [38, 39]. The disulphide bridge that links the heavy and light chain must remain intact on the luminal side of the vesicle until the last stage of L translocation [40]. Once it has reached the cytosolic face of SV membrane, the L chain has to reacquire the native structure in order to cleave its substrate. It has been recently shown that the host chaperone heat shock protein 90 (Hsp90) assists the refolding of the L chain after vesicle membrane translocation as already demonstrated for other bacterial toxins such as Diphteria toxin [41, 42]. L remains attached to the SV until the interchain disulphide bond is reduced in the reducing environment of the cytosol, a crucial step for productive release of the L catalytic subunit, which is common to all the BoNT variants [43].

Step 4: Reduction of the Interchain Disulphide Bond

The interchain S-S bond is exposed to the cytosol after translocation of the L domain, and it is specifically reduced by the NADPH-Thioredoxin reductase-Thioredoxin redox system (Trx-Tx) [43]. This redox system physically interacts with the Hsp90 chaperone on the cytosolic surface of SV and represents the machinery of activation of the L chain [41, 43]. Indeed, inhibitors of the TrxR-Trx redox system prevent the intoxication by BoNTs of neurons in culture and, more importantly, largely prevent the BoNT-induced paralysis in mice in vivo, regardless of the serotype involved [44]. This notion leads to an important translational potential application because these inhibitors are candidates for the prevention of botulism in humans and for the treatment of those forms of botulism, implying a continuous production of toxin molecules such as infant botulism or intestinal botulism [45].

Step 5: Proteolytic Cleavage of SNARE Proteins

The L chains of BoNTs are zinc-dependent metalloproteases specific for members of SNARE family proteins, which form the core complex that mediates fusion of synaptic vesicle membranes to plasma membranes that is essential for neurotransmitter release [46, 47]. The BoNT proteolytic activity is highly specific and directed toward unique peptide bonds within the sequence of their respective SNARE protein targets. BoNT/B, /D, /F, /G cleave VAMP1/2/3, BoNT/A and BoNT/E cleave SNAP-25; and BoNT/C cleaves both SNAP-25 and syntaxin (for reviews see [2, 7]). The L chain of BoNT/X, a recent identified new serotype, cleaves VAMP1/2/3 at a site distinct from the known cleavage sites for all other BoNTs. However, BoNT/X is practically not toxic to mice probably due to its lack of efficient receptor binding [48]. Another BoNT-like toxin, named BoNT/En, was recently identified in the genome of a commensal strain of *Enterococcus faecium* isolated from cow feces. Functional characterization revealed that L/En of this toxin cleaves VAMP1/2/3 at a novel site [49]. Interestingly, L/En is also capable of cleaving SNAP-25 in neurons and the cleavage site is located on the N-terminal part of SNAP-25, which is distinct from all known BoNT cleavage sites, though its cleavage of recombinant SNAP-25 in vitro is not efficient. Similar to BoNT/X, HC/En appears unable to recognize mouse/rat neurons, as BoNT/En is not toxic in cultured neurons or in mice [49]. In most cases, BoNT cleavage results in the loss of a large part of the cytosolic portion of SNARE proteins, thus preventing the formation of the SNARE complex. In contrast, in the case of BoNT/A and BoNT/C, the truncated SNAP25 proteins retain most of their sequences (197 and 198 of 206 amino acid residues, respectively) and are capable of forming stable, though non-functional, SNARE complexes. In any cases the proteolysis of one SNARE protein prevents the formation of a functional SNARE complex and, consequently, the release of neurotransmitter with ensuing neuroparalysis [16, 50]. The exquisite target specificity of botulinum neurotoxins is due to the unique mode of recognition of VAMP, SNAP-25 or syntaxin by the L chain, which involves multiple interactions of the metalloprotease with its substrate including the cleavage site as well as exosites located along the sequence both before and after the hydrolysed peptide bond [51–53].

Distant Effects of BoNTs and Their Implications in Clinical Use

It has been known for a long time that botulinum neurotoxins block acetylcholine release from peripheral nerve terminals and therefore lead to cessation of somatic motor and/or parasympathetic transmission. When locally injected, BoNTs should have only, or mostly, local action and produce long-lasting anticholinergic effects to control various chronic motor and/or autonomic disorders [7, 54, 55]. However, it was experimentally shown that retroaxonal transport of BoNTs does take place, similarly to the related tetanus neurotoxin [56]. Compelling evidence of BoNT/A1 retrotransport to the central nervous system (CNS) was provided by tracing the cleavage of SNAP-25 within CNS neurons after peripheral injection of the toxin, using an antibody very specific for the novel epitope generated by the BoNT/A1 cleavage of SNAP-25 [57, 58]. BoNT/A1 retrograde transport can occur also via sensory neurons, as shown by the injection in the whisker pad, which induces the appearance of truncated SNAP-25 in the trigeminal nucleus caudalis [57, 59] and in the dorsal horn of the spinal cord after subcutaneous or intramuscular injection in the hind limb [60–62]. Moreover, BoNT/A1 can undergo subsequent events of transcytosis and transport to second order neurons, remaining catalytically active [57, 59, 63, 64]. The ability of BoNTs to interfere with sensory transmission both at peripheral and central level has opened new avenues in their clinical application for different pain conditions [65, 66].

Duration of Action of BoNTs

One remarkable aspect of the peripheral neuroparalysis induced by BoNTs is its reversibility, which is an essential aspect of botulism and of the therapeutic use of BoNT. Indeed, the toxin cleaves a SNARE protein as long as it remains intact in the nerve cytosol, but it neither kill the neuron nor it causes axonal degeneration in the intoxicated animal, though the animal may die by respiratory failure. Indeed if a botulism patient is kept under mechanical ventilation and appropriate pharmacological treatments, eventually he/she recovers completely, following the inactivation of the toxin and the replacement of the cleaved SNARE [55]. The duration of the BoNT induced neuroparalysis varies with dose (higher dose equals longer duration), with the animal species (small size mammalians shorter duration), the type of nerve terminal (human skeletal nerve terminals are paralysed for 3–4 months by BoNT/A1 whilst human autonomic cholinergic nerve terminals are paralysed for 12–15 months) and with the serotype of BoNT (type A1 > type B1 >> type E1) [7]. The main determinant of the duration of neuroparalysis is the L chain lifetime within the terminal [67]. BoNT/A1 L chain, which has a very remarkable persistence, has a longer lifetime than that of BoNT/E1 because BoNT/E1 L chain is ubiquitinated and targeted to the ubiquitin-proteasome system, whilst BoNT/A1 L chain escapes the action of the cell degradation system by recruiting de-ubiquitinases, i.e. specialized enzymes that remove polyubiquitin chains [68]. The exceptional length of the paralysis exerted by BoNT/A1 is likely to be supported by effects additional to the L chain degradation. Indeed, there is evidence that the BoNT/A-cleaved SNAP-25, which retains 197 over 206 amino acid residues, is still capable of forming a SNARE heterotrimer with VAMP and syntaxin. This SNARE complex is non-functional in neuroexocytosis but prevents the function of the normal SNARE complex acting as a dominant negative that causes by itself neuroparalysis as long as it is present inside nerve terminals [16, 69]. New understanding of the mechanisms by which these remarkable toxins or their proteolytic products persist within their motor neuron targets will help to develop, on one hand BoNT-based therapeutics with improved persistence properties and therefore longer clinical benefit, and on the other hand BoNT-antidotes which accelerate the toxin degradation and therefore reverse BoNT intoxication.

Future Perspectives for BoNT Medical Use

The structure–activity relationship of the BoNT domains is credited for the selectivity and extreme potency of these molecules, which are regarded as the most potent toxin known to mankind, with an LD50 from 0.1 to 5 ng/Kg depending on the toxin type [70]. At the same time, BoNTs combine potency and specificity with full reversibility, and these unique properties are at the basis of their ever-growing clinical use. The recent understanding of their detailed modular structure and of their multi-step molecular mechanism of neuron intoxication together with advances in the techniques for the production of recombinant proteins has opened up the opportunity to obtain tailor-made therapeutic agents by modifying the binding specificity, affinity, and nerve terminal persistence and thus improving their properties in terms of cell targeting and duration of action [71, 72]. In addition, the identification of many BoNT variants with different biological profiles could potentially represent a natural goldmine to be exploited for new clinical applications.

Acknowledgments Work in the author's laboratory is supported by grants from the University of Padova.

References

1. Rossetto O, Pirazzini M, Montecucco C. Botulinum neurotoxins: genetic, structural and mechanistic insights. Nat Rev Microbiol. 2014;12:535–49.
2. Dong M, Masuyer G, Stenmark P. Botulinum and tetanus neurotoxins. Annu Rev Biochem. 2019;88:811–37.
3. Peck MW, Smith TJ, Anniballi F, Austin JW, Bano L, Bradshaw M, Cuervo P, Cheng LW, Derman Y, Dorner BG, Fisher A, Hill KK, Kalb SR, Korkeala H, Lindstrom M, Lista F, Luquez C, Mazuet C, Pirazzini M, Popoff MR, Rossetto O, Rummel A, Sesardic D, Singh BR, Stringer SC. Historical perspectives and guidelines for botulinum neurotoxin subtype nomenclature. Toxins. 2017;9(1):38.
4. Montecucco C, Rasotto MB. On botulinum neurotoxin variability. MBio. 2015;6:e02131–14.
5. Doxey AC, Mansfield MJ, Montecucco C. Discovery of novel bacterial toxins by genomics and computational biology. Toxicon. 2018;147:2–12.
6. Doxey AC, Mansfield MJ, Lobb B. Exploring the evolution of virulence factors through bioinformatic data mining. mSystems. 2019;21(3):4. pii: e00162-19.
7. Pirazzini M, Rossetto O, Eleopra R, Montecucco C. Botulinum neurotoxins: biology, pharmacology, and toxicology. Pharmacol Rev. 2017;69(2):200–35.
8. Gu S, Rumpel S, Zhou J, Strotmeier J, Bigalke H, Perry K, Shoemaker CB, Rummel A, Jin R. Botulinum neurotoxin is shielded by NTNHA in an interlocked complex. Science. 2012;335(6071):977–98.
9. Simpson LL. The life history of a botulinum toxin molecule. Toxicon. 2013;68:40–59.
10. Fujinaga Y, Sugawara Y, Matsumura T. Uptake of botulinum neurotoxin in the intestine. Curr Top Microbiol Immunol. 2013;364:45–59.
11. Lam KH, Jin R. Architecture of the botulinum neurotoxin complex: a molecular machine for protection and delivery. Curr Opin Struct Biol. 2015;31:89–95.
12. Lacy DB, Tepp W, Cohen AC, DasGupta BR, Stevens RC. Crystal structure of botulinum neurotoxin type A and implications for toxicity. Nat Struct Biol. 1998;5(10):898–902.
13. Swaminathan S, Eswaramoorthy S. Structural analysis of the catalytic and binding sites of Clostridium botulinum neurotoxin B. Nat Struct Biol. 2000;7:693–9.
14. Kumaran D, Eswaramoorthy S, Furey W, Navaza J, Sax M, Swaminathan S. Domain organization in Clostridium botulinum neurotoxin type E is unique: its implication in faster translocation. J Mol Biol. 2009;386:233–45.
15. Swaminathan S. Molecular structures and functional relationships in clostridial neurotoxins. FEBS J. 2011;278(23):4467–85.

16. Pantano S, Montecucco C. The blockade of the neurotransmitter release apparatus by botulinum neurotoxins. Cell Mol Life Sci. 2014;71(5):793–811.
17. Montecucco C. How do tetanus and botulinum toxins bind to neuronal membranes? Trends Biochem Sci. 1986;11:314–7.
18. Rummel A. Double receptor anchorage of botulinum neurotoxins accounts for their exquisite neurospecificity. Curr Top Microbiol Immunol. 2013;364:61–90.
19. Rummel A. Two feet on the membrane: uptake of clostridial neurotoxins. Curr Top Microbiol Immunol. 2017;406:1–37.
20. Hamark C, Berntsson RP, Masuyer G, Henriksson LM, Gustafsson R, Stenmark P, Widmalm G. Glycans confer specificity to the recognition of ganglioside receptors by botulinum neurotoxin a. J Am Chem Soc. 2017;139:218–30.
21. Rummel A, Eichner T, Weil T, Karnath T, Gutcaits A, Mahrhold S, Sandhoff K, Proia RL, Acharya KR, Bigalke H, Binz T. Identification of the protein receptor binding site of botulinum neurotoxins B and G proves the double-receptor concept. Proc Natl Acad Sci U S A. 2007;104:359–64.
22. Peng L, Berntsson RP, Tepp WH, Pitkin RM, Johnson EA, Stenmark P, Dong M. Botulinum neurotoxin D-C uses synaptotagmin I and II as receptors, and human synaptotagmin II is not an effective receptor for type B, D-C and G toxins. J Cell Sci. 2012;125:3233e3242.
23. Strotmeier J, Willjes G, Binz T, Rummel A. Human synaptotagmin-II is not a high affinity receptor for botulinum neurotoxin B and G: increased therapeutic dosage and immunogenicity. FEBS Lett. 2012;586:310–3.
24. Tao L, Peng L, Berntsson RP, Liu SM, Park S, Yu F, Boone C, Palan S, Beard M, Chabrier PE, Stenmark P, Krupp J, Dong M. Engineered botulinum neurotoxin B with improved efficacy for targeting human receptors. Nat Commun. 2017;8(1):53.
25. Pang ZP, Melicoff E, Padgett D, Liu Y, Teich AF, Dickey BF, Lin W, Adachi R, Sudhof TC. Synaptotagmin-2 is essential for survival and contributes to Ca2+ triggering of neurotransmitter release in central and neuromuscular synapses. J Neurosci. 2006;26:13493–504.
26. Li JY, Jahn R, Dahlstrom A. Synaptotagmin I is present mainly in autonomic and sensory neurons of the rat peripheral nervous system. Neuroscience. 1994;63:837–50.
27. Kranz G, Paul A, Voller B, Posch M, Windischberger C, Auff E, Sycha T. Long-term efficacy and respective potencies of botulinum toxin A and B: a randomized, double-blind study. Br J Dermatol. 2011;164:176–81.
28. Yao G, Zhang S, Mahrhold S, Lam KH, Stern D, Bagramyan K, Perry K, Kalkum M, Rummel A, Dong M, Jin R. N-linked glycosylation of SV2 is required for binding and uptake of botulinum neurotoxin A. Nat Struct Mol Biol. 2016;23:656–62.
29. Montecucco C, Zanotti G. Botulinum neurotoxin A1 likes it double sweet. Nat Struct Mol Biol. 2016;23:619–21.
30. Stern D, Weisemann J, Le Blanc A, von Berg L, Mahrhold S, Piesker J, Laue M, Luppa PB, Dorner MB, Dorner BG, Rummel A. A lipid-binding loop of botulinum neurotoxin serotypes B, DC and G is an essential feature to confer their exquisite potency. PLoS Pathog. 2018;14(5):e1007048.
31. Muraro L, Tosatto S, Motterlini L, Rossetto O, Montecucco C. The N-terminal half of the receptor domain of botulinum neurotoxin A binds to microdomains of the plasma membrane. Biochem Biophys Res Commun. 2009;380(1):76–80.
32. Zhang S, Berntsson RP, Tepp WH, Tao L, Johnson EA, Stenmark P, Dong M. Structural basis for the unique ganglioside and cell membrane recognition mechanism of botulinum neurotoxin DC. Nat Commun. 2017;8(1):1637.
33. Montecucco C, Rossetto O, Schiavo G. Presynaptic receptor arrays for clostridial neurotoxins. Trends Microbiol. 2004;12:442–6.
34. Colasante C, Rossetto O, Morbiato L, Pirazzini M, Molgo J, Montecucco C. Botulinum neurotoxin type A is internalized and translocated from small synaptic vesicles at the neuromuscular junction. Mol Neurobiol. 2013;48:120–7.

35. Harper CB, Papadopulos A, Martin S, Matthews DR, Morgan GP, Nguyen TH, Wang T, Nair D, Choquet D, Meunier FA. Botulinum neurotoxin type-A enters a non-recycling pool of synaptic vesicles. Sci Rep. 2016;6:19654.
36. Hughes R, Whaler BC. Influence of nerve-ending activity and of drugs on the rate of paralysis of rat diaphragm preparations by cl. botulinum type a toxin. J Physiol. 1962;160:221–33.
37. Chanaday NL, Cousin MA, Milosevic I, Watanabe S, Morgan JR. The synaptic vesicle cycle revisited: new insights into the modes and mechanisms. J Neurosci. 2019;39(42):8209–16.
38. Montal M. Botulinum neurotoxin: a marvel of protein design. Annu Rev Biochem. 2010;79:591–617.
39. Pirazzini M, Azarnia Tehran D, Leka O, Zanetti G, Rossetto O, Montecucco C. On the translocation of botulinum and tetanus neurotoxins across the membrane of acidic intracellular compartments. Biochim Biophys Acta. 2016;1858:467–74.
40. Fischer A, Montal M. Crucial role of the disulfide bridge between botulinum neurotoxin light and heavy chains in protease translocation across membranes. J Biol Chem. 2007;282:29604–11.
41. Azarnia Tehran D, Pirazzini M, Leka O, Mattarei A, Lista F, Binz T, Rossetto O, Montecucco C. Hsp90 is involved in the entry of clostridial neurotoxins into the cytosol of nerve terminals. Cell Microbiol. 2017;19(2):e12647.
42. Ratts R, Zeng H, Berg EA, Blue C, McComb ME, Costello CE, vanderSpek JC, Murphy JR. The cytosolic entry of diphtheria toxin catalytic domain requires a host cell cytosolic translocation factor complex. J Cell Biol. 2003;160:1139–50.
43. Pirazzini M, Azarnia Tehran D, Zanetti G, Megighian A, Scorzeto M, Fillo S, Shone CC, Binz T, Rossetto O, Lista F, Montecucco C. Thioredoxin and its reductase are present on synaptic vesicles, and their inhibition prevents the paralysis induced by botulinum neurotoxins. Cell Rep. 2014;8:1870–8.
44. Zanetti G, Azarnia Tehran D, Pirazzini M, Binz T, Shone CC, Fillo S, Lista F, Rossetto O, Montecucco C. Inhibition of botulinum neurotoxins interchain disulfide bond reduction prevents the peripheral neuroparalysis of botulism. Biochem Pharmacol. 2015;98(3):522–30.
45. Rossetto O, Pirazzini M, Lista F, Montecucco C. The role of the single interchains disulfide bond in tetanus and botulinum neurotoxins and the development of antitetanus and antibotulism drugs. Cell Microbiol. 2019;21(11):e13037.
46. Jahn R, Scheller RH. SNAREs--engines for membrane fusion. Nat Rev. 2006;7(9):631–43.
47. Sudhof TC, Rothman JE. Membrane fusion: grappling with SNARE and SM proteins. Science. 2009;323(5913):474–7.
48. Zhang S, Masuyer G, Zhang J, Shen Y, Lundin D, et al. Identification and characterization of a novel botulinum neurotoxin. Nat Commun. 2017;8:14130.
49. Zhang S, Lebreton F, Mansfield MJ, Miyashita SI, Zhang J, et al. Identification of a botulinum neurotoxin-like toxin in a commensal strain of Enterococcus faecium. Cell Host Microbe. 2018;23:169–76.e6.
50. Sudhof TC. The molecular machinery of neurotransmitter release (Nobel lecture). Angew Chem Int Ed Engl. 2014;53:12696–717.
51. Rossetto O, Schiavo G, Montecucco C, Poulain B, Deloye F, Lozzi L, Shone CC. SNARE motif and neurotoxins. Nature. 1994;372:415–6.
52. Binz T. Clostridial neurotoxin light chains: devices for SNARE cleavage mediated blockade of neurotransmission. Curr Top Microbiol Immunol. 2013;364:139–57.
53. Chen S. Clostridial neurotoxins: mode of substrate recognition and novel therapy development. Curr Protein Pept Sci. 2014;15:490–503.
54. Dressler D. Clinical applications of botulinum toxin. Curr Opin Microbiol. 2012;15:325–36.
55. Johnson EA, Botulism MC. Handb Clin Neurol. 2008;91:333–68.
56. Mazzocchio R, Caleo M. More than at the neuromuscular synapse: actions of botulinum neurotoxin a in the central nervous system. Neuroscientist. 2015;21:44–61.
57. Antonucci F, Rossi C, Gianfranceschi L, Rossetto O, Caleo M. Longdistance retrograde effects of botulinum neurotoxin A. J Neurosci. 2008;28:3689–96.

58. Restani L, Giribaldi F, Manich M, Bercsenyi K, Menendez G, Rossetto O, Caleo M, Schiavo G. Botulinum neurotoxins A and E undergo retrograde axonal transport in primary motor neurons. PLoS Pathog. 2012;8:e1003087.
59. Matak I, Bach-Rojecky L, Filipovic B, Lackovic Z. Behavioral and immunohistochemical evidence for central antinociceptive activity of botulinum toxin A. Neuroscience. 2011;186:201–7.
60. Marinelli S, Vacca V, Ricordy R, Uggenti C, Tata AM, Luvisetto S, Pavone F. The analgesic effect on neuropathic pain of retrogradely transported botulinum neurotoxin A involves Schwann cells and astrocytes. PLoS One. 2012;7:e47977.
61. Matak I, Riederer P, Lackovic Z. Botulinum toxin's axonal transport from periphery to the spinal cord. Neurochem Int. 2012;61:236–9.
62. Matak I, Lackovic Z. Botulinum toxin A, brain and pain. Prog Neurobiol. 2014;119-120:39–59.
63. Restani L, Antonucci F, Gianfranceschi L, Rossi C, Rossetto O, Caleo M. Evidence for anterograde transport and transcytosis of botulinum neurotoxin A (BoNT/A). J Neurosci. 2011;31:15650–9.
64. Caleo M, Spinelli M, Colosimo F, Matak I, Rossetto O, Lackovic Z, Restani L. Transsynaptic action of botulinum neurotoxin type A at Central Cholinergic Boutons. J Neurosci. 2018;38(48):10329–37.
65. Safarpour Y, Jabbari B. Botulinum toxin treatment of pain syndromes –an evidence based review. Toxicon. 2018;147:120–8.
66. Mittal SO, Jabbari B. Botulinum neurotoxins and cancer-a review of the literature. Toxins. 2020;12(1):32.
67. Shoemaker CB, Oyler GA. Persistence of Botulinum neurotoxin inactivation of nerve function. Curr Top Microbiol Immunol. 2013;364:179–96.
68. Tsai YC, Maditz R, Kuo C-l, Fishman PS, Shoemaker CB, Oyler GA, Weissman AM. Targeting botulinum neurotoxin persistence by the ubiquitin-proteasome system. Proc Natl Acad Sci U S A. 2010;107:16554–9.
69. Megighian A, Zordan M, Pantano S, Scorzeto M, Rigoni M, Zanini D, Rossetto O, Montecucco C. Evidence for a radial SNARE super-complex mediating neurotransmitter release at the Drosophila neuromuscular junction. J Cell Sci. 2013;126:3134–40.
70. Rossetto O, Montecucco C. Tables of toxicity of botulinum and tetanus neurotoxins. Toxins. 2019;11(12):pii:E686.
71. Chen S, Barbieri JT. Engineering botulinum neurotoxin to extend therapeutic intervention. PNAS. 2009;106:9180–4.
72. Sikorra S, Litschko C, Müller C, Thiel N, Galli T, Eichner T, Binz T. Identification and characterization of botulinum neurotoxin a substrate binding pockets and their re-engineering for human SNAP-23. J Mol Biol. 2016;428(2Pt A):372–84.

Chapter 3
Types of Toxins in Commercial Use, Their Similarities and Differences

Khashayar Dashtipour and Paul Spanel

Abstract The clinical application of botulinum toxin currently spans across several medical specialties as new indications continue to be investigated and new products continue to be developed. This chapter discusses similarities and differences among the currently commercially available botulinum toxin products. The mechanism of action of both serotypes, BoNT-A and BoNT-B, is introduced. The clinical indications for each available botulinum toxin product including onabotulinumtoxinA, abobotulinumtoxinA, incobotulinumtoxinA, and rimabotulinumtoxinB are discussed along with potential adverse effects and the potential of developing immunogenicity. Finally, future products such as daxibotulinumtoxinA and praxibotulinumtoxinA with potential for further clinical indications are touched upon.

Keywords OnabotulinumtoxinA · AbobotulinumtoxinA · IncobotulinumtoxinA · RimabotulinumtoxinB · DaxibotulinumtoxinA · PraxibotulinumtoxinA

Introduction

Botulinum toxins (BoNTs) are currently widely used in clinical practice, and their clinical application is ever expanding. There are seven different serotypes of BoNTs; however, only types A and B are available for clinical applications [1, 2]. There is interest to use other serotypes or modifications of these serotypes in order to change the duration of action of the toxin. In this review, the general aspect of BoNTs will be discussed, and then each available toxin will be discussed in detail in regard to their clinical and therapeutic applications. This article will not delve into the cosmetic application of the toxins.

K. Dashtipour (✉) · P. Spanel
Department of Neurology/Movement Disorders, Loma Linda University School of Medicine, Loma Linda, CA, USA
e-mail: kdashtipour@llu.edu

© Springer Nature Switzerland AG 2020   27
B. Jabbari (ed.), *Botulinum Toxin Treatment in Surgery, Dentistry, and Veterinary Medicine*, https://doi.org/10.1007/978-3-030-50691-9_3

BoNT Mechanism of Action and Their Diffusion

The BoNT-A and BoNT-B serotypes are neuromuscular blocking agents, and by blocking the release of acetylcholine at the neuromuscular junction (NMJ), they cause dampening or elimination of muscle overactivity [2–6]. The peak neuromuscular blocking clinical effect of the toxin occurs between 2 and 6 days after administration, and it can last for several months [7]. 7BoNT-A and BoNT-B inhibit the release of acetylcholine into the NMJ without interference with acetylcholine synthesis, uptake, or storage or the propagation of action potentials [6].

In nature, both BoNT-A and BoNT-B serotypes are synthesized as macromolecular protein complexes [6]. These protein complexes are referred to as progenitor toxins and consist of nontoxic accessory proteins (NAP) covalently bonded to the 150 kD neurotoxin [1, 3]. The BoNT-A progenitor toxins vary in molecular weight (300–900 kD) depending on the composition of NAPs and manufacturing process [1, 2, 6]. BoNT-B serotype only forms a 500 kD complex.4 The NAPs can be hemagglutinins (HA17, HA19, HA33, and HA52) or nontoxic–non-HA protein [1, 2, 6]. The NAPs are believed to be chaperones and serve to stabilize and protect the core 150 kD neurotoxin protein from degradation in harsh environments such as acidic PH of the stomach, but the therapeutic function of NAPs is unknown. However, it is clear that the 150 kD neurotoxin must dissociate from NAPs in order to exert pharmacologic effects [1, 2, 6]. The 150 kD core protein must be nicked to a dichain of heavy (100 kD) and light chains (50 kD) to be fully activated [1, 2, 6]. The light and heavy chains are connected through a disulfide bridge and noncovalent bonds.

BoNT formulations contain a variable percentage of "unnicked" toxin (which contributes to the overall protein load).

Upon blocking of the NMJ by BoNT, the binding sites for the toxin diminish, and a booster injection while the muscle is already denervated is not pharmacologically rational. This is due to significant reduction of the toxin uptake into the chemodenervated muscle.

The mechanism of action of BoNT can be described as a four-step process (Fig. 3.1): [1, 8] (1) toxin binding and capture, (2) endosome formation and internalization, (3) active transport of toxin from endosome into cytosol, and (4) cleavage of the acetylcholine neuroexocytosis apparatus (i.e., soluble N-ethylmaleimide-sensitive factor attachment protein receptors [SNAREs]).

Toxin binding and capture involves an array of membrane receptors at the presynaptic motor neuron. Both BoNT-A and BoNT-B enter the neuron by a dual-capture mechanism involving gangliosides (complex glycolipids localized on the outer membrane) and membrane receptors [1, 8]. The BoNT-A binds to the membrane receptor synaptic vesicle protein 2, whereas BoNT-B binds to synaptotagmins I and II [1, 3–6]. The heavy and light chains of the nicked toxin are essential for the toxin activity and each have specific roles. The heavy chain is composed of two domains, HC and HN [1, 3–6]. The HC domain is essential for binding of toxin to the outer membrane receptors and capturing it inside a formed endosome. Once the toxin is inside an endosome, the disulfide bridge is broken, and the catalytic light

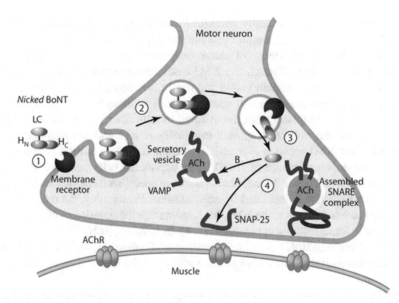

Fig. 3.1 Mechanism of action for botulinum toxins A and B.1–4, 6 Steps 1 and 2: The nicked (cleaved) botulinum neurotoxin (BoNT) is captured at neuronal membrane. Once captured, BoNT receptor binding is irreversible. The nicked BoNT is composed of a light chain (LC) and a heavy chain, which is further composed of two domains (HC and HN). The HC is essential for binding of toxin. On capture and endosome formation, the nicked BoNT disulfide bridge is broken, and the catalytic LC separates from the heavy chain. Step 3: The catalytic LC is released into the cytosol. Step 4: The LC begins to deactivate soluble N-ethylmaleimide-sensitive factor attachment protein receptors (SNAREs). There are different components of the SNARE apparatus, such as synaptosomal-associated protein 25 kD (SNAP-25) and vesicle-associated membrane protein (VAMP, also known as synaptobrevin). One LC will cleave existing and newly synthesized SNAREs, one after another, until the supply is depleted. Botulinum toxin type A catalytically cleaves SNAP-25, which is anchored to the inner layer axonal membrane, and BoNT-B cleaves VAMP, which is embedded within the acetylcholine (ACh) vesicle membrane. Cleavage (deactivation) of SNAP-25 or VAMP results in inhibition of ACh exocytosis, release, and neuromuscular denervation. AChR ACh receptor. (From Chen and Dashtipour 2013 – with reproduced with permission from publisher Wiley and Sons)

chain separates from the heavy chain [1, 3–6]. The catalytic light chain is released from the endosome and enters the axonal cytosol. The heavy chain HN domain is involved in the active transport of light chains from inside the endosome into the axonal cytosolic milieu [1, 3–6].

Upon release of light chains into the cytosol, they begin to deactivate SNARE proteins [1, 3–6]. Within an axon terminal, the light chain cleaves existing and newly synthesized SNAREs, one after another, until the supply is depleted. There are different components of the SNARE apparatus, such as synaptosomal-associated protein 25 kD (SNAP-25) and vesicle-associated membrane protein (VAMP, also known as synaptobrevin) [1, 3–6]. The BoNT-A serotype catalytically cleaves SNAP-25 and BoNT-B cleaves VAMP [1, 3–6]. The SNARE proteins are essential for acetylcholine vesicle docking, exocytosis, and neurotransmitter release [1, 3–6].

The light chain is structurally resistant to inactivation by intracellular protein degradation systems (e.g., ubiquitin-proteasome system), and the slow intracellular removal results in a persistence of pharmacodynamic effects at the NMJ [9]. It is important to note that although the NMJ loses functionality, the motor neuron, NMJ, and muscle fiber remain viable and regain function over time. The disabled axon terminal produces collateral sprouts, which induces the formation of new NMJs and motor endplates with the affected muscle fiber [1, 4]. As the original NMJ recovers, the collateral sprouts eventually retreat and are eliminated. On recovery of the NMJ acetylcholine activity, muscle (hyper) activity is resumed.

The mechanism of action of BoNT at myoepithelial cells (salivary and sweat glands) is not well known. Myoepithelial cells are specialized smooth muscle structures, and contraction is mediated by acetylcholine. Presumably, the mechanism is analogous to what occurs at the NMJ, but it seems that the duration of effect is more prolonged in intraglandular applications [1, 4]. In addition, BoNT-B appears to have a greater effect than BoNT-A in intraglandular applications [1, 4]. This may be due to differences in BoNT kinetics or binding affinity at the neuromyoepithelial effector junction.

BoNT is also known to possess antinociceptive effects, which may be mediated by inhibition of substance P and calcitonin gene-related peptide release [1, 4].

Despite having the same mechanism of action, each BoNT has distinct biologic properties with its own characteristic features. Each toxin has its own unique molecular structure, formulation, potency, and pharmacokinetics. Each toxin exerts its effect at the site of injection and spreads. The diffusion and migration of the BoNT is responsible for its local, distal, and systemic side effects [1, 2].

Multiple studies revealed that central effects can also occur as a consequence of botulinum toxin peripheral injections, possibly due to the retrograde axonal transport to antinociceptive nuclei within the central nervous system [10]. This presumption is based on observations of instances of clinical improvement despite minimal weakness following botulinum toxin injections as well as previous animal and human studies exploring central effects of botulinum toxin [10]. This central effect is believed to occur through retrograde axonal transport of toxin into the CNS or indirect modulation of cortical regions and/or cerebellum. One of the earlier animal studies looking at retrograde transport of botulinum toxin found that 48 hours after injection of radiolabeled botulinum toxin A into the gastrocnemius muscles of cats, there was increased radioactivity in the ventral roots and spinal cord ipsilateral to the side of injection [11]. In a more recent animal study, botulinum toxin A was injected into facial motor neurons of cats, and 3 days later the ipsilateral facial nucleus demonstrated significant amounts of botulinum toxin with Western blot analysis [12]. This evidence has been translated to human studies as well, and one study revealed the reduction of quadriceps H reflex in individuals treated with botulinum toxin to the soleus muscle [13]. This phenomenon resulted from presumed retrograde transport of botulinum toxin exerting effects on Renshaw cells [13]. In addition to the available evidence of retrograde transport resulting in central effects of botulinum toxin, there are several functional MRI studies demonstrating changes in cortical areas and cerebellum following peripheral Botox injection. The proposed central effects of BoNTs raise the possibility of an additional therapeutic impact rather than being attributable to causing additional side effects. However, there is still much to be explored in regard to discovering new applications and therapeutic indications [10].

BoNT for Clinical Application

At the time of this article, only four distinct BoNTs were commercially available for clinical applications (Fig. 3.2). In 2009, the FDA released the updated version of the safety warning on BoNTs with emphasis on the lack of interchangeability among toxins due to difference in units. Another concern of this safety report was about the

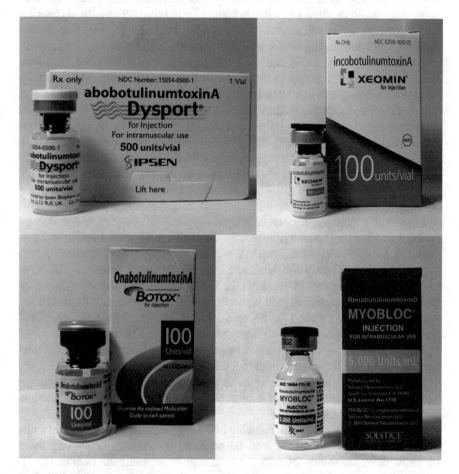

Fig. 3.2   Currently available botulinum toxins in the USA and Europe. (From Chen and Dashtipour 2013, reproduced with permission from Publisher (Wiley and Sons))

spread of the toxin to other body parts and the possibility of unwanted effects as extreme as respiratory failure and death [1, 2].

In recent years, the clinical application of BoNTs has largely expanded beyond neurology and dermatology to numerous subspecialties such as ophthalmology, physical medicine and rehabilitation, dentistry, gynecology, gastroenterology, and urology [1, 2].

The current four formulations of BoNTs do not have the same FDA-approved clinical profile; however, their clinical utility expands beyond their FDA indications. Tables 3.1 and 3.2 summarize the clinical applications of BoNTs and recommended dosing.

Clinicians performing injections should refer to manufacturer suggested dosages for each indication. Factors such as size of muscle being injected, patients' previous response to injections, and type of tissue being targeted need to be taken into consideration as well when deciding on dosage. Studies have been conducted in an effort to establish the dose equivalency among toxin brands. The ratio of onabotulinumtoxinA to incobotulinumtoxinA is reported to be 1:1 [4, 14]. Two studies exploring dose equivalency between onabotulinumtoxinA and abobotulinumtoxinA in the treatment of cervical dystonia (CD) found that ratios of 1:1.7 and 1:2.5 were similar in terms of efficacy and adverse events. However, at a ratio of 1:3, onabotulinumtoxinA was determined to be less efficacious [15, 16].Overall, the conversion ratio between onabotulinumtoxinA and abobotulinumtoxinA of 1:2.5–1:3 is most commonly reported [17]. Conversion ratio for onabotulinumtoxinA/rimabotulinumtoxinB ranges from 1:30 to 1:50. RimabotulinumtoxinB has been reported to have more frequent dry mouth as a side effect and likely has more glandular activity which is also a consideration when deciding on dosing [4]. It is worth noting once again that these conversion ratios are not standardized or globally accepted and deciding on dosage should be based on patients, condition, site of injection, and the past exposure and response to the BoNT.

The conditions for optimal storage are different for incoBoNT-A and other botulinum toxins. OnaBoNT-A, aboBoNT-A, and rimaBoNT-B need to be stored at 2 °C to 8 °C. IncobotulinumtoxinA unopened vials can be stored frozen at −20 °C to −10 °C, refrigerated at 2 °C to 8 °C, or kept at room temperature at 20 °C to 25 °C. RimabotulinumtoxinB is in liquid form and ready to use for injection; however, all other BoNTs need to be reconstituted prior to administration. Only preservative-free normal saline is recommended for reconstitution [1, 2].

Table 3.3 outlines similarities and differences in excipients, packaging, and storage of the four botulinum toxin brands according to manufacturer labeling.

Botulinum toxins have the potential to develop immunogenicity. The concern regarding immunogenicity is important, especially with long-term use and multiple clinical applications of BoNTs.

Multiple factors play a role in inducing immunogenicity, such as the manufacturing process, the antigenic protein load, the presence of accessory proteins, the overall toxin dose, frequency of injections, and prior exposure to BoNTs [1, 2]. Immunogenicity can be primary when there is a lack of response to BoNTs in a toxin-naïve patient, or it can occur as a secondary nonresponsiveness in patients

Table 3.1 Recommended doses of botulinum toxin products for the FDA-approved therapeutic indications

Agent	Indication	Dose
OnabotulinumtoxinA	Axillary hyperhidrosis	50 U per axilla
	Blepharospasm	Blepharospasm: 1.25–2.5 U into the muscles of the upper and lower eyelid (three injection sites) per affected eye
	Strabismus	1.25–5 U into each of three sites per affected eye; dose based on severity of deviation. Total dose should not exceed 25 U per single treatment
	Cervical dystonia	15–150 U per affected muscle based on patient's head/neck/shoulder position, pain localization, muscle hypertrophy; lower dose is recommended for toxin-naïve patients; repeat treatment no more frequently than every 12 weeks Mean dose 236 units, range of 198 units to 300 units
	Chronic migraine prophylaxis	Total dose 155 U divided among seven muscles (total of 31 sites) in head/neck muscles; repeat treatment every 12 weeks
	Upper limb spasticity in adults Upper limb spasticity in pediatrics aged 2–17 years	75 units to 400 units divided among the selected muscles 3–6 units/kg divided among affected muscles
	Lower limb spasticity in adults Lower limb spasticity in pediatrics aged 2–17 years excluding spasticity caused by cerebral palsy	The recommended dose for lower limb spasticity is 300–400 U 4–8 units/kg divided among affected muscles
	Neurogenic detrusor	Total dose of 200 U divided across 30 injection sites in the detrusor muscle (~6.7 U/site); repeat treatment every 42–48 weeks
	Overactive bladder	The recommend dose is 100 U for overactive bladder and is the maximum recommended dose
AbobotulinumtoxinA	Cervical dystonia	Total dose of 500 U divided among affected muscles; repeat treatment every 12–16 weeks; titrate dose in 250 U increments to desired clinical response up to 1000 units
	Upper limb spasticity in adults Upper limb spasticity in pediatrics aged 2 and older excluding spasticity caused by cerebral palsy	500 and 1000 units were divided among selected muscles in the pivotal clinical trial 8–16 units/kg divided among affected muscles

(continued)

Table 3.1 (continued)

Agent	Indication	Dose
	Lower limb spasticity in adults Lower limb spasticity in pediatrics	1000–1500 units divided among affected muscles 10–15 units/kg for unilateral lower limb or 20–30 units/kg for bilateral lower limb injections Maximum of 1000 units
IncobotulinumtoxinA	Blepharospasm	1.25–2.5 U per injection site. For patients previously treated with ONA, INCO dose is the same as previous dose of ONA
	Cervical dystonia	120–240 U divided among affected muscles; repeat treatment no more frequently than every 12 weeks
	Upper limb spasticity	Up to 400 units; repeat no more frequently than every 12 weeks
	Sialorrhea	Recommended total dose is 100 units per treatment consisting of 30 units per parotid gland and 20 units per submandibular gland, no sooner than every 16 weeks
RimabotulinumtoxinB	Cervical dystonia Sialorrhea	Initial recommended dose 2500–5000 U; may be titrated up to 10,000 U based on patient's response; repeat treatment every 12–16 weeks 500 units to 1500 units per parotid gland and 250 units per submandibular gland. No more frequent than every 12 weeks

who have previously responded, but the development of neutralizing antibodies has caused BoNT to be less effective or ineffective. It seems that antigenic protein load is correlated to the protein content of the core toxin (150 kD).

The most recent clinical studies showed almost the same rate of immunogenicity for both toxins: 1.2% for onaBoNT-A and 1.1% for incoBoNT-A [1, 2]. Major differences in immunogenicity among the type A toxin brands is yet to be determined given differences in study populations, assay sensitivity in looking for the presence of neutralizing antibodies, and dose equivalence [18–20]. Serotype B toxin (rimabotulinumtoxinB) appears to be more immunogenic than serotype A with frequency of development of neutralizing antibodies as high as 10–44% [18]. However, the importance of this high percentage of developing antibody with serotype B is not known, and the same rate (10–44%) of clinical unresponsiveness has not been reported. Currently, the standard of care of injecting patients with a frequency of not less than every 3 months and avoiding high doses of toxin in each single injection controls immunogenicity at significantly low levels when compared with older reports. However, in patients with urologic disorders, secondary unresponsiveness may occur due to the fact that the uroepithelium is more sensitive to antigens (e.g., bacterial antigens). Nontoxic accessory proteins (NAPs) do not play a role in the mechanism of action of BoNTs, but the NAPs (e.g., hemagglutinating and non-hemagglutinating proteins) act as adjuvants for the development of neutralizing

Table 3.2 Clinical application of the botulinum toxins

Achalasia	Anal fissure	Benign prostatic hyperplasia	Blepharospasm[a]	Chronic anal fissures	Cervical dystonia[a]	Esophageal dysmotility	Facial esthetics[a]
Hemifacial spasms	Hyperhidrosis[a]	Limb dystonia	Lingual dystonia	Lumbosacral pain and spasms	Migraine[a]	Myofascial pain	Nystagmus
Oromandibular dystonia	Overactive bladder[a]	Palatal myoclonus	Pain syndromes	Pelvic floor spasm	Sialorrhea[a]	Spasticity of upper and lower limb[a]	Spasmodic dysphonia
Strabismus[a]	Stuttering	Temporomandibular joint disorders	Tendinopathies	Tics	Tremors	Vaginismus	Writer's cramp

[a]A current FDA-approved indication

Table 3.3 Summary of botulinum toxin formulations

Toxin name	Toxin serotype	Packaging (units/vial)	Preparation	Excipients	Storage	Storage after reconstitution
OnabotulinumtoxinA (Botox)	Serotype A	100, 200	Vacuum dried powder	HSA, NaCl	Refrigerate 2–8 degrees Celsius	Refrigerate 2–8 degrees Celsius. Use within 24 hours
IncobotulinumtoxinA (Xeomin)	Serotype A	50,100, 200	Lyophilized powder	HSA, sucrose	Frozen, refrigerated, or stored at room temperature	Refrigerate 2–8 degrees Celsius. Use within 24 hours
AbobotulinumtoxinA (Dysport)	Serotype A	300, 500	Lyophilized powder	HSA, lactose	Refrigerate 2–8 degrees Celsius	Refrigerate 2–8 degrees Celsius. Use within 4 hours
RimabotulinumtoxinB (Myobloc)	Serotype B	2500, 5000, 10000	Sterile solution	HSA, NaCl, sodium succinate	Refrigerate 2–8 degrees Celsius	No reconstitution necessary. If solution is further diluted, use within 4 hours

antibodies. In theory, reducing the NAP load may minimize immunoresistance, but this remains an unresolved issue among product comparisons.

A well-known adverse effect involved with therapeutic applications of botulinum toxin involves contiguous spread of toxin to adjacent tissues. This has potential to cause undesirable effects by impacting tissues that were not originally being targeted, for example, eyelid ptosis resulting from the treatment of blepharospasm or dysphagia due to pharyngeal muscle weakness when treating CD. Differences in contiguous spread among the toxin brands have been studied; however, results of these studies have not found significant differences. Variance in contiguous spread among toxin brands is difficult to determine because spread is likely dependent on a variety of factors including injection technique, dosage used, type of target site, level of muscle hyperactivity, postinjection massage, and location of injection within a muscle. Injection techniques that may affect spread of toxin include volume of solution used, injection pressure, and needle size [21, 22].

BoNT Type A

There are currently three commercially available BoNT-As in the United States, onabotulinumtoxinA (onaBoNT-A), abobotulinumtoxinA (aboBoNT-A), and incobotulinumtoxinA (incoBoNT-A). All BoNT-As work by deactivating SNARE proteins by catalytically cleaving synaptosomal-associated membrane protein 25 kD (SNAP-25). This deactivation prevents acetylcholine release. Differences among the three types of BoNT-A include potency, presence or absence of nontoxic accessory proteins, dosing, storage, and FDA-approved indications [1, 2].

OnabotulinumtoxinA

Botox® (Allergan plc, Dublin, Ireland) is the trade name for onaBoNT-A. Originally approved by the FDA in 1989 for clinical use, onaBoNT-A has now been approved by the FDA for all of the following therapeutic conditions: strabismus [23] and blepharospasm [24], CD [25], hyperhidrosis, upper and lower limb spasticity [26], migraine headache [27], overactive bladder, and pediatric spasticity [28]. OnaBoNT-A has been available for clinical use the longest compared to the other type A toxin formulations discussed in this chapter. For this reason, OnaBoNT-A tends to be the toxin of choice among many providers in the United States [2]. OnaBoNT-A requires refrigeration at 2 °C to 8 °C and must be reconstituted in preservative-free normal saline prior to administration. Patients need repeating the injection every 3 months except for overactive bladder when patients receive injection every 6 months [28].

AbobotulinumtoxinA

Dysport® (Ipsen) is the trade name for aboBoNT-A. The FDA has approved the therapeutic application of aboBoNT-A for the following conditions: CD [9, 29], upper and lower limb spasticity in adults, and lower limb spasticity in pediatric patients 2 years of age or older [30]. AboBoNT-A was available in Europe years prior to its approval in the states by FDA. Similar to onaBoNT-A, aboBoNT-A requires refrigeration at 2 °C to 8 °C and must be reconstituted in preservative-free normal saline prior to administration. The typical dosing interval for aboBoNT-A is also about every 3 months [1, 2, 31].

IncobotulinumtoxinA

Xeomin® (Merz) is the trade name for incoBoNT-A. IncoBoNT-A is the most recent BoNT-A to come to the market in the United States. The FDA has approved the application of incoBoNT-A for the following therapeutic conditions: upper limb spasticity [32], CD [33], chronic sialorrhea, and blepharospasm [34]. IncoBoNT-A was manufactured free of potentially immunogenic proteins from clostridia in an attempt to reduce immunogenicity. Unlike the other BoNT-A, incoBoNT-A may be stored at room temperature prior to reconstitution with preservative-free normal saline. Patients tend to require dosing for therapeutic indications once every 3 months [1, 2, 35].

BoNT Type B

There is only one commercial available BoNT-B in the United States, rimabotulinumtoxinB (rimaBoNT-B). Both BoNT-A and BoNT-B work to deactivate SNARE proteins. The one difference between the two toxins is how the deactivation occurs. BoNT-A catalytically cleaves synaptosomal-associated membrane protein 25 kD (SNAP-25). BoNT-B deactivates SNARE by cleaving vesicle-associated membrane protein (VAMP) [1, 2].

RimabotulinumtoxinB

Myobloc® (Solstice Neuroscience) is the trade name for rimaBoNT-B. The FDA has approved rimaBoNT-B for CD [36] and sialorrhea [37]. Unlike the other toxins presented in this article, rimaBoNT-B is the only toxin in a liquid formulation. It seems to be more effective at neuroglandular junctions, lending itself well to use for sialorrhea. The liquid formulation has an acidic pH and causes a stinging pain at the site of injection [1, 2, 22].

Future Products

DaxibotulinumtoxinA (daxiBoNT-A) is a novel BoNT-A product under development by Revance Therapeutics and has the potential to be the first long-acting neuromodulator [23, 36, 38]. DaxiBoNT-A is a purified 150 kDa BoNT-A (RTT150) that is devoid of accessory proteins and formulated with a proprietary stabilizing excipient peptide (RTP004) in a lyophilized powder. The peptide has a backbone of lysines that carry a positive charge which results in the peptide binding electrostatically to the negatively charged core neurotoxin. DaxiBoNT-A is without human serum albumin and is stable at room temperature prior to reconstitution. Preliminary data suggests that injectable daxiBoNT-A at doses of up to 450 U is well tolerated and may offer prolonged efficacy [39]. The median duration of response was 25.3 weeks (95% CI, 20.14–26.14 weeks). There were no serious adverse events, and the most common detected side effects were dysphagia (14%) and injection site erythema (8%). Further studies involving larger numbers of patients are now warranted and underway for cervical dystonia and spasticity.

PraxibotulinumtoxinA (Jeuveau ®) is another BoNT-A product originally developed in South Korea that recently received FDA approval for the cosmetic treatment of glabellar lines based on two randomized multicenter double blinded trials. The product comes as a vacuum dried powder in single-use 100 unit vials [40]. Currently, it has not received FDA approval for any other clinical applications within the United States; however, there is currently an ongoing phase II clinical trial for the treatment of CD.

Acknowledgments We thank Dr. Jessa Koch for her assistance in referencing.

References

1. Chen JJ, Dashtipour K. Abo-, inco-, ona-, and rima-botulinum toxins in clinical therapy: a primer. Pharmacotherapy. 2013;33:304–18.
2. Dashtipour K, Pedouim F. Botulinum toxin: preparations for clinical use, immunogenicity, side effects, and safety profile. Semin Neurol. 2016;36:29–33.
3. Aoki KR, Guyer B. Botulinum toxin type A and other botulinum toxin serotypes: a comparative review of biochemical and pharmacological actions. Eur J Neurol. 2001;8(Suppl 5):21–9.
4. Dressler D, Benecke R. Pharmacology of therapeutic botulinum toxin preparations. Disabil Rehabil. 2007;29:1761–8.
5. Setler PE. Therapeutic use of botulinum toxins: background and history. Clin J Pain. 2002;18:S119–24.
6. Simpson LL. The origin, structure, and pharmacological activity of botulinum toxin. Pharmacol Rev. 1981;33:155–88.

7. Burgen AS, Dickens F, Zatman LJ. The action of botulinum toxin on the neuro-muscular junction. J Physiol. 1949;109:10–24.
8. Wortzman MS, Pickett A. The science and manufacturing behind botulinum neurotoxin type A-ABO in clinical use. Aesthet Surg J. 2009;29:S34–42.
9. Truong D, Brodsky M, Lew M, et al. Long-term efficacy and safety of botulinum toxin type A (Dysport) in cervical dystonia. Parkinsonism Relat Disord. 2010;16:316–23.
10. Weise D, Weise CM, Naumann M. Central effects of botulinum neurotoxin-evidence from human studies. Toxins (Basel). 2019;11:21.
11. Wiegand HEG, Wellhoner H. 125I-labelled botulinum A neurotoxin: pharmacokinetics in cat's after intramuscular injection. Naunyn Schmiedebergs Arch Pharmacol. 1976;292:161–5.
12. Antonucci F, Rossi C, Gianfranceschi L, Rossetto O, Caleo M. Long-distance retrograde effects of botulinum neurotoxin A. J Neurosci. 2008;28:3689–96.
13. Marchand-Pauvert V, Aymard C, Giboin LS, Dominici F, Rossi A, Mazzocchio R. Beyond muscular effects: depression of spinal recurrent inhibition after botulinum neurotoxin A. J Physiol. 2013;591:1017–29.
14. Dressler D, Mander G, Fink K. Measuring the potency labelling of onabotulinumtoxinA (Botox((R))) and incobotulinumtoxinA (Xeomin ((R))) in an LD50 assay. J Neural Transm (Vienna). 2012;119:13–5.
15. Rystedt A, Zetterberg L, Burman J, Nyholm D, Johansson A. A comparison of Botox 100 U/mL and Dysport 100 U/mL using dose conversion ratio 1: 3 and 1: 1.7 in the treatment of cervical dystonia: a double-blind, randomized, crossover trial. Clin Neuropharmacol. 2015;38:170–6.
16. Yun JY, Kim JW, Kim HT, et al. Dysport and Botox at a ratio of 2.5:1 units in cervical dystonia: a double-blind, randomized study. Mov Disord. 2015;30:206–13.
17. Dashtipour K, Chen JJ, Espay AJ, Mari Z, Ondo W. OnabotulinumtoxinA and AbobotulinumtoxinA dose conversion: a systematic literature review. Mov Disord Clin Pract. 2016;3:109–15.
18. Naumann M, Boo LM, Ackerman AH, Gallagher CJ. Immunogenicity of botulinum toxins. J Neural Transm (Vienna). 2013;120:275–90.
19. Pickett A, Perrow K. Formulation composition of botulinum toxins in clinical use. J Drugs Dermatol. 2010;9:1085–91.
20. Pickett A, Rosales RL. New trends in the science of botulinum toxin-A as applied in dystonia. Int J Neurosci. 2011;121(Suppl 1):22–34.
21. Hsu TS, Dover JS, Arndt KA. Effect of volume and concentration on the diffusion of botulinum exotoxin A. Arch Dermatol. 2004;140:1351–4.
22. Ramirez-Castaneda J, Jankovic J, Comella C, Dashtipour K, Fernandez HH, Mari Z. Diffusion, spread, and migration of botulinum toxin. Mov Disord. 2013;28:1775–83.
23. Carruthers JD, Kennedy RA, Bagaric D. Botulinum vs adjustable suture surgery in the treatment of horizontal misalignment in adult patients lacking fusion. Arch Ophthalmol. 1990;108:1432–5.
24. Arthurs B, Flanders M, Codere F, Gauthier S, Dresner S, Stone L. Treatment of blepharospasm with medication, surgery and type A botulinum toxin. Can J Ophthalmol. 1987;22:24–8.
25. Jankovic J, Adler CH, Charles D, et al. Primary results from the cervical dystonia patient registry for observation of onabotulinumtoxina efficacy (CD PROBE). J Neurol Sci. 2015;349:84–93.
26. Wein TEA, Wolfgang J, Ward A, Grace P, Dimitrova R. OnabotulinumtoxinA for the treatment of poststroke distal lower limb spasticity: a randomized trial. PM R. 2018;10:693–703.
27. Dodick DW, Turkel CC, DeGryse RE, et al. OnabotulinumtoxinA for treatment of chronic migraine: pooled results from the double-blind, randomized, placebo-controlled phases of the PREEMPT clinical program. Headache. 2010;50:921–36.
28. A) Bo. [package insert]. In: Allergan I, ed. Irvine, 2017.
29. Truong D, Comella C, Fernandez HH, Ondo WG. Dysport benign essential Blepharospasm study G. Efficacy and safety of purified botulinum toxin type A (Dysport) for the treatment of

benign essential blepharospasm: a randomized, placebo-controlled, phase II trial. Parkinsonism Relat Disord. 2008;14:407–14.

30. Delgado MR, Tilton A, Russman B, et al. AbobotulinumtoxinA for Equinus foot deformity in cerebral palsy: a randomized controlled trial. Pediatrics. 2016;137:e20152830.
31. A) Da. [Prescribing information]. Basking Ridge: Ipsen Biopharmaceuticals, 2017.
32. Elovic EP, Munin MC, Kanovsky P, Hanschmann A, Hiersemenzel R, Marciniak C. Randomized, placebo-controlled trial of incobotulinumtoxina for upper-limb post-stroke spasticity. Muscle Nerve. 2016;53:415–21.
33. Comella CL, Jankovic J, Truong DD, Hanschmann A, Grafe S, Group USXCDS. Efficacy and safety of incobotulinumtoxinA (NT 201, XEOMIN(R), botulinum neurotoxin type A, without accessory proteins) in patients with cervical dystonia. J Neurol Sci. 2011;308:103–9.
34. Jankovic J, Comella C, Hanschmann A, Grafe S. Efficacy and safety of incobotulinumtox-inA (NT 201, Xeomin) in the treatment of blepharospasm-a randomized trial. Mov Disord. 2011;26:1521–8.
35. Xeomin. [package insert]. Raleigh: Merz North America, Inc, 2015.
36. Brashear A, Lew MF, Dykstra DD, et al. Safety and efficacy of NeuroBloc (botulinum toxin type B) in type A-responsive cervical dystonia. Neurology. 1999;53:1439–46.
37. Isaacson SH, Ondo W, Jackson CE, et al. Safety and efficacy of RimabotulinumtoxinB for treatment of Sialorrhea in adults: a randomized clinical trial. JAMA Neurol. 2020;77:461.
38. Myobloc. [package insert]. South San Francisco: Solstics Neurosciences Inc, 2009.
39. Jankovic J, Truong D, Patel AT, et al. Injectable DaxibotulinumtoxinA in cervical dystonia: a phase 2 dose-escalation multicenter study. Mov Disord Clin Pract. 2018;5:273–82.
40. Jeauveau. [package insert]. Santa Barbara: Evolus Inc, 2019.

Chapter 4
Evidence-Based Review of Current Botulinum Toxin Treatment Indications in Medicine

Dhanya Vijayakumar and Joseph Jankovic

Abstract Botulinum neurotoxin (BoNT) has been increasingly used not only as a cosmetic drug but, more importantly, it has emerged as the most versatile therapeutic, utilized in virtually all sub-specialties of medicine. In neurology, there is Level A (effective) evidence for the use of certain serotypes of BoNT in cervical dystonia, chronic migraines, upper- and lower-limb spasticity and Level B (probably effective) evidence in blepharospasm. These levels of recommendation, however, must be interpreted cautiously as they are based only on published randomized, controlled studies and are limited to particular products. United States Food and Drug Administration (US-FDA) approved BoNT for these and other indications, such as focal axillary hyperhidrosis and sialorrhea, but there are a growing number of conditions for which BoNT is used off-label. In addition to focal dystonia, BoNT is also increasingly used to treat tremor and other movement disorders and a variety of neuropathic pain disorders including trigeminal neuralgia, post-herpetic neuralgia, and diabetic neuropathy. In urology, there are several randomized controlled trials supporting the benefits of BoNT in overactive bladder and interstitial cystitis. In gastroenterology, BoNT is used to treat anal fissures and achalasia. Thus, BoNT is the most widely used therapeutic molecule.

Keywords Botulinum toxin · Dystonia · Blepharospasm · Tremor · Spasticity · Pain · Bladder

D. Vijayakumar (✉)
The University of South Carolina School of Medicine Greenville, Prisma Health Upstate, Neuroscience Associates/Department of Internal Medicine, Greenville, SC, USA
e-mail: dhanya.vijayakumar@prismahealth.org

J. Jankovic
Baylor College of Medicine, Baylor St. Luke's Medical Center at the McNair Campus, Houston, TX, USA
e-mail: josephj@bcm.edu

© Springer Nature Switzerland AG 2020   43
B. Jabbari (ed.), *Botulinum Toxin Treatment in Surgery, Dentistry, and Veterinary Medicine*, https://doi.org/10.1007/978-3-030-50691-9_4

Introduction

Botulinum neurotoxin (BoNT) is an exotoxin produced by *Clostridium botulinum* and is the most potent biological toxin [105]. Although the various BoNT products contain only 0.44–5 ng/vial, the estimated lethal dose is 0.09–0.15 μg when BoNT is injected intravenously and 70 μg when ingested; 39.2 g sufficient to eradicate humankind [33]. In addition to the well-defined seven BoNT serotypes (BoNT/A-G), a new mosaic toxin type termed BoNT/HA (also known as BoNT FA or H) was reported [103, 263]. All BoNTs act by inhibiting acetylcholine release at the nerve terminals of striatal and smooth muscles, and exocrine glands, but they also act on other neurotransmitters including adenosine triphosphate, substance P, and calcitonin gene-related peptide and may downregulate sensory receptors, such as transient receptor potential cation channel subfamily V member 1 (TRPV1). The latter mechanism is important in the analgesic's effects of BoNT.

BoNT acts as a zinc proteinase by cleaving neuronal vesicle-associated proteins, collectively called the SNARE (soluble N-ethylmaleimide-sensitive factor attachment protein receptor) complex, thereby preventing the docking and fusion of the vesicles with the presynaptic membrane and thus preventing the release (exocytosis) of acetylcholine into the nerve terminal [142]. Various BoNT serotypes work differently and the sites of cleavage of SNARE complex vary between serotypes. BoNT serotype A, C, and E cleave SNAP-25 (synaptosome-associated protein of 25 kd) while serotypes B, D, F, and G cleave synaptobrevin, also known as VAMP (vesicle-associated membrane protein) [263]. Due to this cleavage, acetylcholine is unable to leave the nerve terminal to initiate contraction in the postsynaptic muscle, resulting in chemodenervation [103]. Of the eight serotypes, only BoNT types A and B are approved for clinical use in the United States. There are three formulations of BoNT type A used in clinical practice in the United States, namely, onabotulinumtoxinA (Botox®), abobotulinumtoxinA (Dysport®), and incobotulinumtoxinA (Xeomin®). BoNT-type B classified as rimabotulinumtoxinB (Myobloc®) is the other neurotoxin available for clinical use in the United States.

In 1977, Dr. Allen Scott first injected BoNT in a patient with strabismus. In October 1981, Dr. Joseph Jankovic first injected a patient with blepharospasm with BoNT, and this was followed by a double-blind controlled study of BoNT in cranial-cervical dystonia including cervical dystonia (CD) and blepharospasm. In 1989, onabotulinumtoxinA (Botox) was the first BoNT product approved by the US Food and Drug Administration (FDA) for the treatment of strabismus, blepharospasm, and cranial nerve VII disorders including hemifacial spasms [105]. Since then, it has been widely adopted for several additional indications in neurology, urology, dermatology, gastroenterology, and pain management/neuro-rehabilitation. BoNT is most frequently used for the treatment of various conditions that involve abnormal, excessive, inappropriate exaggerated muscle contraction, and pain, but its use is expanding to many new and different indications [105].

The duration of benefits from BoNT injections last for about 3–4 months, after which there is a loss of inhibitory effect, likely due to sprouting of new terminals, and eventual loss of effect at the original nerve terminal [193]. Side effects from BoNT vary depending on the area injected and adjacent non-target muscles or glands to which the toxin could spread, resulting in undesired effects such as ptosis, dry eyes with eyelid injections, dysphagia, especially following anterior neck injections, neck weakness, particularly with posterior neck injections, facial asymmetry with injections for hemifacial spasm or facial dystonia, and weakness in the hands with forearm injections for hand dystonia or tremor. In addition to local side effects, about 14% of treatment visits are associated with transient flu-like symptoms [13, 77]. BoNT should be avoided in patients with neuromuscular disorders and motor neuron disease and pregnant or lactating women, although there is no evidence of teratogenicity associated with BoNT therapy [25]. Although EMG, ultrasound, and kinematic guidance can be used for localization, no muscle targeting technique has yet proven to be superior [159, 215, 268].

Neurology

Tremor

The role of BoNT has been studied in different tremor conditions with good success, but BoNT is not yet FDA approved for these tremor indications and its use is off label. Several studies have provided evidence of beneficial effects of BoNT in the treatment of various tremors [148–150, 159].

(a) Dystonic tremor

Dystonic head and neck tremors could be present in patients with CD, voice tremor in spasmodic dysphonia, and dystonic hand tremors in patients with focal dystonia of the upper extremity such as organic writer's cramp, musician's dystonia, and other task-specific tremors. Primary dystonia patients are more likely to have tremor than patients with secondary dystonia including tardive dystonia [169]. Hand tremor has been reported in patients with dystonia affecting other parts of their body and reported the prevalence of postural or kinetic tremor in these patients to range from 14% to 86% [169].

In a retrospective chart review on 91 patients with medically refractory hand tremor treated with botulinum toxin, 31 patients had dystonic tremor. The majority of patients noted a benefit with BoNT injections in the forearm flexor muscles [159]. Other studies have confirmed the efficacy of BoNT in the treatment of essential (ET) and dystonic tremors [104, 148, 159].

(b) Task-specific tremor

Primary writing tremor (PWT) is a type of task-specific movement disorder where tremor occurs predominantly or exclusively while writing. This shares features with ET and dystonia [219, 246]. The lack of adequate response to typical medications used to treat ET like primidone and propranolol, presence of mirror movements typically seen in patients with dystonia, makes this more closely related to dystonia than to ET. PWT causes significant inconvenience to patients in occupations that demand a great deal of writing or enjoy writing as a hobby. Several studies have examined the effects of BoNT on PWT. There are two case series and a case report, which showed beneficial effects of BoNT in this condition [11, 172, 219]. In one of the case series, four out of five patients noted a significant and sustained improvement in tremor during the course of BoNT treatment. In this study, 10–12 units of BoNT/A was injected into flexor carpi radialis, extensor carpi radialis and ulnaris, abductor pollicis longus and extensor digitorum communis [172]. In a case report of a 64-year-old man, retired postal worker, 12.5 units of BoNT type A was injected into flexor carpi radialis under EMG guidance. This resulted in a 75% improvement in the symptoms that sustained for 3 months [219].

(c) Essential tremor
BoNT has been studied in patients with ET resulting in hand tremor, voice tremor, and head tremor. There is a paucity of large trials looking at the efficacy of BoNT for tremors, but BoNT has been used for selected patients who are refractory to medications prior to consideration of more invasive strategies like deep brain stimulation (DBS). The mechanism of BoNT is thought to be from the relaxation of involved muscle groups, or due to altered peripheral or central mechanisms [131].

For ET involving the hands, there were small studies looking at injection of flexor and extensor muscles. These were limited due to side effects of hand weakness noted particularly with extensor muscle injections [109]. In one open label study which enrolled 26 tremor patients of whom 14 had ET, there was significant improvement in the tremor and disability scores of ET patients [234]. Five of the fourteen patients reported moderate-to-marked subjective improvement in functional abilities after BoNT. However, the average reduction in tremor amplitude was less than 25% and the degree of tremor amplitude reduction correlated with patients' subjective impression about tremor benefit [234]. There are a few other open label trials evaluating the efficacy of BoNT in ET hand tremor which have shown significant improvement in tremor subjectively [167, 185, 204] and some using objective tremor [203, 204].

In 1996, Jankovic et al. reported the first randomized double-blind placebo-controlled study to evaluate the effect of BoNT injections in patients with ET hand tremor. Twenty-five patients with moderate–to-severe hand tremor were injected with BoNT, and there was significant improvement in tremor noted on tremor severity rating scales and on accelerometry measurements. Fifty units of BoNT was injected into wrist flexors and extensors with repeat injections in 4 weeks. There was mild and transient weakness of finger and wrist extensors attributed to injections of the extensor carpi radialis and ulnaris muscles [110]. Subsequently, another randomized placebo-controlled study was done involving 133 patients who were injected in the flexors and extensors in two parallel groups of low- and high-dose injections. There was significant improvement in postural tremor in both groups, but there was more weakness in the group injected with higher dose BoNT. There were no major changes in measures of motor tasks and functional disability, possibly due to weakness that resulted after the injections [27]. In a retrospective chart review done in patients with medically refractory tremor, of 53 patients with ET affecting their hands who received BoNT injections, the majority noted improvement in their tremor [159]. As a result of troublesome weakness-associated extensor muscle injections, many investigators tend to avoid injecting these muscles in patients with ET-related hand tremor, but the selection of the muscles and dosage must be individualized [114]. Another randomized double-blind placebo-controlled crossover trial evaluated the efficacy of BoNT in 33 ET patients with hand tremor, with injections customized to individual patients' tremor quality. Between 80 and 120 U of incobotulinumtoxinA was injected between 8 and 14 muscles in the hand and forearm of individual patients. There was significant improvement in Fahn Tolosa Marin tremor rating scales at 4 and 8 weeks. There was no significant hand weakness, but mild weakness was observed in 50% of patients receiving BoNT injections [150].

In ET patients with voice tremor, a minority of patients experience tremor benefit from BoNT injections into the vocal cords. Breathiness of voice is a common side effect seen with BoNT injection into the vocal cord. In a study which included 34 patients, 16 noted improvement in their voice tremor after BoNT injections into thyroarytenoid muscle [222]. In another study, EMG-guided injections were performed depending on the type of tremor, with thyroarytenoid injections performed for horizontal tremor, and strap muscle injections for vertical laryngeal tremor. For mixed tremor type, injections were performed based on the tremor type that was dominant/more severe. If both vertical and horizontal tremors were equally severe, strap muscles were injected first with thyroartytenoid injection done 2 weeks later. Starting doses of 1 unit was injected into the thyroarytenoid muscle with higher doses less than 10 units used for strap muscles and other adjacent neck muscles injected in this study. All 16 patients who received injections in this series had tremor benefit from BoNT; hoarseness was the only side effect observed, mostly following injections to the thyroarytenoid muscle [93]. Another small open label crossover study looked into BoNT injection into vocalis muscle either unilaterally or bilaterally. This was a small study in 10 patients with essential voice tremor, with EMG guided injections of 15 units into the left vocalis (unilaterally) with cross over to the bilateral vocalis injection arm (2.5 units into each vocalis) of the study after 16 or 18 weeks or vice versa. Only 3 of the 10 patients had objective reduction in voice tremor with bilateral injections and 2 of 9 patients who received unilateral injection. Breathiness and reduced vocal effort were seen, but 8 of the 10 patients chose to get re-injected at the end of the study [255]. In 15 patients with ET resulting in voice tremor, BoNT was injected into thyroarytenoid or into the cricothyroid or thyrohoid muscles; there was significant improvement in voice tremor based on subjective evaluation and also based on perceptual evaluation of recorded speech samples [97]. There is a small study by Ludlow et al. in 1989, another study by Brin et al. in 1992 and a case report by Warrick et al. in 2000, all of which showed efficacy of BoNT in the treatment of voice tremor. A prospective randomized trial over 6 weeks involving 13 ET patients with voice tremor showed that there was improvement in voice tremor in all patients over the observed period with dysphagia and breathiness being the most common side effects [3]. Based on these studies, an evidence-based review suggested level 1 recommendation for the use of BoNT in ET affecting the voice [179].

About 30–40% of ET patients with head tremor do not respond well to medications. There was one small double-blind placebo-controlled trial by Pahwa et al. in 1995 assessing BoNT in 10 patients with head tremor. In this study, 40 units were injected into bilateral sternocleidomastoid muscles and 60 units into bilateral splenius capiti muscles, with subsequent crossover into the placebo group. There was over mild-to-moderate improvement in 50% of the patients compared to 10% improvement noted in the placebo group [168]. Transient, non-disabling, neck weakness is the most common side effect observed with this pattern of injection. Several patients with essential tremor also have concomitant CD and dystonic tremor affecting their head. BoNT appears to work better for dystonic head tremors than for ET associated head tremor [130].

In a study involving 43 patients of which 13 had head tremor due to ET without dystonic component, and the remaining had head tremor secondary to CD, BoNT was injected into neck muscles with dosing individualized based on neck position and visible and palpable tremor oscillation. A mean dose of 400 units of abobotulinumtoxinA was split between the two splenius capiti muscles in patients with ET head tremor. There was significant improvement in tremor, based on accelerometry analysis in both groups of patients with head tremor from ET and from CD [259]. In a study involving 51 patients with disabling tremor, 8 of whom had ET related head tremor, there was significant improvement in tremor with BoNT injections [109].

(d) Parkinson-associated rest tremor

The rest tremor in Parkinson's disease (PD) tends to be responsive to levodopa, but in some patients there is insufficient tremor control or side effects with medication titration which limits tremor control. In these patients, BoNT could be used for better tremor control with muscle selection individualized based on the nature of the tremor depending on the predominant movement (flexion-extension, pronation supination or ulnar-radial deviation type), and the predominant joint involved (finger tremor, wrist tremor or elbow tremor) [160].

In a randomized double-blind placebo-controlled cross-over study, 30 patients received BoNT injections into the hand and forearm muscles. Patients were injected customized to their tremor rather than a standard protocol. Between 2.5 and 20 units of BoNT/A was injected in different muscles, including lumbricals, flexor carpi radialis, flexor carpi ulnaris, flexor digitorum superficialis, pronator, biceps, triceps, extensor carpi radialis, extensor carpi ulnaris, extensor digitorum, flexor pollicis brevis, flexor digitorum profundus, abductor pollicis brevis, brachioradialis, supinator, and opponens pollicis. There was a significant improvement in the tremor on tremor severity scale and improvement in patients' impression of change and an improved ability to do activities at home, without much weakness as side effect [149].

In an open label study, 28 patients were injected with BoNT for PD tremor using kinematic measures to personalize muscle selection for injection. There was significant decrease in Unified Parkinson's Disease Rating Scale (UPDRS) rest tremor scores and Fahn-Tolosa-Marin tremor severity scores. Ten patients experienced mild weakness which did not affect activities of daily living [187, 203]. In another 3-month open label study in 7 patients with PD-related upper-limb tremor, with kinematic assessment of tremor done pre and post injections, there was significant improvement in kinematic assessments of static and functional tasks at 2 and 3 months. There was also significant improvement in the UPDRS tremor scores and spiral drawings [186]. In another open label study in 26 patients, 12 of whom had PD; there was over 50% reduction in tremor in 2 patients and moderate-to-marked subjective improvement in functional benefit in 5 patients after BoNT injections. However, the average tremor reduction was less than 25% by quantitative measures [234]. In a prospective study in 187 patients with tremor, 15 patients with tremor due to Parkinson's disease, BoNT injections were done under EMG guidance with booster injections given if needed for optimum tremor control. In this study, there was an average BoNT efficacy of 35.7% for PD tremor. There was marked subjective improvement in tremor along with significant reduction in tremor amplitude of over 50% in 2 of 15 patients with PD tremor [185].

(e) Jaw tremor
Jaw tremor could be seen as part of the tremor spectrum in patients with ET, dystonic tremor, PD, task specific tremor and also in other neurologic conditions such as hereditary geniospasm. Patients with jaw tremor as part of ET typically have more widespread severe tremor and a long history of having ET. There is some thought that jaw tremor may be a marker of subsequent development of PD in these patients [132]. Jaw tremor is more common in PD than in ET patients, with prevalence in ET estimated to be between 7.5% and 18% [96]. Jaw tremor could also be a dystonic tremor in the setting of dystonia. In patients with bothersome jaw tremor, refractory to medical therapy, BoNT should be considered as a therapeutic option.

In a case report about a woman with position specific jaw tremor, likely dystonic in nature, where there was improvement in tremor after BoNT injections [228]. In a case series of 7 patients with jaw tremor in the setting of dystonia, one patient had BoNT injection for jaw tremor and noted improvement in the tremor. Others in this series did not receive injection and received oral medications with inadequate benefit [206].

In a pilot study involving three patients with jaw tremor due to PD, who were injected with onabotulinumtoxinA, there was significant improvement in jaw tremor in all 3 patients at 4 and 9 weeks post injection. Between 30 and 100 units of abobotulinumtoxinA was injected in the masseter bilaterally with mentalis muscle included in one of the patients. There were no side effects including no dry mouth [207].

(f) Holmes tremor
Holmes tremor, also called rubral, mesencephalic, or thalamic tremor, is a slow (2–5 Hz tremor), high-amplitude tremor, present at rest, worse with action. This often occurs after lesions affecting the thalamus, brainstem, or cerebellum. Usual

etiology of the lesion includes vascular lesions, demyelinating disorders, head trauma, AV malformations, or neoplasms [63, 188].

A case report of a 29-year-old male patient with Holmes tremor after pontine hemorrhage describes marked improvement in tremor after BoNT injection. BoNT was injected into the 2nd, 3rd, 4th flexor digitorum superficialis and 40 units in the extensor pollicis longus using ultrasound guidance. There was sustained improvement at the 4- and 9-week follow-up. There was some improvement noted in the activities of daily living [4].

(g) Cerebellar tremor

Lesions in the deep cerebellar nuclei (dentate, globose, or emboliform) or in the brachium conjunctivum (superior cerebellar peduncle), which contains fibers crossing over to the contralateral ventrolateral thalamus, could result in a cerebellar intention tremor. These deep cerebellar lesions cause intension tremor on the ipsilateral extremity. This is often an irregular 3–5 Hz tremor, affecting proximal more than distal muscle groups [63].

A retrospective analysis about the effect of BoNT on cerebellar tremor in 14 patients before and 1 month after injections, showed that there was improvement in tremor after BoNT injection into the agonist muscles alone. Antagonist muscles were avoided to prevent limb weakness. However, in this study, in addition to patients with cerebellar tremor from stroke, multiple sclerosis, and spinocerebellar ataxia, some ET patients were also included [243].

A small pilot study looked at the effect of BoNT in five patients with cerebellar tremor from multiple sclerosis and found no significant improvement in tremor with BoNT injection, but there was a trend toward improvement on some of the tremor ratings. Two of these five patients were injected again 2 months from first injection. There was worsening of pre-existing weakness that limited the use of BoNT in these patients [41].

(h) Palatal myoclonus (tremor)

Palatal myoclonus or tremor could either be primary/essential palatal myoclonus or secondary due to lesions in the Guillian-Mollaret triangle or the dentato-rubro-olivary network. Essential palatal myoclonus is due to repetitive contraction of the tensor veli palatini muscle, innervated by the trigeminal nerve, which results in rhythmic opening of the eustachian tube. Secondary palatal myoclonus is due to contraction of the levator veli palatini and results in repetitive palatal elevation [12]. This ear clicking and palatal myoclonus could be bothersome and distracting to patients.

There are several case reports which show efficacy of BoNT in palatal myoclonus [45, 49, 129, 214, 252]. BoNT is injected trans-palatal into the aponeurosis of the tensor veli palatini muscle.

In a case series of five patients with palatal myoclonus who received BoNT injections, four reported complete resolution of symptoms. One patient reported transient dysphagia and weak voice. BoNT was injected into the soft palate at the posteromedial aspect of maxillary tuberosity, where tensor veli palitini and levator veli palitini insert. Starting doses between 5 and 15 units of abobotulinumtoxinA were used in this study [178].

Other Parkinsonian Disorders

There are many symptoms experienced by patients with PD that may be amenable to BoNT therapy including blepharospasm, anterocollis, camptocormia, foot dystonia, hand and jaw tremor, sialorrhea, seborrhea, overactive bladder, and constipation [32, 104, 106, 111]. In addition to utilizing BoNT in the treatment of PD-related symptoms, there is emerging research on the role of BoNT in the central nervous system that may have relevance to the treatment of neurodegenerative disorders such as PD. For example BoNT/B when injected in the brains of animal models has been shown to block the transynaptic transmission of alpha-synuclein [164].

Freezing of gait (FoG)

There have been several studies suggesting the use of BoNT in FoG, but the results have been inconsistent [271]. This initially came about after a patient who received BoNT for off dystonia in the foot reported improvement in FoG [82, 84]. This was studied further in a pilot study of ten PD patients with FoG where three patients reported marked improvement in FoG, while two had no benefit, and one patient who was injected in a blinded manner had no improvement with saline injections and marked improvement after BoNT injection in calf muscles. Between 100 and 300 units of onabotulinumtoxinA was injected into the lateral and medial heads of gastrocnemius and into the soleus in this study. One or both legs were injected [83]. In another study involving 20 patients with PD of whom 10 had FoG, there was improvement in FoG after BoNT injection into the tensor fascia latae. Eight of the ten patients had significant improvement in FoG scores [240]. However, in a prospective double-blind placebo-controlled trial testing this concept further in 11 patients, 6 patients received 150 units of onabotulinumtoxinA injections and 5 received saline injections into the calves of both legs. There was no significant improvement in FoG in either group with leg weakness and falls, resulting in early termination of the study [92].

In a study involving 14 PD patients with FoG, 9 were injected with 5000 units of rimabotulinumtoxinB into the gastrocnemius-soleus complex of the predominantly affected leg. Five patients received placebo. There was marked improvement in symptoms in one patient, minimal improvement in two patients, unchanged symptoms in nine patients, and two patients with minimal worsening of symptoms. No significant differences in UPDRS scores between treatment and placebo groups were found [69].

Levodopa-induced Dyskinesia

Levodopa-induced dyskinesia (LID) occurs in over 90% of patients treated with levodopa for over 15 years, although the prevalence varies from study to study. Peak dose dyskinesia is the most common form of LID, followed by wearing off dystonia, both of which could benefit from BoNT injections as a treatment option [244]. In a randomized double-blind crossover study of 12 patients with medication refractory levodopa-induced cervical dyskinesia, 200 units of BoNT was injected in the neck muscles (bilateral sternocleidomastoid, splenius capitis, trapezius). Of these 12 patients, 8 were randomized and only 4 completed the study before it was voluntarily terminated due to safety concerns, predominantly due to excessive neck weakness. There was a trend towards reduced On time with LID in the BoNT group compared to baseline, and reduced dyskinesia on self-reported dyskinesia and pain related to dyskinesia [65]. There are other studies demonstrating the utility of BoNT in the treatment of various forms of LID [106].

Axial Dystonia (anterocollis, camptocormia, Pisa syndrome)
See section "Dystonia"
   Constipation: see section "Gastroenterology"
   Hyperhidrosis: see section "Autonomic Disorders"

Dystonia

Dystonia is a movement disorder characterized by sustained or intermittent muscle contraction, resulting in abnormal repetitive movements, posture or both [5]. Dystonic movements are often patterned, initiated, or worsened with voluntary action and associated with overflow activation of involved muscles. Dystonia can be classified based on several factors including the age of onset, body distribution, temporal pattern, and also based on associated symptoms as part of a systemic condition. Dystonia could also be classified based on etiology. Based on body distribution, dystonia could be classified as focal, segmental, hemidystonia, multifocal, and generalized dystonia [5]. BoNT has become the mainstay treatment for focal and segmental dystonia. Muscle selection and adequate dosing are also important factors to determine efficacy, as in other dystonic conditions. BoNT has been noted to be an effective and safe treatment option for long term use [116].

(a) Blepharospasm and apraxia of eyelid opening
Blepharospasm is a type of focal cranial dystonia resulting in repetitive involuntary forceful eyelid closure, often associated with dystonia of other adjacent areas like neck, jaw, and facial muscles. Since BoNT was approved by the FDA in 1989, for the treatment of blepharospasm, this has become the mainstay of treatment for this form of focal dystonia [245]. Based on 2016 Practice Guidelines from the American Academy of Neurology [217], onabotulinumtoxinA and incobotulinumtoxinA have level B evidence (probably effective) and abobotulinumtoxinA has level C evidence (possibly effective) for use in the treatment of blepharospasm. OnabotulinumtoxinA and incobotulinumtoxinA are FDA approved in the United States for the treatment of blepharospasm; abobotulinumtoxinA is approved for the treatment of blepharospasm in Europe.

   A randomized, double-blind, placebo-controlled multicenter trial evaluated the safety and efficacy of incobotulinumtoxinA in 109 patients in a 2:1 ratio for treatment to placebo, and found a significant difference in the Jankovic Rating Scale (JRS) in favor of the BoNT group [107]. There was also clinically relevant improvement in symptoms and in functional impairment assessed using the

Blepharospasm Disability Index (BSDI) and patient and physicians' global assessments. Ptosis and dry eyes were the few noted adverse effects.

There have been randomized, double-blind studies and split face studies (injecting different BoNT products to either side of the face) comparing different BoNT products which did not find significant difference between these toxins for use in blepharospasm [217]. A randomized double-blind trial compared incobotulinumtoxinA (Xeomin®) to onabotulinumtoxinA (Botox®) in patients with blepharospasm. Both BoNT products reduced scores on JRS, BSDI, and Patient Global Assessment (PGA) scales with no significant difference between the two products but with a tendency toward greater improvement with onabotulinumtoxinA [249]. Similarly, there are studies comparing incobotulinumtoxinA (Xeomin®) to onabotulinumtoxinA (Botox®) [192] and abobotulinumtoxinA (Dysport®) to onabotulinumtoxin A (Botox®) [162] with no significant difference in benefits seen between the two products.

Studies evaluating the long-term use of BoNT in patients with blepharospasm noted that the benefits persist for several decades of treatment [40, 217, 237]. A study in 128 patients who were receiving abobotulinumtoxinA or onabotulinumtoxinA had maintained benefit at 15 years [18, 189].

Frowning as a result of frontal dystonia, in the absence of blepharospasm, could also be treated using BoNT. A case series on two patients who had facial frowning reported an improvement in symptoms after BoNT injections. Corrugator and nasalis were the main muscles injected in these patients with improvement in facial frowning [99]. We have also used BoNT in the treatment of levodopa-induced dyskinesia, manifested by repetitive frontalis contractions [106].

Apraxia of eyelid opening
Apraxia of eyelid opening refers to the inability to open the eyelid in the absence of paralysis, sensory loss, or other disorders affecting language or alertness. This is often seen co-existing in patients with blepharospasm, Parkinson's disease, atypical parkinsonian syndromes, especially in progressive supranuclear palsy (PSP). The mechanism of "apraxia of eyelid opening" is not well understood, but it is probably not a true apraxia and more likely related to a dystonia phenomenon, inhibition of levator palpebrae, or other mechanisms [61].

Smaller studies have shown improvement in apraxia of eyelid opening after BoNT injections, especially if associated with blepharospasm. Injection of the pretarsal portion of the orbicularis oculi seems to be critical to help with apraxia of eyelid opening [102]. There have been several case reports on the benefit of BoNT in apraxia of eyelid opening [68, 126, 180].

One study noted benefits of BoNT in 32 patients with apraxia of lid opening, of which 3 patients had primary apraxia of eyelid opening, 20 with associated blepharospasm, 7 with PSP, and 2 with dystonic parkinsonian syndrome. Injections to the junction of preseptal and pretarsal portion of palpebral orbicularis oculi yielded best results. 83% of patients had improvement in symptoms after BoNT injections on a rating scale administered pre-and post-BoNT injections [119].

Another study looked into the effect of BoNT in 10 patients with apraxia of eyelid opening, where 8 of 10 had improvement in eyelid opening after BoNT injections. Between 20 and 30 units were used per eye injected at two sites at the junction of orbital and preseptal orbicularis oculi, compared to 10–20 units injected at one site at the middle of the upper lid close to the eyelash line. Injection of BoNT close to the pretarsal portion of orbicularis oculi resulted in improvement whereas injections to the preseptal and orbital portions did not yield the same benefit [53].

Ten patients with apraxia of eyelid opening associated with blepharospasm had BoNT injections and the lid opening parameters were compared to normal eyelid opening parameters obtained from 12 healthy control subjects. There was improvement in all lid opening measurements after BoNT injections [73].

(b) Cervical dystonia

Cervical dystonia (CD) is the most common isolated focal dystonia affecting the muscles of the neck and shoulders. BoNT is the first line treatment of CD. There are several good-quality studies that show the benefit of BoNT in CD. The 2008 American Academy of Neurology (AAN) evidence-based review identified 7 Class I studies showing the effect of BoNT in CD [215]. These have been listed and described briefly in Table 4.1.

The 2016 AAN Practice Guideline Update reviewed the evidence and listed level A (effective) evidence for the use of abobotulinumtoxinA and rimabotulinumtoxinB in patients with CD and level B (probably effective) evidence for the use of onabotulinumtoxinA and incobotulinumtoxinA in CD. These are based on 15 randomized double-blind clinical trials, listed in Table 4.1. All the formulations are approved for use in CD in the US [217].

Although anterocollis is often excluded from clinical trials of CD, some patients benefit from BoNT injections into the anterior scalene muscles, sternocleidomastoid muscles, and submental complex [106].

(c) Camptocormia

Camptocormia refers to an abnormal forward flexion in the thoracolumbar region, of more than 45°, apparent while standing or walking, but resolves in supine position. This is seen in PD patients with longer disease duration and severity, estimated to have prevalence between 3% and 17% in PD patients [59, 256].

In a case series studying 16 patients with camptocormia from different etiology, 9 patients were injected with BoNT for camptocormia. Between 300 and 600 units of onabotulinumtoxinA was injected in the rectus abdominus muscle. Of these 9 patients, 4 had marked improvement in symptoms lasting for about 3 months [10].

An open label study in 10 patients with camptocormia looked into the effect of ultrasound-guided injection of 100–300 units of incobotulinumtoxinA injected into either the rectus abdominus muscle or iliopsoas muscle based on whether the flexion was at the hip or lower trunk. There was no significant improvement in posture with these injections [72].

A case series of 4 patients with camptocormia, due to PD in 3 patients and one patient with MSA-P, evaluated changes in camptocormia after injecting 500–1500 units of abobotulinumtoxin A to bilateral iliopsoas using ultrasound

Table 4.1 Evidence-based review of the use of BoNT

Indication	Study	Results	BoNT injection pattern	Comments
Neurology:				
Essential tremor	Jankovic et al. [110]: Randomized double-blind placebo-controlled study in 25 patients with hand tremor	Significant improvement in tremor severity rating scale in BoNT-injected patients compared to placebo	50 units of Botox into wrist flexors and extensors of dominant limb Additional 100 units in 4 weeks for non-responders	Some degree of finger weakness in all patients
	Brin et al. [27]: Randomized placebo-controlled study involving 133 patients	Significant hand tremor improvement in the low-and high-dose BoNT groups compared to placebo	Low-dose group: 15 units into flexor carpi radialis and ulnaris; 10 units into extensor carpi radialis and ulnaris High-dose group: 30 units into flexors and 20 units into extensors	More weakness in the high-dose group (30% in low-dose and 70% in high-dose group)
	Pahwa et al. [168]: Double-blind placebo-controlled crossover study assessing head tremor in 10 patients	50% had moderate to marked improvement compared to 10% in placebo group in blinded raters' tremor scales 50% patients had moderate to marked subjective improvement compared to 30% in placebo group	40 units of Botox in each sternocleidomastoid and 60 units in splenius capiti	No statistical difference between the groups based on accelerometry
	Wissel et al. [259]: Study involving 14 patients with ET head tremor without dystonia and 29 with head tremor due to CD	Subjective improvement in 100% of ET patients and in 90% of CD patients Significant improvement in head tremor based on accelerometry analysis and clinical evaluation	Mean doses of 400 units of Dysport divided between bilateral splenius capiti muscles in ET patients Mean dose of 500 units in CD patients with muscle selection based on neck position	Local pain, neck weakness and dysphagia were side effects

(continued)

Table 4.1 (continued)

Indication	Study	Results	BoNT injection pattern	Comments
	Hertegård et al. [97]: Study in 15 patients with ET voice tremor	Significant subjective and perceptual improvement in voice tremor	Between 0.6 and 7.5 units of BoNT injected into thyroarytenoid muscle or in some patients, into the cricothyroid or thyrohyoid muscle under EMG guidance	Acoustic evaluations showed that during sustained vowel phonation, there was a significant decrease in fundamental frequency variation after BoNT injection compared to pre-injection.
Cervical dystonia (CD)	Greene et al. [91]: Double-blind placebo-controlled parallel design study in 55 patients with CD	61% patients injected with BoNT improved statistically in severity of torticollis, pain, disability and degree of head turning In an open-label extension of the study with higher doses of BoNT, 74% patients had improvement	Between 30 and 250 units were injected in total (mean dose of 118 units) Between 15 and 55 units were injected to individual muscles including trapezius, SCM, and splenius capitis	
	Poewe et al. [184]: Randomized prospective multicenter double-blind placebo-controlled trial in 75 patients with CD who received abobotulinumtoxinA (Dysport®)	79% patients reported subjective improvement Postural head deviation rated using modified Tsui scale was significant at week 4 in the 500 and 1000 units Dysport® group compared to placebo	A total dose of 250, 500 or 1000 units of Dysport® was divided between one splenius capitis and contralateral sternocleidomastoid muscle	39% with dysphagia in the 1000 units Dysport® group, but 10% of patients in the placebo group also had dysphagia Neck weakness was present in 56% patients in the 1000 units group, which was significantly more than in the placebo group

Brans et al. [23]: Prospective randomized double-blind trial in 64 patients comparing abobotulinumtoxinA (Dysport®) to oral trihexyphenidyl with 32 patients in each group. BoNT or placebo injections at entry to the study and repeated in 8 weeks	Significant improvement in disability score on Toronto Western Spasmodic Torticollis Rating Scale (TWSTRS-Disability), Tsui scale and General Health Perception subscale in favor of BoNT	Mean dose of Dysport® was 292 units in the first session (week 0) and 262 units in the second session (week 8) Mean dose of trihexyphenidyl was 16.25 mg	Adverse effects were significantly less in the BoNT group compared to trihexyphenidyl group
Lew et al. [127]: Randomized multicenter, double-blind, placebo-controlled 4-arm parallel group study in 122 patients with cervical dystonia who received botulinum toxin type B at 2500, 5000, or 10,000 units vs placebo	Significant improvement in TWSTRS – Total, Severity, Disability, and Pain scores at week 4 The proportion of patients that responded increased with increased doses of BoNT	Four arms included botulinum toxin type B at 2500, 5000, or 10,000 units vs placebo	Noted a dose response to AE (dry mouth and dysphagia) with higher doses causing more AE
Brashear et al. [24]: Randomized multicenter, double-blind, placebo-controlled trial in 109 patients with three groups, including placebo, 5000 and 10,000 units of BoNT-B	Improvement in pain, disability and severity of CD on TWSTRS in BoNT B compared to placebo with most improvement noted in the 10,000 units group	5000 or 10,000 units of BoNT B compared to placebo injected into 2–4 muscles including levator, scalene, splenius capitis, SCM, semispinalis capitis, or trapezius	AE were mild
Brin et al. [26]: Double-blind placebo-controlled trial of BoNT-B in 77 BoNT-A-resistant patients (38 placebo, 39 active)	Improvement in severity, disability, and pain scores on TWSTRS in the BoNT-B-treated group	Placebo vs 10,000 units of BoNT B into 2–4 involved muscles	Dry mouth and dysphagia were AE seen
Truong et al. [236]: Multicenter double-blind placebo-controlled trial of abobotulinumtoxinA (Dysport®) in 80 patients	Significant improvement in symptoms quantified by reduction in TWSTRS total score in the Dysport® group 38% patients showed positive response in the Dysport® group	500 units of Dysport® vs placebo	Mean duration of benefit was 18.5 weeks

(continued)

Table 4.1 (continued)

Indication	Study	Results	BoNT injection pattern	Comments
	Odergren et al. [163]: Double-blind, randomized, parallel group study in 73 patients to compare dose equivalence between onabotulinumtoxinA (Botox®) and abobotulinumtoxinA (Dysport®) with 38 patients in Dysport® group and 35 in Botox® group	Substantial improvement in Tsui score in both groups by week 2 Similar response in terms of efficacy and duration of response	Mean dose of 477 units of Dysport® and 152 units of Botox® into clinically determined muscles	In patients with rotational CD, patients treated with Botox® or Dysport® in 3 times the dose of Botox® had successful treatment of symptoms
	Comella et al. [43]: Multicenter, randomized double-blind parallel arm study in 139 patients randomized to BoNT-A or BoNT-B toxin	Improved TWSTRS score in both groups	Maximum dose received in the BoNT-A group was 250 units and in BoNT-B group was 10,000 units into muscles clinically determined by physician	The dose ration used was 1 U of BoNT-A to at least 40 units of BoNT-B
	Tintner et al. [233]: Randomized double-blind trial in 20 patients who were randomized to receive BoNT-A or BoNT-B (11 patients BoNT-A and 9 patients BoNT-B)	Improved TWSTRS severity, pain, and disability score in BoNT A and B compared to baseline scores pre-injection No significant difference in efficacy between BoNT-A and BoNT-B	BoNT-A (Botox®) dose: 227 ± 83 BoNT-B (Myobloc®) dose: 12,083 ± 5899	Less saliva production and increased constipation in BoNT-B group compared to BoNT-A group No other difference in autonomic function between the BoNT-A and BoNT-B groups
	Pappert et al. [173]: Randomized, double-blind, parallel group study in 111 patients (55 BoNT-A and 56 BoNT-B) comparing BoNT-A to BoNT-B	Improvement in TWSTRS Score in BoNT-A and BoNT-B groups with similar duration of benefit	BoNT-A 150 units BoNT-B 10,000 units injected into 2–4 neck or shoulder muscles clinically determined by a blinded physician	Mild dry mouth was more common with BoNT B than with BoNT A No difference in moderate to severe dry mouth

Study	Efficacy	Dose	Adverse events
Comella et al. [44]: Prospective, randomized, double-blind, placebo-controlled, multicenter clinical trial of incobotulinumtoxinA (Xeomin®) in 233 patients (219 completed the study)	Significantly improved TWSTRS score compared to placebo at 120 U and 240 U	Xeomin®: 120 units or 240 units vs placebo	Dysphagia, neck pain, and mild neck weakness were AE noted; slightly more AE at 240 U dose compared to 120 U
Charles et al. [35]: Double-blind, prospective, randomized, placebo-controlled trial in 170 patients (82 placebo and 88 BoNT-A) who received onabotulinumtoxinA or placebo in a 10-week study period (period 2). This was preceded by a 10-week open label study (period 1) in 214 patients, of whom 170 were randomized in period 2 of the study	Significant improvement in Cervical Dystonia Severity Scale and Physician Global assessment scale at 6 weeks	OnabotulinumtoxinA Period 1 (open label): Mean dose was 241 units (between 95 and 360 U) Period 2 (blinded placebo-controlled): Mean dose 236 units (95–360 units)	Rhinitis and dysphagia were significantly more in the BoNTA group compared to placebo Large number of drop outs: 37 of 170 due to lack of efficacy Two patients seroconverted from neutralizing Ab negative to positive status during the study but remained clinically responsive to BoNT
Evidente et al. [66]: Randomized, double-blind, placebo-controlled multicenter trial of incobotulinumtoxinA (Xeomin®) in 214 patients injected with 120 or 240 U injected at a flexible interval of ≥6 weeks over a treatment period of 48 weeks followed by 20 weeks observation period; Of these, 169 patients completed the study	Both 120 U and 240 U doses resulted in significant improvement in TWSTRS total score, severity, disability, and pain scores	IncobotulinumtoxinA 120 U or 240 U vs placebo	Dysphagia was the most common AE (23.4% in 240 U group and 12.6% in the 120 U group)

(continued)

Table 4.1 (continued)

Indication	Study	Results	BoNT injection pattern	Comments
	Yun et al. [267]: Randomized, double-blind, multicenter, parallel group crossover study in 103 patients. 94 completed the study. Patients received Botox® or Dysport® and were followed for 16 weeks followed by 4 week washout period before crossover to the other group	No statistical difference between Botox® and Dysport® at a conversion ratio 2.5:1 based on TWSTRS, Clinical Global Impression, and Patient Global Impression Mean changes in Tsui score tended to favor Botox®, but was not statistically significant	Botox® 200 units Dysport® 500 units Dysport®: Botox® ratio 2.5:1	No significant difference in AE between the groups
	Rystedt et al. [199]: Double-blind, randomized crossover study in 46 patients who received Botox® in 2 different doses and Dysport® using conversion ratios of 1:3 and 1:1.7	No significant difference between Botox® and Dysport® at 1:1.7 conversion ratio Median TWSTRS score was 1.96 points higher for Botox® at 1:3 ratio (not statistically significant). There was a statistically significant shorter duration of benefit for Botox® at 12 weeks when this 1:3 low dose was used	Botox®: Dysport® ratio 1: 3 and 1:1.7	When using 1:3 dose, patient assessments showed suboptimal benefit from Botox® Dose conversion of Botox®: Dysport® may be lower than 1:3
	Poewe et al. [183]: Randomized, double-blind, multicenter, placebo-controlled trial in 369 patients who were randomized to receive abobotulinumtoxinA dry formulation, and solution compared to placebo	AbobotulinumtoxinA 500 units in dry and solution formulation were superior to placebo based on TWSTRS score	AbobotulinumtoxinA 500 units in dry formulation and in solution formulation	Dysphagia and injection-site pain were similar between dry freeze dried formulation and solution formulation
	Yi et al. [264]: Randomized double-blind, placebo-controlled crossover study in 16 patients with CD secondary to dyskinetic cerebral palsy	Significant improvement in TWSTRS score in BoNT-A group compared to placebo (saline) at week 4	Median dose of BoNT-A: 145 U Mean dose: 139.7 U	There was improvement in pain and disability subscores Dysphagia was transient and improved within 2 weeks

Lew et al. [128]: Multicenter, randomized double-blind placebo-controlled trial of abobotulinumtoxinA (Dysport®) at 500 units/2 ml dilution compared to placebo in 134 patients of which 129 completed the study (84 patients Dysport® and 45 placebo)	Significant improvement in TWSTRS score in BoNT group compared to placeo	500 U of Dysport® in toxin naive patients Between 250 and 500 units of Dysport® at a conversion ratio of 2.5:1 to their previous Botox® dose	Dysphagia, neck pain, neck weakness, headaches were AE
Parkinson's disease hand rest tremor Mittal et al. [149]: Randomized double-blind placebo-controlled crossover study in 30 patients with hand rest tremor	Significant improvement in tremor based on tremor rating scales and subjective patient impression	Between 2.5 and 20 units per muscle of incobotulinumtoxinA was injected in the forearm and hand muscles individualized based on tremor Between 85 and 110 units of incobotulinumtoxinA in a single patient	
PD freezing of gait Gurevich et al. [92]: Double-blind placebo-controlled trial involving 11 PD patients with FoG, 6 of whom received BoNT and 5 received saline	Significant improvement in FoG after BoNT injection	OnabotulinumtoxinA between 100 and 300 units injected divided between the gastrocnemius and soleus of one or both legs	
Fernandez et al. [69]: Randomized, double-blind, placebo-controlled trial in 14 PD patients with FoG who received BoNT (n = 9) or placebo (n = 5)	No significant difference between BoNT group and placebo	RimabotulinumtoxinB 5000 U to the gastrocnemius-soleus complex of predominantly affected leg involved in FoG	
Camptocormia Case series only available			
Pisa syndrome Tassorelli et al. [229]: Double-blind, randomized placebo-controlled trial of 26 patients, 13 who received BoNT injections and 13 received saline injections	Significant improvement in posture, pain, and range of motion in patients who received BoNT injection	50–200 units of incobotulinumtoxinA injected with EMG guidance into either iliopsoas, rectus abdominis, or thoracic or lumbar paravertebral muscles	

(continued)

Table 4.1 (continued)

Indication	Study	Results	BoNT injection pattern	Comments
	Artusi et al. [9]: Open label pilot study of 15 patients, 13 of whom completed follow-up assessments	11 of 13 patients had over 40% improvement in trunk posture, while all had improvement in pain and discomfort	Between 50 and 75 units of onabotulinumtoxinA injected in paraspinal muscles using US and EMG guidance Between 25 and 50 units injected in the non-paraspinal muscles	No significant adverse events or complications
Levodopa-induced dyskinesia	Espay et al. [65]: Randomized double-blind placebo-controlled crossover study of 12 patients, of whom 8 were randomized	Study prematurely terminated due to safety concerns Only 4 patients completed the study There was a trend towards improved ON time without dyskinesia Reduction in self-reported dyskinesia	200 units of onabotulinumtoxinA injected in the neck muscles (25 units in each sternocleidomastoid, 50 units in each splenius capiti, 25 units in each trapezius)	Excessive neck weakness and dysphagia were noted, which led to termination of the study
Dystonic tremor	Data is from retrospective studies			
Sialorrhea	Mancini et al. [136]: Double-blind placebo-controlled trial to evaluate the effect of Dysport® on drooling in 20 patients with parkinsonism	Average secretion of saliva was significantly lower in the BoNT group compared to placebo	450 units of Dysport® into the parotid and submandibular glands under ultrasound guidance	No side effects in either group
	Ondo et al. [165]: Randomized, double-blind, placebo-controlled parallel group study in 16 PD patients	Significant improvement in the BoNT group in Visual Analog Scale, global impression of change, Drooling Rating Scale, Drooling Severity and Frequency Scale	BoNT-B 1000 units into each parotid and 250 U into submandibular gland vs pH matched placebo	AE was mild and included dry mouth
	Lagalla et al. [123]: Double-blind placebo-controlled trial in 32 patients, 16 of whom received BoNT	Significant improvement in drooling, ADLs, and decreased saliva weight	50 units of onabotulinumtoxinA injected in each parotid gland	

	Lagalla et al. [124]: Randomized, double-blind, placebo-controlled trial in 36 PD patients with drooling	Significant improvement in all measures of sialorrhea a month after BoNT injection	BoNT-B 4000 units vs placebo	Benefits lasted 19.2 weeks ±6.3 weeks
	Stone and O'Leary [221]: Systematic review	2 of 5 studies included in this review showed benefit of BoNT in sialorrhea, but all included studies were small studies		Not high-powered studies included
	Chinnapongse et al. [37]: Multicenter, randomized, double-blind placebo-controlled trial in 54 patients who received BoNT-B at 1500 U, 2500 U, 3500 units compared to placebo	Significant improvement in the Drooling Frequency and Severity Scale in a dose-related manner at week 4	BoNT-B at 1500 U, 2500 U, 3500 units	Dry mouth was more common in the BoNT group compared to placebo
	Narayanaswami et al. [154]: Randomized, double-blind placebo-controlled crossover study in 9 patients injected with incobotulinumtoxinA into parotid (20 units) and submandibular glands (30 units)	No significant change in saliva weight one month post injection	IncobotulinumtoxinA 20 units into parotid and 30 units into submandibular glands bilaterally	Doses used could have resulted in this outcome
Hyperhidrosis	Naumann and Lowe [156]: multicenter, randomized, double-blind, placebo-controlled, parallel group study in 307 patients with axillary hyperhidrosis	At 4 weeks, 94% of patients in BoNT group had responded, which was significantly better than the placebo group	Botox® 50 U per axilla or placebo	
	Heckmann et al. [95]: Multicenter, randomized double-blind placebo-controlled trial in 145 patients with axillary hyperhidrosis who received BoNT or placebo. Placebo group received 100 U of BoNT two weeks later.	Mean sweat production dropped significantly	Dysport® 200 U Placebo group received 100 U two weeks later	

(continued)

Table 4.1 (continued)

Indication	Study	Results	BoNT injection pattern	Comments
	Schnider et al. [208]: Randomized, double-blind, placebo-controlled trial in 11 patients with palmar hyperhidrosis who received BoNT in one palm with placebo in the other	Mean sweat production dropped significantly (26–31%) between weeks 4 and 13	Dysport® 120 U per palm with placebo in contralateral palm	
	Lowe et al. [133]: Randomized double-blind placebo-controlled trial in 19 patients with palmar hyperhidrosis who received BoNT in one palm and placebo in the other	Significant reduction in palmar hyperhidrosis	OnabotulinumtoxinA 100 U in one palm and placebo in the other	No decrease in grip strength
Palatal myoclonus	Mostly case reports and case series available	No double-blind placebo-controlled studies available		
Oromandibular dystonia (OMD)	Tan and Jankovic [226]: Prospective study in 162 patients, majority with primary oromandibular dystonia, with jaw closing dystonia being the most common type	67.9% patients reported definite functional improvement after BoNT injections. Mean duration of response: 16.4 weeks	Between 25 and 100 units in masseter muscle (Mean dose 54.2 units). Between 10 and 200 units in submental complex (mean dose 28.6)	Complication rate was low. Dysarthria and dysphagia were some of the reported AE
	Most studies for OMD are case series or observational studies			
Cerebellar tremor	Data is mostly from retrospective and pilot studies			
Tics	Marras et al. [141]: Randomized double-blind placebo-controlled crossover study of onabotulinumtoxinA in 20 patients with tics, 18 of whom completed the study	There was improved tic frequency and urge leading up to the tic. Patients, however, did not notice an improvement in their tics	Doses were individualized to patients based on the type of tic	Disability burden of the targeted tic should be taken into account when deciding about BoNT injections
	Other studies for this condition are smaller open label trials			

Blepharospasm	Jankovic and Orman [108]: Double-blind, placebo-controlled, prospective, crossover study in 12 patients	All patients had improvement in blepharospasm	25 units of onabotulinumtoxinA/eye and if ineffective 50 units/eye	Blurred vision, tearing, ptosis, ecchymosis were some noted adverse effects
	Girlanda et al. [85]: Compared BoNT injection in one eye with saline injection in the other in 6 patients	Bilateral improvement in blepharospasm symptoms with unilateral BoNT injection	20 units of onabotulinumtoxinA/eye	Small cohort
	Nüssgens and Roggenkämper [162]: Double-blind study in 212 patients with blepharospasm who received either onabotulinumtoxin A or abobotulinumtoxin A at separate visits with the comparison of benefit	Similar benefits with similar duration of action for both formulation of BoNT (about 8 weeks)	Botox® average dose: 45 units Dysport® average dose: 182 units	The bioequivalence of onaB: aboB (Botox®: Dysport®) was found to be 1:4 in this study
	Roggenkämper et al. [192]: Randomized, double-blind, prospective, parallel study in 300 patients comparing Botox® to Xeomin®	There was improvement in symptoms in both groups quantified using JRS No significant difference in safety and efficacy of Botox® compared to Xeomin®	≤35 units/eye or 70 units total Botox® average dose: 40.8 units Xeomin® average dose: 39.6 units	Larger cohort
	Truong et al. [235]: Large multicenter, randomized, placebo-controlled trial evaluating the safety and efficacy of abobotulinumtoxinA (Dysport®) compared to placebo in 120 patients	Reduced frequency and intensity of spasms and improvement in functional ability Best balance between safety and efficacy was seen at 80 U of Dysport®/eye	abobotulinumtoxinA doses of 40 U, 80 U and 120 U	Blurred vision and ptosis were observed with higher doses There were a high number of withdrawals (35 patients) but this was more in the placebo group due to lack of benefit

(continued)

Table 4.1 (continued)

Indication	Study	Results	BoNT injection pattern	Comments
	Wabbels et al. [249]: Randomized, double-blind, parallel group study comparing incobotulinumtoxinA (Xeomin®) to onabotulinumtoxinA (Botox®) in 65 patients	Improved symptoms with both products, quantified using JRS, BSDI and PGA No significant difference in benefits with Xeomin® and Botox®	Doses individualized to patients (≥20 U/eye)	Trend toward greater improvement with Botox® than Xeomin®
	Jankovic et al. [107]: Randomized, double-blind placebo-controlled multicenter trial in 109 patients with blepharospasm	Significant improvement in the severity of blepharospasm assessed by JRS and in functional impairment, assessed by blepharospasm disability index (BSDI), and patient and physician evaluation of global effect	IncobotulinumtoxinA dosing was individual specific, not to exceed 50 units per eye	Ptosis and dry eyes were some noted adverse effects
	Truong et al. [237]: Open label extension of Jankovic et al. [107] study of Xeomin® in 102 patients for 69 weeks	Significant improvement in JRS, BSDI	Xeomin® individually dosed	Ptosis and dry eyes were most common AE noted
	Saad and Gourdeau [200]: Randomized, double-blind, prospective split face study in 48 patients	Similar improvement between Xeomin® and Botox® using JRS and BSDI to quantify improvement	Average 20 units/eye of Xeomin® or Botox®	
Apraxia of eyelid opening	Forget et al. [73]: Pilot study in 10 patients with apraxia of eyelid opening associated with blepharospasm	Improved lid opening measures post BoNT injection and reduction in functional impairment	4–5 units of Botox® in the orbicularis oculi with 3 injections in the pretarsal portion (medial and lateral upper lid and lateral lower lid) and 4th injection in the external canthus	

Synkinesis	Borodic et al. [21]: Randomized double-blind placebo-controlled trial in 30 patients with chronic facial palsy, 15 of whom received onabotulinumtoxinA injections to the side with synkinesis compared to 15 patients who received placebo	There was reduction in the synkinesis based on videotape and blinded physician examination and improved quality of life, vision, and social interaction Improved vertical palpebral fissure distance, synkinesis physician grading scale in the BoNT group compared to placebo	BoNT was quantified using Schantz-Kautter method of "LD 50" determination. 2.5 LD 50 units per 0.1 cc was injected to four injection points in the periocular areas avoiding the medial lower lid and mid upper lid to avoid side effects	Increased incidence of exposure keratitis in the BoNT group compared to placebo group
	do Nascimento Remigio et al. [57]: Randomized comparative study analyzing the effects of onabotulinumtoxinA and abobotulinumtoxinA in 55 patients with chronic facial nerve palsy; 25 patients received onabotulinumtoxinA and 30 patients received abobotulinumtoxinA	Both toxins improved facial symmetry	A dose conversion ratio of 1:3 was used for onabotulinumtoxinA to abobotulinumtoxinA BoNT was injected to the non-paralyzed side of the face	
	Monini et al. [152]: Randomized placebo-controlled trial in 20 patients with synkinesis after recovery from facial palsy; 10 patients received BoNT followed by neuromuscular retraining therapy (NMRT) compared to 10 patients who received NMRT alone	Significant improvement in synkinesis in BoNT group compared to placebo group that received NMRT only	Between 10 and 40 units were injected	
Hemifacial spasm	Yoshimura et al. [265]: Prospective blinded, placebo-controlled crossover study in 11 patients	Subjective improvement in 79% and objective improvement in 84% patients	3 different graded doses between 2.5 and 10 U	Facial weakness was seen in 97% after injection Ptosis, diplopia, and facial bruising were other adverse effects

(continued)

Table 4.1 (continued)

Indication	Study	Results	BoNT injection pattern	Comments
	Sampaio et al. [205]: Randomized, single-blind, parallel group study in 49 patients with HFS, 22 received Botox® and 27 received Dysport®	Similar improvement with Botox® and Dysport®	17.5 units of Botox® 70 units of Dysport®	Single-blinded study (investigator was not blinded)
	Park et al. [175]: started as a placebo-controlled study, and then later switched to an open trial, in 101 patients	98.6% had significant improvement in symptoms	Mean dose of Botox® used in a patient with HFS: 13.5 units 71% of patients with HFS received between 7.5 and 20 units	Dry eye, facial weakness and ptosis were the adverse
Pain:				
Trigeminal neuralgia	Zhang et al. [270]: Randomized double-blind placebo-controlled trial in 84 patients with trigeminal neuralgia	Significantly better response rate with BoNT compared to placebo Response rate was 70.4% for the 25 U group, 86.2% for 75 U group, and 32.1% for placebo group	BoNT/A 25 U and 75 U vs placebo intradermal or submucosal Injection was submucosal if pain involved oral mucosa	
	Wu et al. [260]: Randomized double-blind placebo-controlled trial in 40 patients	Significant improvement in pain intensity and pain attacks and more response rate in BoNT group Response rate in BoNT group was 68.18% and 15% in placebo group	Intradermal and/or submucosal injection of 75 U of BoNT/A in the dermatome of pain symptoms; submucosal injections done if pain was in the oral mucosa	
	Zúñiga et al. [272]: Randomized double-blind placebo-controlled trial in 36 patients	Significant improvement in Visual Analog Scale (VAS) at 3 months in the BoNT group	BoNT/A 50 U subcutaneous injection in the involved distribution Additional 10 U BoNT A vs placebo intramuscular injection in the ipsilateral masseter if pain involved was in the third branch of trigeminal nerve	

Post-herpetic neuralgia	Xiao et al. [261]: Randomized double-blind placebo-controlled trial in 60 patients who received BoNT, lidocaine, or placebo	Significant decrease in pain scores at day 7 and month 3 in the BoNT group compared to lidocaine and placebo. Percent of patients on opiods was least post treatment in the BoNT group	BoNT/A less than 200 U in the involved dermatome	VAS scores improved in all three groups post treatment compared to pre
	Apalla et al. [8]: Randomized double-blind placebo-controlled parallel group study in 30 patients	Significant improvement in VAS pain scores in BoNT group compared to placebo	BoNT/A 5 U per site in a chessboard pattern	
Diabetic neuropathy	Ghasemi et al. [78]: Randomized double-blind placebo-controlled trial in 40 patients with diabetic neuropathy, 20 patients BoNT and 20 patients placebo	Reduction in neuropathic pain scores compared to placebo	BoNT/A 100 U distributed between 12 sites at 8–10 U per site on the dorsum of the foot	
	Yuan et al. [266]: Randomized double-blind placebo-controlled crossover trial in 18 patients	Significant reduction in VAS pain score in the BoNT group. 44.4% patients had reduction in VAS scores in BoNT group with no similar effect in the placebo group	50 U per foot intradermal injections of BoNT/A with 4 U per site	There was transient improvement in sleep quality in the BoNT group

Neuro-rehabilitation:

Upper-limb spasticity	There are smaller DB PC trials earlier than 2009, that are not included in this table			
	Kaňovský et al. [115]: Multicenter, double-blind, randomized-controlled trial in 148 patients with upper-limb spasticity post stroke	Statistically improved tone and disability in BoNT group	Xeomin® dose ≤400 units Median dose: 320 U	

(continued)

Table 4.1 (continued)

Indication	Study	Results	BoNT injection pattern	Comments
	Simpson et al. [216]: Multicenter, randomized, double-blind, placebo-controlled, parallel group study in 60 patients with upper-limb spasticity post stroke or from traumatic brain injury with 3 arms, BoNT injection group, Tizanidine, and placebo	BoNT reduced tone more than tizanidine	OnabotulinumtoxinA 50 units each to flexor carpi radialis and ulnaris Remaining muscles were injected with doses at the discretion of the physician; Max dose 500 U	Higher incidence of AE in Tizanidine group
	McCrory et al. [143]: Multicenter, randomized, double-blind, placebo-controlled trial in 96 patients with upper-limb spasticity, who were treated with BoNT compared to placebo	BoNT group had significant reduction in spasticity However, quality of life, mood, disability, and caregiver burden did not differ between the groups	AbobotulinumtoxinA 750–1000 U initial Repeat 500–1000 U in 12 weeks	
	Turner-Stokes et al. [238]: Secondary analysis of McCrory et al. [143] study	Significant treatment effect	Dysport® 500–1000 U	
	Kaji et al. [112]: Multicenter, randomized, double-blind, placebo-controlled trial in 109 patients with post-stroke upper-limb spasticity who were randomized to get a low- or high-dose BoNT compared to placebo	Significant improvement in spasticity in the higher dose BoNT group	BoNT-A Low-dose group: 120–150 U High-dose group: 200–240 U	
	Cousins et al. [47]: Randomized double-blind placebo-controlled trial in 30 patients with upper-limb spasticity post stroke, 21 of whom completed the study. Half or quarter of the standard doses were used in the active arms of the study	No benefit for active treatment compared to control On subgroup analysis, both treatment groups had improvement in functional gain compared to placebo	OnabotulinumtoxinA Half or quarter of the standard doses of BoNT vs placebo Standard doses identified in this study: 100 units for biceps brachii; 60 units for brachialis, 50 U brachioradialis, 50 units flexor digitorum superficialis, 50 units flexor digitorum profundus	No serious AE Inadequate dosing likely resulted in the observed result

Shaw et al. [211]: Multicenter, randomized trial in 333 patients with upper-limb spasticity with one group who received BoNT-A and therapy; the second group received therapy only	Significant improvement in tone in the BoNT group at 1 month and improved arm strength at 3 months; No significant differences between the groups in arm function at 1 month	Dysport® Median dose 200–300 U	No significant AE
Hesse et al. [98]: Single-blind, randomized pilot study in 18 patients with upper extremity spasticity with group A receiving BoNT-A injection into wrist and finger flexors compared to group B receiving no injection followed by aggressive rehab in both groups	Significant improvement in finger flexor stiffness in BoNT-injected group compared to the other group, and improved disability scores	IncobotulinumtoxinA 150 units into superficial and deep finger flexors (100 units) using ultrasound guidance and wrist flexors (50 units)	
Rosales et al. [195]: Multicenter, randomized, placebo-controlled trial in 163 patients with upper-limb spasticity injected with BoNT or placebo (80 patient received BoNT and 83 received placebo)	Significant improvement in Modified Ashworth Scale (MAS) scores in BoNT group The Functional Motor Assessment Scale did not show significant differences between the groups	Dysport® 500 U to wrist and elbow mover muscles	
Lam et al. [125]: Randomized, double-blind placebo-controlled trial in 55 patients with upper-limb spasticity who received BoNT injections or saline as placebo	Significant improvement in Carer Burden Scale in BoNT group, MAS scores and passive range of motion at the joints	Dysport Max dose 100 U Doses individualized to patient needs	

(continued)

Table 4.1 (continued)

Indication	Study	Results	BoNT injection pattern	Comments
	Marciniak et al. [140]: Randomized double-blind placebo-controlled trial in 21 post-stroke patients with shoulder spasticity that received BoNT injections vs placebo	BoNT and placebo groups had no difference in pain scores at 4 weeks Significant improvement in hygiene score on Disability Assessment Scale in the BoNT group	OnabotulinumtoxinA 140–200 U into pectoralis major with or without injections to teres major	
	Gracies et al. [88]: Randomized double-blind placebo-controlled trial in 24 hemiparetic patients who received two different doses of BoNT-B	Both BoNT groups improvement in elbow function compared to placebo Higher dose of BoNT-B improved patient perceived stiffness, pain and functioning	RimabotulinumtoxinB 10,000 U (2500 U into elbow flexors) Or 15,000 U (5000 U into elbow flexors)	No AE
	Ward et al. [254]: Prospective double-blind study in 273 patients with focal post-stroke spasticity, followed by open-label extension in 225 patients. Patients randomized to BoNT or placebo along with standard of care treatment	No significant changes in principal active functional goal achievement between the BoNT group and placebo Significant improvement in passive function in BoNT group compared to placebo	OnabotulinumtoxinA max dose 800 U	No major AE
	Gracies et al. [89]: Multicenter, double-blind, randomized, placebo-controlled trial in 243 patients with upper-limb spasticity from stroke or brain injury	Mean changes in MAS was significant in both the BoNT groups compared to placebo Change in PGA scores were significant in BoNT groups compared to placebo	AbobotulinumtoxinA 500 U, 1000 U vs placebo injected into the most hypertonic muscle among elbow, wrist, and finger flexors (primary target muscles) and at least 2 other muscle groups	No serious treatment-related AE; mild muscle weakness was the AE

	Elovic et al. [64]: Randomized, placebo-controlled trial randomized to 2:1 ratio of incobotulinumtoxinA: placebo in 259 patients with post-stroke spasticity	Significant improvement in upper-limb spasticity and associated disability. BoNT resulted in larger improvement in Ashworth Scale compared to placebo	IncobotulinumtoxinA 400 U in a fixed dose pattern. Flexed elbow 200 U. Flexed wrist 150 U. Clenched fist 100 U	Mild/moderate AE reported in BoNT group, dry mouth being the most common
	Rosales et al. [194]: Randomized, double-blind, placebo-controlled trial in 163 patients with upper-limb spasticity	BoNT significantly improved MAS scores; BoNT group had sustained improvement in upper-limb spasticity when combined with rehabilitation	AbobotulinumtoxinA 500 units (200 units to biceps brachii; 100 units to brachioradialis, 100 U flexor carpi radialis and 100 U flexor carpi ulnaris) Vs placebo	No significant AE
Lower-limb spasticity	Richardson et al. [191]: Prospective, randomized, double-blind, placebo-controlled parallel group study in 52 patients with hypertonia in upper and lower extremity injected with BoNT or placebo	Significant improvement in Ashworth Scale, passive range of motion, Rivermead scores for lower limb and subjective rating of problem severity in the BoNT group compared to placebo	OnabotulinumtoxinA injected with EMG guidance into clinically determined muscles in the upper or lower extremity	Pain at injection site for 4 patients
	Hyman et al. [101]: Prospective, randomized, double-blind, placebo-controlled dose ranging study in 74 patients	Primary efficacy variable (passive hip abduction and distance between the knees) improved for BoNT and placebo group. Improvement in distance between the knees was significantly better in the 1500 U Dysport group. Muscle tone improved in the BoNT groups only	Dysport® 500 U, 1000 U and 1500 U	Twice as much AE in the higher BoNT dose than lower doses with muscle weakness being a common AE

(continued)

Table 4.1 (continued)

Indication	Study	Results	BoNT injection pattern	Comments
	Pittock et al. [182]: Randomized, double-blind, placebo-controlled trial of three doses of Dysport® in 234 patients with spastic equinovarus deformity post stroke	Small but significant improvement in calf spasticity, limb pain and reduction in the use of walking aids in the BoNT group 2 min walking distance and stepping rate improved significantly in all groups including placebo without significant differences between groups	Dysport® 500 U, 1000 U and 1500 U	
	Verplancke et al. [242]: Prospective, randomized double-blind, placebo-controlled trial in 35 patients with lower-limb spasticity	Significant improvement in MAS scores in BoNT group and significant improvement in Glasgow Outcome Scale (GOS)	OnabotulinumtoxinA 200 units per leg (100 units to gastrocnemius and 100 units soleus) Vs saline placebo	Flu-like illness in one patient in the BoNT group 3 deaths (none in the BoNT group; unrelated to treatment intervention) and 4 were withdrawn from the study
	Gusev et al. [94]: Multinational, randomized, double-blind, placebo-controlled trial in 55 patients who received BoNT or placebo injections into adductor muscle of each leg	Significant pain reduction in BoNT groups Trend in favor of BoNT for other endpoints without statistical significance	Dysport® 500–750 U into adductor muscles of each leg with dose adjustment based on spasticity severity, patient size, and prior BoNT exposure	

Kaji et al. [113]: Multicenter, randomized, double-blind, placebo-controlled parallel group study in 120 post-stroke patients with lower-limb spasticity randomized to receive BoNT or placebo injections	Significant improvement in spasticity in BoNT group Significant change in MAS in BoNT group compared to placebo	OnabotulinumtoxinA 300 U to ankle plantar flexors or invertors	
Maanum et al. [134]: Single center, randomized, double-blind, placebo-controlled trial in 66 patients with spastic cerebral palsy where patients received BoNT or placebo injections	No significant differences between groups in primary outcome sagittal kinematics of knee, ankle and hip; and health-related quality of life Improvement in self-reported muscle stiffness/spasticity in BoNT group	OnabotulinumtoxinA with EMG guidance into clinically determined muscles Semimembranosus, semitendinosus, biceps femoris, flexor digitorum brevis, flexor digitorum longus were muscles injected	
Dunne et al. [60]: Randomized, double-blind placebo-controlled trial in 85 patients with lower-limb spasticity, followed by open label extension	No difference between BoNT groups with different doses No difference in hypertonia between groups Significant improvement in spasm frequency, pain reduction, active dorsiflexion, and gait quality in BoNT group compared to placebo	OnabotulinumtoxinA 200 U or 300 U	No significant difference in AE between groups

(continued)

Table 4.1 (continued)

Indication	Study	Results	BoNT injection pattern	Comments
	Fietzek et al. [71]: Single-center, double-blind, randomized, placebo-controlled trial in 52 patients with lower-limb spasticity, followed by open label extension of the study	BoNT group with lower MAS compared to placebo During open label extension, there was a further decline in muscle tone in patients previously in the placebo group. Overall patients that received BoNT in the first cycle had lower MAS scores	OnabotulinumtoxinA 230 units (60 units medial gastrocnemius, 30 U later gastrocnemius, 70 units soleus and 70 U tibialis posterior) 230 U: Unilateral 460 U: Bilateral injections Vs saline as placebo	No major AE
	Tao et al. [227]: Randomized, double-blind, placebo-controlled trial in 23 patients with lower-limb spasticity	Significant improvement in gait analysis measures in BoNT treated group	OnabotulinumtoxinA 200 units (100 units in medial and lateral gastrocnemius, 50 units soleus and 50 units tibialis posterior) vs saline placebo	No major AE
	Ding et al. [55]: Randomized blinded study in 80 post-stroke patients with one group who received BoNT and another group who received BoNT and stimulation by a spasmodic muscle therapeutic instrument. The stimulation is thought to improve muscle spasms.	Muscle tension reduced significantly in both groups after BoNT injection. MAS reduced significantly in both groups after BoNT injection. Motor function of lower extremities improved after BoNT + use of therapeutic instrument	OnabotulinumtoxinA 350 U injected with 50–100 U per muscle under ultrasound guidance	
	Gracies et al. [90]: Multicenter, randomized, double-blind placebo-controlled trial in 381 patients with chronic hemiparesis who received one lower-limb injection with BoNT or placebo. This was followed by an open extension study	After a single BoNT injection, there were improved MAS scores and muscle tone. After repeat BoNT injections in the open label phase, there was improved walking speed	Dysport® 1000 U, 1500 U or placebo	

Gracies et al. [90]: Post hoc analysis of Gracies et al. [90] study comparing upper and lower extremity BoNT to lower extremity only BoNT injections in 127 patients	Simultaneous upper and lower extremity BoNT injections does not hamper walking speed improvement compared to BoNT injections in the lower limbs only	AbobotulinumtoxinA 1000 U, 1500 U in lower extremities for cycle 1 and 3. Optional upper extremity injection with 500 U and lower extremity 1000 units from cycle 3 onward	Treating lower-limb spasticity with BoNT also improved postural sway/ balance
Kerzoncuf et al. [118]: Multicenter, prospective, randomized, double-blind, placebo-controlled study in 40 post-stroke patients with lower-limb spasticity where 19 patients received BoNT and 21 placebo (physiologic serum)	Spasticity decreased significantly in the BoNT group. During dual task, there was a significant improvement in sway area in the BoNT group	OnabotulinumtoxinA up to 300 units. Mean dose 227 U. Main muscles injected were gastrocnemius and soleus	
Baricich et al. [16]: Randomized, single blind pilot study in 30 patients where one group was given electrical stimulation to antagonistic muscles after BoNT injection of flexor muscles for patients with spastic equinus foot	Significant reduction in muscle tone and ankle range of motion in both groups. No significant difference between the groups receiving only BoNT vs BoNT + electrical stimulation	OnabotulinumtoxinA: Between 50 and 120 U for each muscle under ultrasound guidance. Gastrocnemius and soleus were the muscles injected	
Urology:			
Overactive bladder (OAB)	Sahai et al. [201]: Randomized, double-blind, placebo-controlled trial in 34 patients with OAB who received BoNT injections (n = 16) or placebo (n = 18)	Significant increase in maximum cystometric capacity (MCC) at weeks 4 and 12 in BoNT group compared to placebo. Significant improvement in quality of life	BoNT-A 200 U or placebo	Extension study showed that BoNT benefits lasted at least 24 weeks

(continued)

Table 4.1 (continued)

Indication	Study	Results	BoNT injection pattern	Comments
	Dmochowski et al. [56]: Double-blind, randomized, placebo-controlled trial of BoNT in 313 patients with OAB who received intradetrusor injections of BoNT or placebo	Improved durable efficacy for all BoNT group over 100 U for primary and secondary measures including urinary incontinence free patients. Doses greater than 150 U contributed minimal additional or clinically relevant improvement in symptoms	OnabotulinumtoxinA 50 U, 100 U, 150 U, 200 U or 300 U or placebo	There was a significant increase in UTI and urinary retention in the BoNT group compared to placebo
	Rovner et al. [196]: Randomized, double-blind, placebo-controlled trial in 313 patients with OAB and urinary urge incontinence with or without detrusor overactivity, who received intradetrusor injections of BoNT (269 patients) vs placebo (44 patients)	Changes in MCC with BoNT >100 U was superior to placebo at week 12 Dose-dependent increase in MCC was seen for 150 U, 200 U, and 300 U	OnabotulinumtoxinA 50 U, 100 U, 150 U, 200 U, and 300 U	Doses >100 U were commonly associated with post-void residual urine volumes >200 ml
	Cruz et al. [48]: Multicenter, randomized, double-blind, placebo-controlled trial in 275 patients with urinary incontinence due to neurogenic detrusor overactivity secondary to multiple sclerosis or spinal cord injury, who received BoNT injections 200 U (92 patients), 300 U (91 patients), or placebo (92 patients)	BoNT 200 U and 300 U significantly reduced urinary incontinence at week 6 compared to placebo	OnabotulinumtoxinA 200 U, 300 U, or placebo intradetrusor injections at 30 sites	Urinary tract infections (UTI) and urinary retention were AE seen

Tincello et al. [232]: Multicenter, randomized, double-blind, placebo-controlled trial in 240 patients with OAB, 122 received BoNT, and 118 placebo	Median voiding frequency was lower in BoNT group compared to placebo. Continence was more common in BoNT group compared to placebo	OnabotulinumtoxinA 200 U or placebo	UTI and voiding difficulty requiring self-catheterization was more common in the BoNT group
Denys et al. [54]: Prospective, randomized, double-blind, placebo-controlled trial in 99 patients with idiopathic overactive bladder who received BoNT injections at three different doses or placebo	3 months after BoNT injection, there was >50% improvement in 65% patients who received 100 U and in 56% who received 150 U; >75% improvement in 40% patients of both 100 U and 150 U groups	Onabotulinumtoxin A 50 U, 100 U or 150 U	100 U showed reasonable efficacy with less risk of high post-void residual
Chapple et al. [34]: Multicenter, randomized, double-blind, placebo-controlled trial in 548 patients, 277 of whom received BoNT and 271 placebo	BoNT significantly decreased urinary incontinence episodes per day at week 12. All other OAB symptoms were reduced in the BoNT group compared to placebo	OnabotulinumtoxinA 100 U injected at 20 sites intradetrusor	
Chuang et al. [38]: Prospective, randomized, double-blind, two center study in 62 patients, 31 of whom received a single intravesical application of liposomal-BoNT and 31 patients received placebo	Statistically significant improvement in micturition frequency per 3 days. Reduced urgency severity scores in BoNT group compared to placebo	Catheter intravesical installation of 200 U of liposomal onabotulinumtoxinA	Lipo-BoNT installation was not associated with increased urinary retention

(continued)

Table 4.1 (continued)

Indication	Study	Results	BoNT injection pattern	Comments
	Nitti et al. [161]: Randomized, multicenter, placebo-controlled trial in 557 patients, 280 patients received BoNT injections, 277 received placebo	At 12 weeks, there was a 3–4 fold decrease in mean frequency of urinary incontinence in the BoNT group compared to placebo. BoNT group had significant improvement in all OAB symptoms and multiple measures of quality of life compared to placebo	OnabotulinumtoxinA 100 U into the detrusor muscle	
	de Sá Dantas Bezerra et al. [51]: Prospective randomized, single-blinded study in 21 female patients with overactive bladder, who received intravesical injections with two different doses of BoNT	Maximum cistometric capacity increased in both BoNT groups without significant difference between the groups. Patients were better or much better in 70% patients who received 300 U and in 88.9% who received 500 U at 12 weeks	AbobotulinumtoxinA 300 or 500 U Injected into 30 sites, avoiding the trigone	
	Schurch et al. [209]: Randomized, double-blind, placebo-controlled trial in 23 patients with neurogenic detrusor overactivity, who received BoNT 200 U or 300 U vs placebo	Significant decrease in urinary frequency; with no significant difference between 200 U and 300 U groups	OnabotulinumtoxinA 200 U or 300 U	No significant AE
	Ghei et al. [79]: Randomized, double-blind, placebo-controlled crossover study in 20 patients with neurogenic and non-neurogenic detrusor overactivity	Significant differences in the urinary frequency, changes in voided volume, and episodes of incontinence in the BoNT group compared to placebo	Myobloc® 5000 U or placebo through cystoscope	4 patients with urinary retention

Interstitial cystitis (IC)/painful bladder syndrome (PBS)	Kuo and Chancellor [120]: Prospective, randomized, placebo-controlled trial in 67 patients with IC/PBS who received BoNT injections at 200 U (n = 15), 100 U (n = 29) followed by hydrodistention (HD), or placebo (n = 23) followed by HD	IC symptoms score reduced in all three groups. Pain reduction visual analogue scale, functional bladder capacity, and cystometric bladder capacity increased significantly in BoNT+HD group compared to HD only at 3 months	OnabotulinumtoxinA 100 U or 200 U
	El-Bahnasy et al. [62]: Randomized controlled trial in 36 patients with IC who either received intravesical bacillus Calmette-Guerin (BCG) (n = 16) or BoNT (n = 16)	Global IC survey improved in 71% in BCG group and in 92% in the BoNT group. BoNT group had statistically significant improvement in all parameters including nocturia, pelvic pain, urgency, and dysuria compared to BCG group	BoNT-A 300 U
	Taha et al. [225]: Randomized controlled trial in 28 women with IC/PBS who were randomized to BoNT (n = 14) or Pentosan polysulfate sodium (PPS) (n = 14)	BoNT group had significant improvement over placebo in all parameters compared including global PBS/IC survey, decrease in daily void, urgency, nocturia, pelvic pain, and dysuria	Cystoscopic intravesical injection of BoNT-A 300 U in 30 points including trigone
	Gottsch et al. [87]: Randomized, double-blind, placebo-controlled trial in 20 women with IC/PBS who received BoNT (n = 9) or placebo (n = 11)	No improvement in female modified Chronic Prostatitis Symptom Index or other symptom indices between BoNT and placebo groups	BoNT-A 50 U injected peri-urethrally

(continued)

Table 4.1 (continued)

Indication	Study	Results	BoNT injection pattern	Comments
	Kasyan and Pushkar [117]: Randomized controlled trial in 32 women with IC/PBS who were randomized to BoNT (n = 15) or placebo who got standard hydrodistention (n = 17)	BoNT-A had similar efficacy to hydrodistention in IC	BoNT-A 100 U injected into the trigone of the bladder using a flexible needle through a cystoscope	
	Manning et al. [137]: Double-blind, randomized, placebo-controlled trial in 50 women, randomized to receive HD, HD + saline or abobotulinumtoxinA	BoNT was not associated with significant increase in total O-Leary Sant questionnaire (OLS) score	AbobotulinumtoxinA 500 U intravesical	12 patients had UTI treated during the follow-up period, which confounded the results
	Kuo et al. [121]: Multicenter, randomized, placebo-controlled, double-blind study in 60 IC/PBS patients randomized in a 2:1 ratio of HD + BoNT (n = 40): saline (n = 20)	Significant reduction in pain in the BoNT group compared to placebo cystometric bladder capacity increased in the BoNT group	BoNT-A 100 U	AE did not differ significantly between groups
	Chuang and Kuo [39]: Randomized, two-center, double-blind, placebo-controlled trial in patients with IC/PBS who received intravesical liposomal botulinum toxin (n = 31), BoNT injection (n = 28) or placebo (n = 31)	Improved pain scores and OLS score in all 3 groups No difference in improvement between the groups	Intravesical liposomal botulinum toxin OnabotulinumtoxinA 200 U	No significant AE
	Pinto et al. [181]: Single-center, randomized, double-blind, placebo-controlled pilot trial in 19 women with IC/PBS who received trigonal injections of BoNT (n = 10) or placebo (n = 9)	Significant pain reduction in BoNT group compared to placebo at week 12 Significant improvement in OLS score and quality of life in BoNT group compared to placebo	OnabotulinumtoxinA 100 U injected in trigone at 10 sites	
Detrusor sphincter dyssynergia	Gallien et al. [76]: Randomized, double-blind, placebo-controlled trial in 86 patients with MS	No difference in post-voiding residual urine volume (PRUV)	OnabotulinumtoxinA 100 U as single transperineal injection into the sphincter	

	de Sèze et al. [52]: Randomized, double-blind, placebo-controlled trial in 13 patients with urinary retention from detrusor sphincter dyssynergia, who received transperineal injections of BoNT or lidocaine	Significant mean decrease of PRUV in the BoNT group	OnabotulinumtoxinA 100 U as single transperineal injection into the sphincter Or lidocaine	
Otolaryngology:				
Laryngeal dystonia	Data is based on observational studies and retrospective chart reviews			
Spasmodic dysphonia	Data is based on observational studies and retrospective chart reviews			
Gastroenterology:				
Achalasia	Mikaeli et al. [146]: Prospective, randomized, single-blinded, placebo-controlled trial in 40 patients with achalasia who were randomized to receive BoNT ($n = 20$) or pneumatic dilatation ($n = 20$)	12-month remission rate was significantly higher for pneumatic dilatation group than patients receiving single injection of BoNT	Dysport® 200 U	Efficacy of a single pneumatic dilatation is similar to two BoNT injections
	Bansal et al. [14]: Randomized, double-blind study in 34 patients with achalasia randomized to receive BoNT ($n = 16$) or Witzel balloon dilatation ($n = 18$)	Initial therapy with Witzel procedure is associated with better long-term outcome than a single BoNT injection	Botox® 80 U into lower esophageal sphincter (LES)	Due to risk of perforation with Witzel, BoNT remains a possible alternative
	Mikaeli et al. [145]: Randomized controlled trial in 54 patients with achalasia randomized to receive BoNT one month before pneumatic dilatation ($n = 27$) or pneumatic dilatation alone ($n = 27$)	One-year remission rate was 77% in BoNT group compared to 62% in pneumatic dilatation group Injection of BoNT before dilatation does not significant enhance the efficacy of pneumatic dilatation	Dysport® 400 U in LES	

(continued)

Table 4.1 (continued)

Indication	Study	Results	BoNT injection pattern	Comments
	Zaninotto et al. [269]: Randomized controlled trial in patients with achalasia randomized to receive BoNT ($n = 40$) or laparoscopic myotomy ($n = 40$)	After 6 months, results were comparable between the groups	Botox® 100 U injected in the LES; Patients with a good response received a second round of injection	
	Zaninotto et al. [269]: Randomized trial in 37 patients with achalasia who were randomized to receive laparoscopic myotomy ($n = 20$) or two injections of BoNT one month apart ($n = 17$)	Probability of being asymptomatic 2 years later was 34% for BoNT and 90% for myotomy No significant difference in cost effectiveness between these two groups over 2 years	Two injections of Botox® 100 U injected one month apart	
Anal fissure	Brisinda et al. [29]: Randomized, placebo-controlled trial in 50 patients injected with BoNT or nitroglycerin application twice daily	96% patients in the BoNT group had healing of anal fissure at 2 months compared to 60% in the placebo group, which was statistically significant	OnabotulinumtoxinA 20 U 9 patients in the nitroglycerin group crossed over to the BoNT group due to lack of benefit; 1 patient in BoNT group crossed over to nitroglycerin group due to lack of benefit	
	De Nardi et al. [50]: Randomized controlled trial in 30 patients who received either BoNT ($n = 15$) or 0.2% glycerine trinitrate (GTN) ointment three times daily at the anal margin	12 patients in GTN group and 11 patients in BoNT group had relief in symptoms at one month visit; no significant difference between the groups	OnabotulinumtoxinA 20 U into the internal anal sphincter on each side of anterior midline	No incontinence in either group
	Brisinda et al. [28]: Randomized controlled trial in 100 patients, who were randomized to receive BoNT (30 U Botox® or 90 U Dysport®) or 0.2% nitroglycerin ointment	92% patients (46 of 50 patients) in BoNT group and 70% patients in nitroglycerin group (35 of 50 patients) had healed anal fissures at 2 months. 12 patients from nitroglycerin group and 4 from BoNT group crossed over to the other group due to inadequate benefit	30 U Botox® or 90 U Dysport® injected into internal anal sphincter	Mild incontinence and flatus in BoNT group that lasted 3 weeks Mild headache in nitroglycerin group

4 Evidence-Based Review of Current Botulinum Toxin Treatment Indications… 85

	Results	Dosing	Notes
Festen et al. [70]: Randomized blinded trial in 108 patients with anal fissure, randomized to get BoNT injection and placebo ointment or placebo injection and isosorbide dinitrate (ISDN) ointment	14 of 37 patients in BoNT group and 21 of 36 patients in ISDN group had healing of anal fissure after 4 months; BoNT not found to have an advantage over ISDN	OnabotulinumtoxinA 10 U to each side of anterior midline in the internal anal sphincter (20 units total)	
Berkel et al. [19]: Multicenter randomized clinical trial in 60 patients with anal fissure who received either BoNT or ISDN ointment	Significant improvement in healing of anal fissure in BoNT group over ISDN group at 9 weeks (18 of 27 patients in Dysport group and 11 of 33 patients in ISDN group had healing of anal fissure)	Dysport® 60 U 30 U on each side of the anterior midline of the internal anal sphincter	Recurrence rate in both groups is high; 28% of Dysport group and 50% in ISDN group had recurrence of fissure in a year
Abd Elhady et al. [2]: Randomized controlled parallel group study in 160 patients with chronic anal fissure who were divided into 4 treatment groups (n = 40 each group), including treatment by lateral internal sphincterotomy, local diltiazem ointment, local GNT ointment, and BoNT injections into internal anal sphincter	Mean time to healing was not statistically different between the groups. Mean time to pain relief was significantly lower in the BoNT group compared to diltiazem and local GNT group. Mean time to pain relief was lower in the BoNT group compared to sphincterotomy group but the difference was not statistically significant. Most patients refused to continue medical therapy and were referred for lateral sphincterotomy	OnabotulinumtoxinA 20 U to each side (40 U total) of anterior midline of the internal anal sphincter	Recurrence rate after BoNT was 52.5% while recurrence rate in sphincterotomy group was 10%
Gastroparesis	Data is from case series		
Constipation	Data is from open label trials		

guidance. There was subtle improvement in two patients, worsening of posture in one, and marked worsening in one patient. At the highest doses, all patients complained of mild hip weakness [247].

Another study in two patients where 300 units of BoNT was injected in the rectus abdominis with CT guidance showed no improvement in symptoms after BoNT injection [42].

A case report of a single patient with camptocormia, who had insufficient benefit in trunk posture and pain after rectus abdominis injection, was injected with 200 units of onabotulinumtoxinA in the external oblique on one side and rectus abdominis on the other side. This led to an improvement in trunk posture and improvement in pain. This patient had a partial resection of rectus abdominis on one side for breast cancer reconstruction surgery [257]. This was based on the observation in a previous study where injection of lidocaine into external oblique muscles in patients with camptocormia resulted in an improvement in posture and pain in 8 of 12 patients [75].

(d) Pisa syndrome

Pisa syndrome refers to the marked lateral flexion of the trunk, of more than 10°, improves with lying down, and with passive manipulation. This is estimated to have a prevalence of about 8% in PD patients with longer disease duration [59], and in patients with atypical parkinsonian syndromes.

In a randomized placebo-controlled trial involving 26 patients, 13 patients received BoNT injections while the remaining 13 received saline injections for camptocormia. Between 50 and 200 units of incobotulinumtoxinA was injected using EMG guidance into iliopsoas, rectus abdominis, thoracic, or lumbar paravertebral muscles. There was significant improvement in trunk posture in the patients injected with BoNT and also in pain and range of motion [229].

In an open label pilot study of the effect of BoNT in Pisa syndrome, 13 of 15 patients initially enrolled completed follow-up assessments, and of these, 11 patients had at least 40% improvement in posture, and all patients had improvement in pain/ discomfort. Between 50 and 75 units of onabotulinumtoxinA was injected into the paraspinal muscles under ultrasound or EMG guidance, and between 25 and 50 units injected in the non-paraspinal muscles with pathologic hyperactivity on EMG [9].

Hemifacial Spasm (HFS)

HFS is characterized by unilateral, involuntary clonic contraction of muscles innervated by the seventh cranial nerve. This is often due to an aberrant vascular loop compressing the exiting nerve root [262]. Secondary HFS could occur when seventh cranial nerve is damaged due to tumor, infection, Bell's palsy, or demyelinating causes. HFS is primary in 79% patients and secondary in 21% [116].

There is level C (possibly effective) recommendation for the use of BoNT in HFS. The evidence for the use of BoNT is not optimal but the initial open label studies showed significant degree of benefit and this has discouraged larger controlled studies for this condition [215]. However, BoNT has become the mainstay first-line treatment for HFS and both primary and secondary HFS respond well to BoNT injection [116]. Pretarsal injections have been noted to be more beneficial to help the eyelid spasms in HFS than preseptal injections [31].

An open trial studied the effects of BoNT in 101 patients with HFS. Of 144 treatments, 98.6% had significant improvement in symptoms. This study initially started as a double-blind study with 8 patients randomized to receive BoNT and 4 patients in the placebo arm received saline injections. Due to the benefits noted with BoNT, the remaining patients were studied in an open trial and all patients treated with BoNT received benefit after the first injection for HFS. Patients with suboptimal benefit received repeat injections 7–10 days after the first round of BoNT [175]. This practice is generally discouraged due to concern for immunoresistance with injections repeated less than 3 weeks apart [17]. Dry eye, facial weakness, and ptosis were the adverse effects noted.

A prospective, placebo-controlled blinded study in 11 patients with HFS showed subjective improvement in 79% and objective improvement in 84% after BoNT injections [265].

In a single-blinded randomized parallel group study comparing two BoNT products, onabotulinumtoxinA (Botox®) and abobotulinumtoxinA (Dysport®) were studied in 49 patients with HFS. Similar improvement was noted with the two BoNT products with a slightly higher number of patients needing booster injections with Dysport® than with Botox®. A conversion ratio of 4:1 was used for Dysport®: Botox® to estimate an equivalent potency [205]. In a study of BoNT in blepharospasm and HFS, 28 patients with HFS had improvement in symptoms with the injection of BoNT to pretarsal orbicularis oculi [31]. In a retrospective chart, review of 32 patients injected with BoNT for blepharospasm and HFS, 11 patients had HFS. There was improvement in symptoms with BoNT injections, and these persisted with repeat treatments over the course of 10 years. A slightly higher dose was needed for similar benefits over time [1].

Synkinesis

Aberrant regeneration of the facial nerve after facial nerve injury or paralysis from a variety of etiologies could result in abnormal movement of facial muscles called synkinesis. The involved muscles could include eyelid and upper or lower facial muscles. BoNT can treat these abnormal movements to restore facial symmetry in these patients.

A double-blind multicenter placebo-controlled trial evaluated the use of BoNT in 30 patients with synkinesis and an additional 6 patients in an open label pilot study design. Etiology of facial paralysis for patients in this study included chronic Bell's palsy in 20 patients, post-acoustic neuroma surgery in 4 patients, Ramsey-Hunt syndrome in 4 patients and one patient after mastoiditis and another after meningioma resection. BoNT/A injected to the synkinetic side suppressed the degree of abnormal movements associated with different facial movements in both study designs. In the double-blind placebo-controlled study, 15 patients received BoNT injections and were compared to 15 patients who received placebo. In this study, there was reduction in the synkinetic movements based on videotape and blinded physician examination and improvement in quality of life, vision, social interaction, and self-perception of facial asymmetry [21].

Another study compared onabotulinumtoxinA to abobotulinumtoxinA in facial synkinesis by injecting BoNT to the non-paralyzed side of the face using a dose conversion ratio of 1:3, which is the most commonly used conversion ratio. After randomization, 25 patients received onabotulinumtoxinA and 30 patients received abobotulinumtoxinA with doses individualized to the patients. Both toxins showed an improvement in facial asymmetry after injections using subjective and objective assessments. Facial symmetry was assessed subjectively by independent evaluation by two plastic surgeons on a four-point scale, and objective evaluation included Clinical Score for Facial Palsy and Facial Disability index [57].

A randomized placebo-controlled trial in 20 patients with facial palsy followed by synkinesis evaluated the effects of BoNT in these patients. Ten were randomized to receive BoNT followed by neuromuscular retraining therapy (NMRT), which is an exercise program to improve synkinesis, compared to 10 patients who received NMRT alone. There was significant improvement in synkinesis in the BoNT group compared to placebo [46, 152].

Another randomized single-blind three-arm comparison clinical trial compared three different BoNT types, onabotulinumtoxinA, abobotulinumtoxinA, and incobotulinumtoxinA, in 28 patients with facial synkinesis. Of these, 6 patients were enrolled multiple times. Of a total of 38 treatment visits, 15 were onabotulinumtoxinA, 13 abobotulinumtoxinA, and 10 incobotulinumtoxinA injection visits. There was no significant difference in SAQ score improvement between the three toxin groups, implying similar efficacy of these toxins for facial synkinesis up to 4 weeks. At 4 weeks, incobotulinumtoxinA had less effect on SAQ scores compared to onabotulinumtoxinA, probably due to shorter duration of action. Higher doses may be needed to allow for longer duration of benefit when using incobotulinumtoxinA for facial synkinesis [231].

In addition to these randomized clinical trials, there are multiple other open label studies showing benefits of BoNT in synkinesis.

A prospective cohort study in 23 patients who received BoNT injections for facial synkinesis showed improvement in synkinesis after injections. Some of these patients got injections to the buccinator muscle, which is thought to be a symptomatic muscle in synkinesis. Although all patients who received BoNT injections had improved synkinesis, patients who received injections to the buccinator had greater improvement in post-injection scores and greater difference between the pre- and post-injection scores on the Synkinesis Assessment Questionnaire (SAQ). Buccinator injections were performed, using EMG guidance, below the dentate line in the buccal mucosa anterior to the level of Stenson's duct [176].

Another prospective cohort study in 99 patients with facial synkinesis who received BoNT injections showed that there was significant improvement in synkinesis after BoNT injections. Bell's palsy and facial paralysis after resection of vestibular schwannoma were the main etiology preceding facial synkinesis in these patients. A group of 6 muscles including corrugator, orbicularis oculi superioris, orbicularis oculi inferioris, risorius, mentalis, and platysma were injected in these patients. SAQ was used to assess symptoms pre and post injections. Higher doses of BoNT injections resulted in increased improvement in SAQ scores [212].

In a cohort of 51 patients who received BoNT injections, SAQ was administered pre and post injections. There was significant improvement in SAQ scores and improvement in scores for every question on the SAQ post onabotulinumtoxinA injection compared to the pre scores [158].

Orofacial and Oromandibular Dystonia

Orofacial/oromandibular dystonia (OMD) refers to dystonic contraction of the facial muscles along with pharyngeal, laryngeal, and masticatory muscles [116]. This could accompany dystonia in the neck as part of cranial cervical dystonia. There are numerous case reports and case series describing the benefit of BoNT in OMD, but there is paucity of well-designed, placebo-controlled trials [144, 151]. Jaw closing dystonia with or without bruxism tends to be more responsive to BoNT than jaw opening dystonia [218, 226]. In a double-blind, placebo-controlled trial of 23 patients with sleep bruxism treated with BoNT/A injections into masseter and temporalis (60 and 40 units each, respectively) or placebo, the clinical global impression and the visual analog scale favored the BoNT/A group [166].

A prospective, longitudinal, observational case series evaluated 30 patients with focal facial dystonia pre and post BoNT injections using Abnormal Involuntary Movement Scale (AIMS). BoNT doses between 3 and 100 units were used (mean dose 27.4 units). There was improvement in the AIMS score and the percentage of improvement depended on the dose injected, the area affected, and the etiology. However, among patients with facial dystonia, this study included 11 patients with HFS and 7 patients with facial paralysis, all inappropriately listed under the facial dystonia class [197].

In a large prospective open label study looking at the safety and efficacy of BoNT in OMD, 162 patients with OMD had Botox® injections in either the masseter or the submental complex or both muscle groups. Jaw closing dystonia was the most common type in this study and the majority had primary/idiopathic dystonia. 110 of the 162 patients had a global improvement of ≥3 on a scale where 4 means complete resolution/marked improvement of symptoms [226].

A cross-sectional survey of 23 patients, 5 with OMD, showed that patients with OMD had benefits noted on the Glasgow Benefit Inventory (GBI). This questionnaire evaluates quality of life after otolaryngologic interventions, in this case, BoNT for spasmodic dysphonia and OMD. The benefit was less than what was noted in patients with spasmodic dysphonia (SD), but there was not a significant difference between the groups. All patients with SD and OMD noticed benefits after BoNT injections [20].

Another similar study in 12 patients with jaw opening OMD, using GBI scores pre and post BoNT injections showed a significant improvement in quality of life after BoNT injections. Doses of 40 units or more were injected into the lateral pterygoid muscles bilaterally with an additional midline injection of 10 units into the submental complex for patients with suboptimal benefit despite dose increase to the lateral pterygoid muscles. There was significant reduction in the GBI scores after BoNT injections. There were no major adverse effects [36].

Neuro-rehabilitation: Spasticity

BoNT has level A evidence of efficacy in patients with upper- and lower-limb spasticity [105]. There are several reports which show a significant reduction in post-stroke spasticity in patients receiving BoNT. There is also improved pain with reduced spasticity in these patients. However, a meta-analysis of six studies reported no significant improvement in functional status or change in disability after BoNT injections. However, there was a trend toward reduced spasticity-related pain [194]. The AAN Practice Update in 2016 and a meta-analysis by Sun et al. in 2019 lists several randomized placebo-controlled trials which show the efficacy and safety of BoNT in patients with upper- and lower-limb spasticity [217, 223]. Some of these studies, along with a brief description, are listed in Table 4.1. BoNT injections in patients with spasticity should occur in conjunction with aggressive neurorehabilitation for improved functional status and reduced disability in this patient population.

Tics

There are not many studies providing good-quality evidence for this indication, but BoNT injections continue to be a strategy that is considered when tics are at danger of causing secondary complications or if there are isolated simple tics affecting one body segment which is not responding well to medications [131, 230]. For example, with whiplash tics, which are forceful and repetitive, there is a risk of cervical myelopathy and cord injury if left untreated or inadequately treated. With forceful repetitive eye blinking tics, there could be functional blindness, which could limit driving or potentially result in harmful situations. BoNT injections into the vocal cords have been found to be very effective in the treatment of troublesome phonic tics, including coprolalia [122]. There are reports on the efficacy of BoNT in reducing tic frequency and severity, and this is also thought to reduce the premonitory urge associated with both motor and phonic tics. A small randomized double-blind placebo-controlled cross-over study involving 18 patients with tics, noted a significant improvement in tic frequency and the urge leading up to the tic. However, this study interestingly noted that the patients did not appreciate any improvement in their tics. This discrepancy between the lack of adequate benefit noted by the patients and significant tic reduction observed by the examiner was thought to be due to presence of other tics in muscle groups that were not injected [141].

A Cochrane review which looked into the utility of BoNT for the treatment of motor and phonic tics was able to only find one study that met their selection criteria [170]. This is the study mentioned above by Marras et al. in 2001. The overall beneficial effect of BoNT was deemed to be uncertain by the Cochrane review [170].

There are other small open label studies where there has been improved patient-reported tic control after BoNT injection. In an open label study of BoNT in 35 patients with tics, 29 patients reported an improvement in tics after BoNT injections, and 21 of 25 patients with a premonitory urge noted an improvement in this urge after BoNT injections [122].

Autonomic Disorders

(a) Sialorrhea

Sialorrhea may accompany several neurological disorders including PD, atypical parkinsonian conditions, amyotrophic lateral sclerosis (ALS), and cerebral palsy. Sialorrhea results in social embarrassment for the patient and family members and in addition could result in tissue breakdown where saliva pools in the neck or result in fungal infections from drooling and constant moisture. BoNT works by inhibiting acetylcholine release at the parasympathetic ganglion, thereby reducing saliva secretion [100]. In these patients, drooling is often thought to be due to decreased swallowing more than due to overproduction of saliva [157].

There are several randomized controlled trials showing efficacy of BoNT in sialorrhea [123, 179, 221]. Injections are typically done in the parotid gland and submandibular glands, with benefits lasting between 3 and 6 months, with injections repeated for benefit maintenance. Both BoNT type A and B could be used for injections with benefit in sialorrhea [214].

Over 50% patients with ALS have problems with sialorrhea and trouble handling the secretions. Trouble swallowing saliva due to bulbar involvement contributes to this symptom. About 20% patients have sialorrhea despite the use of anticholinergics or have side effects limiting the use of oral medications. A systematic review of five small studies in 28 patients showed positive benefit of BoNT on sialorrhea in this patient population [221]. This review included 5 small studies, two of which showed reduction in sialorrhea after BoNT-A injection [80, 258], one study showed no change in the number of tissue papers used and no subjective effect on sialorrhea [210], another showed some improvement based on QoL questions in 5 patients [138], and the last included study showed 30% reduction in daily tissue use and improvement in drooling impact score in over half the patients with bulbar ALS [241].

Between 40% and 80% patients with PD have sialorrhea. BoNT is thought to probably be safe and effective for treating drooling in patients with PD [157]. Oropharyngeal dysphagia due to bradykinesia is thought to cause sialorrhea. A double-blind placebo-controlled trial of the use of BoNT in sialorrhea in 32 PD patients showed that there was significant improvement in sialorrhea when assessed a month after injecting 50 units of BoNT in each parotid when compared to placebo [123]. Another double-blind study involving 20 parkinsonian patients, 14 with PD and 6 with multiple system atrophy (MSA), showed significant improvement in sialorrhea starting a week after injecting 145 units of BoNT in bilateral parotid glands and 80 units in each submandibular gland [136]. Another double-blind placebo-controlled trial in 54 patients also showed improved salivation after BoNT injection [37]. A list of double-blind placebo-controlled trials evaluating the use of BoNT in patients with sialorrhea has been listed in Table 4.1.

BoNT has been studied for sialorrhea from other etiology as well. In pediatric population with neurologic impairment, Dohar, J retrospectively looked at the effect of BoNT for sialorrhea in a long-term study which showed persistent benefit of BoNT over time in 112 children over the study period of 9 years [58].

(b) Hyperhidrosis
Sweating abnormalities could be seen in patients with PD with prevalence as high as 60%. Injection of BoNT is thought to work by inhibiting acetylcholine at the parasympathetic nerve terminals [250]. The use of BoNT in these patients is based on studies done on patients with essential hyperhidrosis.

Primary focal hyperhidrosis is a disorder of excessive sweating which could be localized to the axilla, palms, soles, or forehead. Based on the 2008 AAN review, BoNT is established to be safe and effective in axillary hyperhidrosis and is probably safe and effective for use in patients with palmar hyperhidrosis [157]. A list of randomized controlled trials that led to these recommendations is briefly described in Table 4.1.

Otolaryngology

BoNT is the preferred treatment for laryngeal dystonia/spasmodic dysphonia (SD), a form of focal dystonia affecting the larynx and vocal cords resulting in a strained effortful voice or irregular, interrupted speech during spasms of vocal cords [198]. There are three main different subtypes are adductor SD, abductor SD, and mixed SD. Abductor SD is characterized by a breathy voice and breaks in speech due to inappropriate glottal opening during speech. The posterior cricoarytenoid muscles are the main muscles involved in abductor SD. In Adductor SD, there is a strained quality to the voice and speech interruptions due to excessive glottal closure [213]. Injection of BoNT into thyroarytenoid muscle improves the symptoms of adductor spasmodic dysphonia [153]. In a survey of 70 physicians who inject patients with SD, where they collectively injected over 4000 patients with SD over the prior year.

In this survey, the physicians self-reported that the majority used EMG to inject the thyroarytenoid or throarytenoid-lateral cricoarytenoid muscle complex or for adductor SD via transcricothyroid membrane approach. A substantial majority (87%) preferred to start with bilateral injections. For abductor SD, 92% targeted the posterior cricoarytenoid muscle alone, 31 physicians (51%) preferred the anterior transcricoid injection approach, and 67% used EMG guidance for the injections [213].

A prospective, observational study in 30 patients with laryngeal dystonia (LD), with or without accompanying jaw dystonia, evaluated the effect of BoNT in patients with LD using oromandibular dystonia questionnaire-25 (OMDQ-25). This study noted a significant reduction in the OMDQ-25 scores after BoNT injections at 4 and 8 weeks post injection. No major adverse effects were observed. A consistent, measurable improvement in quality of life was noted after BoNT injections in LD patients with the injection of genioglossus and other muscles in the oromandibular region [155].

A cross-sectional survey of 23 patients, 18 with SD and 5 with OMD, showed that patients with SD had significant benefit in symptoms noted after BoNT injections when quantified on the Glasgow Benefit Inventory. The benefit was higher in the SD group than patients with OMD [20].

The dose of BoNT required for adductor spasmodic dysphonia typically tends to reduce over time. A retrospective chart review in the charts of 44 patients who were on BoNT treatment for adductor Spasmodic Dysphonia showed that over time, patients received less BoNT doses over a course of 10 years with maintained benefit [22]. Similar results were noted by another study where the BoNT doses required reduced over time when patients were observed for a 20-year period. Unilateral or bilateral thyroarytenoid muscles were injected in these patients [153].

A retrospective study of 8 patients with adductor SD as part of Meige syndrome, who received BoNT injections under EMG guidance had clinically relevant improvement noted after injections [177].

A retrospective chart review in 32 patients with adductor spasmodic dysphonia, who received EMG-guided intracordal BoNT injections, were performed. Doses of BoNT injected ranged from 2.74 U to 3.85 U, with mean dose of 3.64 U. There was significant improvement in voice quality after 1 month and this stabilized after 3 months [139].

Urology

Overactive bladder affects 12–17% of the general population at some point in life, of which about a third experience urge incontinence [161]. BoNT chemodenervation is the third-line treatment for overactive bladder (OAB) in patients that have refractory symptoms despite behavioral and pharmacologic treatment [224].

Mechanism of action for the benefit is thought to be secondary to blockage of synaptic release of acetylcholine, resulting in paralysis of detrusor muscle, and relaxation and improvement in symptoms of overactive bladder. There is, however, increasing evidence that BoNT has effects on afferent nerve terminals as well. There is now high-quality evidence for the efficacious use of BoNT in detrusor overactivity. Effects from BoNT last about 8–11 months before injections have to be repeated [171]. Urinary retention is a possible adverse effect, and patients may need to self-catheterize for urinary retention, if this happens.

In an open label study in 20 PD patients with overactive bladder, 100 units of onabotulinumtoxinA was injected into submucosal intradetrusor. This resulted in improved bladder symptoms at 1 and 3 months, and 50% decreased incontinence episodes over 6 months. 57% had moderate to marked improvement [7].

In another open label study of onabotulinumtoxinA in 24 PD patients with OAB, 100 units of onabotulinumtoxinA was injected into bladder wall and trigone. In this study, 79.2% patients had improved symptoms of OAB at 4 weeks, and 29.1% had resolution of urge incontinence [248].

A large randomized placebo-controlled clinical trial in 557 patients with OAB, 280 of who received BoNT injections for urge incontinence refractory to anticholinergic medications, about 65% of BoNT-treated patients had improvement in symptoms. The rate of urinary retention in these patients was 5.4% [161].

In a prospective randomized single-blinded trial in 21 female patients with OAB who had failed first-line and second-line therapies, abobotulinumtoxinA was injected at two doses of 300 U and 500 U. Intravesical injections were done at 30 sites, avoiding the trigone. At 12 weeks, there was significant improvement in 91% patients in both groups. Patients were better or much better in 70% patients who received 300 U and in 88.9% patients who received 500 U BoNT injections at 12 weeks; and in 50% who received 300 U and in 100% at 500 U at 24 weeks. Intravesical injections of 500 U improved quality of life and symptoms for longer periods of time than 300 U [51].

There are several other trials which demonstrated the benefits of BoNT for overactive bladder, some of which are listed in Table 4.1.

BoNT has also been used to treat interstitial cystitis (IC)/bladder painful syndrome. Several randomized controlled trials (RCT) have evaluated the efficacy of BoNT in IC, some of which have been described briefly in Table 4.1.

Gastroenterology

(a) Esophageal motility disorders
BoNT has been used for the treatment of spastic esophageal motility disorders and achalasia. BoNT provides short-term symptom relief in patients who are considered high risk for more invasive surgical treatment options like myotomy or esophageal dilatation [239]. BoNT is considered less efficacious than the surgical alternatives [190] but could be considered in high-risk surgical candidates. About 70–90% of patients notice improvement in symptoms within a month of injection; but over half requires repeat injections within 6–24 months [239].

There are several randomized controlled trials that evaluated the benefits of BoNT in achalasia. A meta-analysis that evaluated this deemed that there were better remission rate and reduced relapse rate in patients that received pneumatic dilatation when compared to BoNT injections [253]. Several of these RCTs are included in Table 4.1.

In patients with nonachalasia spastic dysmotility disorders, BoNT may improve dysphagia symptoms, based on small retrospective studies [220].

(b) Anal fissure

Anal fissure is a linear ulceration in the anal canal, affecting especially young adults, resulting in pain and bleeding after defecation. Chronic anal fissure is a fissure that persists after 4–12 weeks of treatment. BoNT injection into the internal anal sphincter or intersphincteric groove is a minimally invasive procedure that results in symptom release, often for 3 months. Flatus (18%) and fecal incontinence (5% of patients) are possible side effects with less of a risk of fecal incontinence when compared to the other surgical interventions including lateral internal sphincterotomy (LIS), which is first-line surgery for medically refractory anal fissure [15]. Three meta-analysis showed that LIS is superior to BoNT for anal fissure, but there is less of a risk of fecal incontinence with BoNT injections compared to LIS [15]. In a retrospective observational study of 128 patients treated with BoNT over 5 years, 46.6% of patients had complete response, 23.9% had partial response, and 29.5% were refractory. Complete response was defined by symptomatic improvement along with anal fissure healing, while partial response including symptomatic improvement without fissure healing and refractory patients had neither symptomatic improvement or fissure resolution [15]. Reported dosages of BoNT vary between 20 and 100 units injected into the internal anal sphincter, under the anal fissure, on both sides of the fissure, or circumferential injections, with no one method deemed superior to another [15, 86, 251].

A meta-analysis identified six randomized controlled trials evaluating the effect of BoNT in chronic anal fissure which showed that BoNT has fewer side effects than topical nitrates, but there is no difference in fissure healing or recurrence [202]. These studies are briefly described in Table 4.1.

(c) Internal anal sphincter achalasia

Internal anal sphincter achalasia is a condition similar to Hirschsprung disease but with ganglion cells preserved. BoNT has been studied in this condition. A meta-analysis that looked at 16 prospective and retrospective studies deemed posterior myectomy to be a more efficacious procedure than interspincteric BoNT in patients with internal anal sphincter achalasia [74].

(d) Constipation

There are a few open label studies looking into the utility of BoNT for constipation [111]. In an open label involving 10 patients, onabotulinum toxin A was injected into the puborectalis muscle; there was reduced rectal tone while straining [6]. In another study involving 18 patients, where 100 units of onabotulinum toxin A was injected at two sites on the puborectalis muscle, there was subjective symptomatic improvement in 10 patients at 2 months and in 8 patients at 1 month post injection. There was also a significant reduction in the straining pressure [30].

(e) Gastroparesis

Pyloric sphincter dysfunction could result in delayed gastric emptying and lead to idiopathic and diabetic gastroparesis; and relaxation of this using BoNT has been postulated to improve gastroparesis. There are some case reports and case series on the use of BoNT for gastroparesis.

In a case series of two patients with PD who had gastroparesis diagnosed by gastroenterologist via gastric emptying study (GES), both received 100 U of BoNT into the pyloric sphincter via endoscopy and was followed for 4–8 weeks. The first patient had complete resolution of abdominal discomfort and nausea at 5 weeks and a repeat GES was "within normal limits." The second patient had complete resolution of nausea and abdominal discomfort after 2 months from injection and repeat GES was normal [81].

In another case series of ten patients with idiopathic gastroparesis not responding to medications, 80–100 U of BoNT was injected into the pyloric sphincter. There was significant improvement in mean solid gastric retention 4 weeks after injections and significant improvement in symptoms as well after BoNT injections [147].

In a case series of six patients with diabetic gastroparesis and an abnormal solid phase gastric emptying study, injection of 100 U of BoNT into the pyloric sphincter improved symptoms. There was mean improvement of 55% in subjective symptoms by 2 weeks, with improvement maintained at 6 weeks [67].

Pain Medicine

BoNT has been found to have an effect on many peripheral and central mechanisms of pain and has been studied in multiple conditions associated with pain [142]. At the peripheral nerve endings, BoNT inhibits the secretion of pain modulators like substance P, calcitonin gene–related peptide (CGRP), glutamate from nerve endings, and dorsal root ganglion; reduces local inflammation at the nerve endings; and is also thought to potentially have a regenerative effect on injured nerves [142, 174]. Currently, chronic migraine is the only FDA-approved pain condition for which BoNT is approved. BoNT is also approved for use in spasticity and could help relieve spasticity-related pain. BoNT has also been observed to reduce pain associated with dystonia. BoNT has been studied in painful temporomandibular disorders in several RCTs, but the level of evidence was low and insufficient to support the use of BoNT for this condition. However, BoNT was well tolerated without significant increase in adverse effects [135]. BoNT is being studied for use in neuropathic pain conditions and considered effective in the treatment of conditions including post-herpetic neuralgia, diabetic neuropathy, trigeminal neuralgia, and intractable neuropathic pain [174]. There are smaller studies showing a beneficial role of BoNT in occipital neuralgia, carpal tunnel syndrome, phantom limb pain, and some randomized controlled trials showing a beneficial role of BoNT in spinal cord injury–related neuropathic pain and central post-stroke pain [174]. The possible role for BoNT in pain management is being increasingly recognized and studied. Evidence for a few of these indications is briefly discussed below. Other pain conditions will be discussed in further detail in a separate chapter.

(a) Trigeminal neuralgia

A randomized double-blind placebo-controlled trial in 84 patients who received submucosal and intradermal injections of BoNT/A at two doses of 25 U and 75 U showed that patients had reduced pain, with patient reports of being "much improved" or "very much improved." The response rate was 70.4% for the 25 U group and 86.2% for 75 U group, significantly higher than the placebo group at 32.1% [270].

In another randomized double-blind placebo-controlled trial in 42 patients who received intradermal and/or submucosal injections of BoNT/A compared to placebo, there was significant improvement in pain intensity and pain attacks at week 1. There were significantly more responders in the BoNT injection group (68.18%) than in placebo group (15%) [260].

Another randomized double-blind placebo-controlled trial in 36 patients compared patients who received placebo to patients who received subcutaneous injections of BoNT in the affected area, along with an additional intramuscular injection of 10 U BoNT or placebo in the ipsilateral masseter of patients with involvement of the third branch of the trigeminal nerve. Three months after injection, there was significant improvement in the visual analog scale (VAS) of pain in the BoNT group when compared to placebo [272].

(b) Post-herpetic neuralgia

In a randomized double-blind placebo-controlled trial in 60 patients who received BoNT, lidocaine, or placebo in the affected dermatome. Doses less than 200 U of BoNT/A were used based on individualized patient dosing. There was significant decrease in pain scores at week 1 and at 3 months compared to the lidocaine and placebo groups [261].

In another randomized double-blind placebo-controlled parallel group trial in 30 patients who received BoNT vs placebo, 13 patients had over 50% reduction in VAS score [8].

(c) Diabetic neuropathy

In a randomized double-blind placebo-controlled trial in 40 patients, 20 of whom received intradermal injections on the dorsum of the foot (total of 12 sites with 8–10 u per site), there was a reduction in neuropathic pain score compared to placebo [78].

In another randomized double-blind placebo-controlled crossover trial in 18 patients who received intradermal injections (4 U per site, 50 U per foot) of BoNT vs placebo, 44.4% had a reduction in VAS scores within 3 months with no similar response in the placebo group [266].

References

1. Ababneh OH, Cetinkaya A, Kulwin DR. Long-term efficacy and safety of botulinum toxin A injections to treat blepharospasm and hemifacial spasm. Clin Exp Ophthalmol. 2014;42:254–61. https://doi.org/10.1111/ceo.12165.
2. Abd Elhady HM, Othman IH, Hablus MA, et al. Long-term prospective randomised clinical and manometric comparison between surgical and chemical sphincterotomy for treatment of chronic anal fissure. S Afr J Surg. 2009;47:112–4.
3. Adler CH, Bansberg SF, Hentz JG, et al. Botulinum toxin type A for treating voice tremor. Arch Neurol. 2004;61:1416–20. https://doi.org/10.1001/archneur.61.9.1416.
4. Ahn S-Y, Kim D-A, Park Y-O, Shin J-H. Effect of ultrasonography-guided botulinum toxin type A injection in holmes' tremor secondary to pontine hemorrhage: case report. Ann Rehabil Med. 2014;38:694–7. https://doi.org/10.5535/arm.2014.38.5.694.
5. Albanese A, Bhatia K, Bressman SB, et al. Phenomenology and classification of dystonia: a consensus update. Mov Disord. 2013;28:863–73. https://doi.org/10.1002/mds.25475.
6. Albanese A, Brisinda G, Bentivoglio AR, Maria G. Treatment of outlet obstruction constipation in Parkinson's disease with botulinum neurotoxin A. Am J Gastroenterol. 2003;98:1439–40. https://doi.org/10.1111/j.1572-0241.2003.07514.x.
7. Anderson RU, Orenberg EK, Glowe P. OnabotulinumtoxinA office treatment for neurogenic bladder incontinence in Parkinson's disease. Urology. 2014;83:22–7. https://doi.org/10.1016/j.urology.2013.09.017.
8. Apalla Z, Sotiriou E, Lallas A, et al. Botulinum toxin A in postherpetic neuralgia. Clin J Pain. 2013;29:857–64. https://doi.org/10.1097/AJP.0b013e31827a72d2.
9. Artusi CA, Bortolani S, Merola A, et al. Botulinum toxin for Pisa syndrome: an MRI-, ultrasound- and electromyography-guided pilot study. Parkinsonism Relat Disord. 2019;62:231–5. https://doi.org/10.1016/j.parkreldis.2018.11.003.
10. Azher SN, Jankovic J. Camptocormia: pathogenesis, classification, and response to therapy. Neurology. 2005;65:355–9. https://doi.org/10.1212/01.wnl.0000171857.09079.9f.
11. Bain PG, Findley LJ, Britton TC, et al. Primary writing tremor. Brain. 1995;118:1461–72. https://doi.org/10.1093/brain/118.6.1461.
12. Baizabal-Carvallo JF, Cardoso F, Jankovic J. Myorhythmia: phenomenology, etiology, and treatment. Mov Disord. 2015;30:171–9. https://doi.org/10.1002/mds.26093.
13. Baizabal-Carvallo JF, Jankovic J, Feld J. Flu-like symptoms and associated immunological response following therapy with botulinum toxins. Neurotox Res. 2013;24:298–306. https://doi.org/10.1007/s12640-013-9400-9.
14. Bansal R, Nostrant TT, Scheiman JM, et al. Intrasphincteric botulinum toxin versus pneumatic balloon dilation for treatment of primary achalasia. J Clin Gastroenterol. 2003;36:209–14. https://doi.org/10.1097/00004836-200303000-00005.
15. Barbeiro S, Atalaia-Martins C, Marcos P, et al. Long-term outcomes of botulinum toxin in the treatment of chronic anal fissure: 5 years of follow-up. United European Gastroenterol J. 2017;5:293–7. https://doi.org/10.1177/2050640616656708.
16. Baricich A, Picelli A, Carda S, et al. Electrical stimulation of antagonist muscles after botulinum toxin type A for post-stroke spastic equinus foot. A randomized single-blind pilot study. Ann Phys Rehabil Med. 2019;62:214–9. https://doi.org/10.1016/j.rehab.2019.06.002.
17. Bellows S, Jankovic J. Immunogenicity associated with botulinum toxin treatment. Toxins (Basel). 2019;11:491. https://doi.org/10.3390/toxins11090491.
18. Bentivoglio AR, Fasano A, Ialongo T, et al. Fifteen-year experience in treating blepharospasm with Botox or Dysport: same toxin, two drugs. Neurotox Res. 2009;15:224–31. https://doi.org/10.1007/s12640-009-9023-3.
19. Berkel AEM, Rosman C, Koop R, et al. Isosorbide dinitrate ointment vs botulinum toxin A (Dysport) as the primary treatment for chronic anal fissure: a randomized multicentre study. Color Dis. 2014;16:O360–6. https://doi.org/10.1111/codi.12615.

20. Bhattacharyya N, Tarsy D. Impact on quality of life of botulinum toxin treatments for spasmodic dysphonia and oromandibular dystonia. Arch Otolaryngol Head Neck Surg. 2001;127:389–92. https://doi.org/10.1001/archotol.127.4.389.

21. Borodic G, Bartley M, Slattery W, et al. Botulinum toxin for aberrant facial nerve regeneration: double-blind, placebo-controlled trial using subjective endpoints. Plast Reconstr Surg. 2005;116:36–43. https://doi.org/10.1097/01.PRS.0000169689.27829.C4.

22. Bradley JP, Barrow EM, Hapner ER, et al. Botulinum toxin-A dosing trends for adductor spasmodic dysphonia at a single institution over 10 years. J Voice. 2017;31:363–5. https://doi.org/10.1016/j.jvoice.2016.09.022.

23. Brans JW, Lindeboom R, Snoek JW, et al. Botulinum toxin versus trihexyphenidyl in cervical dystonia: a prospective, randomized, double-blind controlled trial. Neurology. 1996;46:1066–72. https://doi.org/10.1212/wnl.46.4.1066.

24. Brashear A, Lew MF, Dykstra DD, et al. Safety and efficacy of NeuroBloc (botulinum toxin type B) in type A-responsive cervical dystonia. Neurology. 1999;53:1439–46. https://doi.org/10.1212/wnl.53.7.1439.

25. Brin MF, Kirby RS, Slavotinek A, et al. Pregnancy outcomes following exposure to onabotulinumtoxinA. Pharmacoepidemiol Drug Saf. 2016;25:179–87. https://doi.org/10.1002/pds.3920.

26. Brin MF, Lew MF, Adler CH, et al. Safety and efficacy of NeuroBloc (botulinum toxin type B) in type A-resistant cervical dystonia. Neurology. 1999;53:1431–8. https://doi.org/10.1212/wnl.53.7.1431.

27. Brin MF, Lyons KE, Doucette J, et al. A randomized, double masked, controlled trial of botulinum toxin type A in essential hand tremor. Neurology. 2001;56:1523–8. https://doi.org/10.1212/wnl.56.11.1523.

28. Brisinda G, Cadeddu F, Brandara F, et al. Randomized clinical trial comparing botulinum toxin injections with 0·2 per cent nitroglycerin ointment for chronic anal fissure. Br J Surg. 2007;94:162–7. https://doi.org/10.1002/bjs.5514.

29. Brisinda G, Maria G, Bentivoglio AR, et al. A comparison of injections of botulinum toxin and topical nitroglycerin ointment for the treatment of chronic anal fissure. N Engl J Med. 1999;341:65–9. https://doi.org/10.1056/NEJM199907083410201.

30. Cadeddu F, Bentivoglio AR, Brandara F, et al. Outlet type constipation in Parkinson's disease: results of botulinum toxin treatment. Aliment Pharmacol Ther. 2005;22:997–1003. https://doi.org/10.1111/j.1365-2036.2005.02669.x.

31. Cakmur R, Ozturk V, Uzunel F, et al. Comparison of preseptal and pretarsal injections of botulinum toxin in the treatment of blepharospasm and hemifacial spasm. J Neurol. 2002;249:64–8. https://doi.org/10.1007/pl00007849.

32. Cardoso F. Botulinum toxin in parkinsonism: the when, how, and which for botulinum toxin injections. Toxicon. 2018;147:107–10. https://doi.org/10.1016/j.toxicon.2017.08.018.

33. Cenciarelli O, Riley PW, Baka A. Biosecurity threat posed by botulinum toxin. Toxins (Basel). 2019;11:681. https://doi.org/10.3390/toxins11120681.

34. Chapple C, Sievert K-D, MacDiarmid S, et al. OnabotulinumtoxinA 100 U significantly improves all idiopathic overactive bladder symptoms and quality of life in patients with overactive bladder and urinary incontinence: a randomised, double-blind, placebo-controlled trial. Eur Urol. 2013;64:249–56. https://doi.org/10.1016/j.eururo.2013.04.001.

35. Charles D, Brashear A, Hauser RA, et al. Efficacy, tolerability, and immunogenicity of OnabotulinumtoxinA in a randomized, double-blind, placebo-controlled trial for cervical dystonia. Clin Neuropharmacol. 2012;35:208–14. https://doi.org/10.1097/WNF.0b013e31826538c7.

36. Charous SJ, Cornelia CL, Fan W. Jaw-opening dystonia: quality of life after botulinum toxin injections. Ear Nose Throat J. 2011;90:E9–E12. https://doi.org/10.1177/014556131109000210.

37. Chinnapongse R, Gullo K, Nemeth P, et al. Safety and efficacy of botulinum toxin type B for treatment of sialorrhea in Parkinson's disease: a prospective double-blind trial. Mov Disord. 2012;27:219–26. https://doi.org/10.1002/mds.23929.

38. Chuang Y-C, Kaufmann JH, Chancellor DD, et al. Bladder instillation of liposome encapsulated onabotulinumtoxina improves overactive bladder symptoms: a prospective, multicenter, double-blind, randomized trial. J Urol. 2014;192:1743–9. https://doi.org/10.1016/j.juro.2014.07.008.
39. Chuang Y-C, Kuo H-C. A prospective, multicenter, double-blind, randomized trial of bladder instillation of liposome formulation OnabotulinumtoxinA for interstitial cystitis/bladder pain syndrome. J Urol. 2017;198:376–82. https://doi.org/10.1016/j.juro.2017.02.021.
40. Cillino S, Raimondi G, Guépratte N, et al. Long-term efficacy of botulinum toxin A for treatment of blepharospasm, hemifacial spasm, and spastic entropion: a multicentre study using two drug-dose escalation indexes. Eye (Lond). 2010;24:600–7. https://doi.org/10.1038/eye.2009.192.
41. Clarke CE. Botulinum toxin type A in cerebellar tremor caused by multiple sclerosis. Eur J Neurol. 1997;4:68–71. https://doi.org/10.1111/j.1468-1331.1997.tb00301.x.
42. Colosimo C, Salvatori FM. Injection of the iliopsoas muscle with botulinum toxin in camptocormia. Mov Disord. 2009;24:316–7. https://doi.org/10.1002/mds.22249.
43. Comella CL, Jankovic J, Shannon KM, et al. Comparison of botulinum toxin serotypes A and B for the treatment of cervical dystonia. Neurology. 2005;65:1423–9. https://doi.org/10.1212/01.wnl.0000183055.81056.5c.
44. Comella CL, Jankovic J, Truong DD, et al. Efficacy and safety of incobotulinumtoxinA (NT 201, XEOMIN®, botulinum neurotoxin type A, without accessory proteins) in patients with cervical dystonia. J Neurol Sci. 2011;308:103–9. https://doi.org/10.1016/j.jns.2011.05.041.
45. Conill Tobías N, de Paula Vernetta C, García Callejo FJ, Marco Algarra J. Mioclonía palatal como causa de acúfeno objetivo. Uso de toxina botulínica: a propósito de un caso. Acta Otorrinolaringol Esp. 2012;63:391–2. https://doi.org/10.1016/j.otorri.2011.02.004.
46. Cooper L, Lui M, Nduka C. Botulinum toxin treatment for facial palsy: a systematic review. J Plast Reconstr Aesthet Surg. 2017;70:833–41. https://doi.org/10.1016/j.bjps.2017.01.009.
47. Cousins E, Ward A, Roffe C, et al. Does low-dose botulinum toxin help the recovery of arm function when given early after stroke? A phase II randomized controlled pilot study to estimate effect size. Clin Rehabil. 2010;24:501–13. https://doi.org/10.1177/0269215509358945.
48. Cruz F, Herschorn S, Aliotta P, et al. Efficacy and safety of OnabotulinumtoxinA in patients with urinary incontinence due to neurogenic detrusor overactivity: a randomised, double-blind, placebo-controlled trial. Eur Urol. 2011;60:742–50. https://doi.org/10.1016/j.eururo.2011.07.002.
49. Dang J, Carol Liu Y-C. Treatment of objective tinnitus with transpalatal Botox® injection in a pediatric patient with middle ear myoclonus: a case report. Int J Pediatr Otorhinolaryngol. 2019;116:22–4. https://doi.org/10.1016/j.ijporl.2018.09.024.
50. De Nardi P, Ortolano E, Radaelli G, Staudacher C. Comparison of glycerine trinitrate and botulinum toxin-a for the treatment of chronic anal fissure: long-term results. Dis Colon Rectum. 2006;49:427–32. https://doi.org/10.1007/s10350-005-0287-2.
51. de Sá Dantas Bezerra D, de Toledo LGM, da Silva Carramão S, et al. A prospective randomized clinical trial comparing two doses of AbobotulinumtoxinA for idiopathic overactive bladder. Neurourol Urodyn. 2018;38:nau.23884. https://doi.org/10.1002/nau.23884.
52. de Sèze M, Petit H, Gallien P, et al. Botulinum a toxin and detrusor sphincter dyssynergia: a double-blind lidocaine-controlled study in 13 patients with spinal cord disease. Eur Urol. 2002;42:56–62. https://doi.org/10.1016/S0302-2838(02)00209-9.
53. Defazio G, Livrea P, Lamberti P, et al. Isolated so-called apraxia of eyelid opening: report of 10 cases and a review of the literature. Eur Neurol. 1998;39:204–10. https://doi.org/10.1159/000007935.
54. Denys P, Le Normand L, Ghout I, et al. Efficacy and safety of low doses of onabotulinumtoxinA for the treatment of refractory idiopathic overactive bladder: a multicentre, double-blind, randomised, placebo-controlled dose-ranging study. Eur Urol. 2012;61:520–9. https://doi.org/10.1016/j.eururo.2011.10.028.

55. Ding X, Huang L, Wang Q, et al. Clinical study of botulinum toxin A injection combined with spasmodic muscle therapeutic instrument on lower limb spasticity in patients with stroke. Exp Ther Med. 2017;13:3319–26. https://doi.org/10.3892/etm.2017.4376.
56. Dmochowski R, Chapple C, Nitti VW, et al. Efficacy and safety of onabotulinumtoxinA for idiopathic overactive bladder: a double-blind, placebo controlled, randomized, dose ranging trial. J Urol. 2010;184:2416–22. https://doi.org/10.1016/j.juro.2010.08.021.
57. do Nascimento Remigio AF, Salles AG, de Faria JCM, Ferreira MC. Comparison of the efficacy of OnabotulinumtoxinA and AbobotulinumtoxinA at the 1. Plast Reconstr Surg. 2015;135:239–49. https://doi.org/10.1097/PRS.0000000000000800.
58. Dohar JE. Sialorrhea & aspiration control – a minimally invasive strategy uncomplicated by anticholinergic drug tolerance or tachyphylaxis. Int J Pediatr Otorhinolaryngol. 2019;116:97–101. https://doi.org/10.1016/j.ijporl.2018.10.035.
59. Doherty KM, van de Warrenburg BP, Peralta MC, et al. Postural deformities in Parkinson's disease. Lancet Neurol. 2011;10:538–49. https://doi.org/10.1016/S1474-4422(11)70067-9.
60. Dunne JW, Gracies J-M, Hayes M, et al. A prospective, multicentre, randomized, double-blind, placebo-controlled trial of onabotulinumtoxinA to treat plantarflexor/invertor overactivity after stroke. Clin Rehabil. 2012;26:787–97. https://doi.org/10.1177/0269215511432016.
61. Dutton JJ, Fowler AM. Botulinum toxin in ophthalmology. Surv Ophthalmol. 2007;52:13–31.
62. El-Bahnasy AE, Farahat YA, El-Bendary M, et al. A randomized controlled trail of bacillus Calmette-Guerin and botulinum toxin-A for the treatment of refractory interstitial cystitis. UroToday Int J. 2008;02. https://doi.org/10.3834/uij.1944-5784.2008.12.06.
63. Elble RJ. Tremor: clinical features, pathophysiology, and treatment. Neurol Clin N Am. 2009;27:679–95. https://doi.org/10.1016/j.ncl.2009.04.003.
64. Elovic EP, Munin MC, Kaňovský P, et al. Randomized, placebo-controlled trial of incobotulinumtoxina for upper-limb post-stroke spasticity. Muscle Nerve. 2016;53:415–21. https://doi.org/10.1002/mus.24776.
65. Espay AJ, Vaughan JE, Shukla R, et al. Botulinum toxin type A for Levodopa-induced cervical dyskinesias in Parkinson's disease: unfavorable risk-benefit ratio. Mov Disord. 2011;26:913–4. https://doi.org/10.1002/mds.23522.
66. Evidente VGH, Fernandez HH, LeDoux MS, et al. A randomized, double-blind study of repeated incobotulinumtoxinA (Xeomin®) in cervical dystonia. J Neural Transm. 2013;120:1699–707. https://doi.org/10.1007/s00702-013-1048-3.
67. Ezzeddine D, Jit R, Katz N, et al. Pyloric injection of botulinum toxin for treatment of diabetic gastroparesis. Gastrointest Endosc. 2002;55:920–3. https://doi.org/10.1067/mge.2002.124739.
68. Fernández E, Latasiewicz M, Pelegrin L, et al. Botulinum toxin for treating unilateral apraxia of eyelid opening in a patient with congenital myotonia. Arq Bras Oftalmol. 2017;80:330–1. https://doi.org/10.5935/0004-2749.20170081.
69. Fernandez HH, Lannon MC, Trieschmann ME, Friedman JH. Botulinum toxin type B for gait freezing in Parkinson's disease. Med Sci Monit. 2004;10:CR282–4.
70. Festen S, Gisbertz SS, van Schaagen F, Gerhards MF. Blinded randomized clinical trial of botulinum toxin versus isosorbide dinitrate ointment for treatment of anal fissure. Br J Surg. 2009;96:1393–9. https://doi.org/10.1002/bjs.6747.
71. Fietzek UM, Kossmehl P, Schelosky L, et al. Early botulinum toxin treatment for spastic pes equinovarus--a randomized double-blind placebo-controlled study. Eur J Neurol. 2014;21:1089–95. https://doi.org/10.1111/ene.12381.
72. Fietzek UM, Schroeteler FE, Ceballos-Baumann AO. Goal attainment after treatment of parkinsonian camptocormia with botulinum toxin. Mov Disord. 2009;24:2027–8. https://doi.org/10.1002/mds.22676.
73. Forget R, Tozlovanu V, Iancu A, Boghen D. Botulinum toxin improves lid opening delays in blepharospasm-associated apraxia of lid opening. Neurology. 2002;58:1843–6. https://doi.org/10.1212/wnl.58.12.1843.

74. Friedmacher F, Puri P. Comparison of posterior internal anal sphincter myectomy and intrasphincteric botulinum toxin injection for treatment of internal anal sphincter achalasia: a meta-analysis. Pediatr Surg Int. 2012;28:765–71. https://doi.org/10.1007/s00383-012-3123-5.
75. Furusawa Y, Mukai Y, Kawazoe T, et al. Long-term effect of repeated lidocaine injections into the external oblique for upper camptocormia in Parkinson's disease. Parkinsonism Relat Disord. 2013;19:350–4. https://doi.org/10.1016/j.parkreldis.2012.09.008.
76. Gallien P, Reymann J-M, Amarenco G, et al. Placebo controlled, randomised, double blind study of the effects of botulinum A toxin on detrusor sphincter dyssynergia in multiple sclerosis patients. J Neurol Neurosurg Psychiatry. 2005;76:1670–6. https://doi.org/10.1136/jnnp.2004.045765.
77. George EB, Cotton AC, Shneyder N, Jinnah HA. A strategy for managing flu-like symptoms after botulinum toxin injections. J Neurol. 2018;265:1932–3. https://doi.org/10.1007/s00415-018-8934-4.
78. Ghasemi M, Ansari M, Basiri K, Shaigannejad V. The effects of intradermal botulinum toxin type A injections on pain symptoms of patients with diabetic neuropathy. J Res Med Sci. 2014;19:106–11.
79. Ghei M, Maraj BH, Miller R, et al. Effects of botulinum toxin B on refractory detrusor overactivity: a randomized, double-blind, placebo controlled, crossover trial. J Urol. 2005;174:1873–7; discussion 1877. https://doi.org/10.1097/01.ju.0000177477.83991.88.
80. Giess R, Naumann M, Werner E, et al. Injections of botulinum toxin A into the salivary glands improve sialorrhoea in amyotrophic lateral sclerosis. J Neurol Neurosurg Psychiatry. 2000;69:121–3. https://doi.org/10.1136/jnnp.69.1.121.
81. Gil RA, Hwynn N, Fabian T, et al. Botulinum toxin type A for the treatment of gastroparesis in Parkinson's disease patients. Parkinsonism Relat Disord. 2011;17:285–7. https://doi.org/10.1016/j.parkreldis.2011.01.007.
82. Giladi N. Medical treatment of freezing of gait. Mov Disord. 2008;23:S482–8. https://doi.org/10.1002/mds.21914.
83. Giladi N, Gurevich T, Shabtai H, et al. The effect of botulinum toxin injections to the calf muscles on freezing of gait in parkinsonism: a pilot study. J Neurol. 2001;248:572–6.
84. Giladi N, Honigman S. Botulinum toxin injections to one leg alleviate freezing of gait in a patient with Parkinson's disease. Mov Disord. 1997;12:1085–6. https://doi.org/10.1002/mds.870120641.
85. Girlanda P, Quartarone A, Sinicropi S, et al. Unilateral injection of botulinum toxin in blepharospasm: single fiber electromyography and blink reflex study. Mov Disord. 1996;11:27–31. https://doi.org/10.1002/mds.870110107.
86. Glover PH, Tang S, Whatley JZ, et al. High-dose circumferential chemodenervation of the internal anal sphincter: a new treatment modality for uncomplicated chronic anal fissure: a retrospective cohort study (with video). Int J Surg. 2015;23:1–4. https://doi.org/10.1016/j.ijsu.2015.08.076.
87. Gottsch HP, Miller JL, Yang CC, Berger RE. A pilot study of botulinum toxin for interstitial cystitis/painful bladder syndrome. Neurourol Urodyn. 2011;30:93–6. https://doi.org/10.1002/nau.20946.
88. Gracies J-M, Bayle N, Goldberg S, Simpson DM. Botulinum toxin type B in the spastic arm: a randomized, double-blind, placebo-controlled, preliminary study. Arch Phys Med Rehabil. 2014;95:1303–11. https://doi.org/10.1016/j.apmr.2014.03.016.
89. Gracies J-M, Brashear A, Jech R, et al. Safety and efficacy of abobotulinumtoxinA for hemiparesis in adults with upper limb spasticity after stroke or traumatic brain injury: a double-blind randomised controlled trial. Lancet Neurol. 2015;14:992–1001. https://doi.org/10.1016/S1474-4422(15)00216-1.
90. Gracies J-M, Esquenazi A, Brashear A, et al. Efficacy and safety of abobotulinumtoxinA in spastic lower limb. Neurology. 2017;89:2245–53. https://doi.org/10.1212/WNL.0000000000004687.

91. Greene P, Kang U, Fahn S, et al. Double-blind, placebo-controlled trial of botulinum toxin injections for the treatment of spasmodic torticollis. Neurology. 1990;40:1213. https://doi.org/10.1212/WNL.40.8.1213.

92. Gurevich T, Peretz C, Moore O, et al. The effect of injecting botulinum toxin type A into the calf muscles on freezing of gait in Parkinson's disease: a double blind placebo-controlled pilot study. Mov Disord. 2007;22:880–3. https://doi.org/10.1002/mds.21396.

93. Gurey LE, Sinclair CF, Blitzer A. A new paradigm for the management of essential vocal tremor with botulinum toxin. Laryngoscope. 2013;123:2497–501. https://doi.org/10.1002/lary.24073.

94. Gusev YI, Banach M, Simonow A, et al. Efficacy and safety of botulinum type A toxin in adductor spasticity due to multiple sclerosis. J Musculoskelet Pain. 2008;16:175–88. https://doi.org/10.1080/10582450802161952.

95. Heckmann M, Ceballos-Baumann AO, Plewig G, Hyperhidrosis Study Group. Botulinum toxin A for axillary hyperhidrosis (excessive sweating). N Engl J Med. 2001;344:488–93. https://doi.org/10.1056/NEJM200102153440704.

96. Hernandez NC, Louis ED. Jaw tremor resulting in broken teeth: on the essential tremor spectrum. Tremor Other Hyperkinet Mov (N Y). 2015;5:354. https://doi.org/10.7916/D8T15339.

97. Hertegård S, Granqvist S, Lindestad P-Å. Botulinum toxin injections for essential voice tremor. Ann Otol Rhinol Laryngol. 2000;109:204–9. https://doi.org/10.1177/000348940010900216.

98. Hesse S, Mach H, Fröhlich S, et al. An early botulinum toxin A treatment in subacute stroke patients may prevent a disabling finger flexor stiffness six months later: a randomized controlled trial. Clin Rehabil. 2012;26:237–45. https://doi.org/10.1177/0269215511421355.

99. Hirota N, Hirota M, Mezaki T. Dystonic frowning without blepharospasm. Parkinsonism Relat Disord. 2008;14:579–80. https://doi.org/10.1016/j.parkreldis.2007.12.001.

100. Hosp C, Naumann M, Hamm H. Botulinum toxin treatment of autonomic disorders: focal hyperhidrosis and Sialorrhea. Semin Neurol. 2016;36:020–8. https://doi.org/10.1055/s-0035-1571214.

101. Hyman N, Barnes M, Bhakta B, et al. Botulinum toxin (Dysport(R)) treatment of hip adductor spasticity in multiple sclerosis: a prospective, randomised, double blind, placebo controlled, dose ranging study. J Neurol Neurosurg Psychiatry. 2000;68:707–12. https://doi.org/10.1136/jnnp.68.6.707.

102. Inoue K, Rogers JD. Botulinum toxin injection into Riolan's muscle: somatosensory 'trick'. Eur Neurol. 2007;58:138–41. https://doi.org/10.1159/000104713.

103. Intiso D, Basciani M, Santamato A, et al. Botulinum toxin type A for the treatment of neuropathic pain in neuro-rehabilitation. Toxins (Basel). 2015;7:2454–80. https://doi.org/10.3390/toxins7072454.

104. Jankovic J. Disease-oriented approach to botulinum toxin use. Toxicon. 2009;54:614–23. https://doi.org/10.1016/j.toxicon.2008.11.013.

105. Jankovic J. Botulinum toxin: state of the art. Mov Disord. 2017;32:1131–8. https://doi.org/10.1002/mds.27072.

106. Jankovic J. An update on new and unique uses of botulinum toxin in movement disorders. Toxicon. 2018;147:84–8. https://doi.org/10.1016/j.toxicon.2017.09.003.

107. Jankovic J, Comella C, Hanschmann A, Grafe S. Efficacy and safety of incobotulinumtoxinA (NT 201, Xeomin) in the treatment of blepharospasm-a randomized trial. Mov Disord. 2011;26:1521–8. https://doi.org/10.1002/mds.23658.

108. Jankovic J, Orman J. Botulinum A toxin for cranial-cervical dystonia: a double-blind, placebo-controlled study. Neurology. 1987;37:616–23.

109. Jankovic J, Schwartz K. Botulinum toxin treatment of tremors. Neurology. 1991;41:1185. https://doi.org/10.1212/WNL.41.8.1185.

110. Jankovic J, Schwartz K, Clemence W, et al. A randomized, double-blind, placebo-controlled study to evaluate botulinum toxin type A in essential hand tremor. Mov Disord. 1996;11:250–6. https://doi.org/10.1002/mds.870110306.

111. Jocson A, Lew M. Use of botulinum toxin in Parkinson's disease. 2019. https://doi.org/10.1016/j.parkreldis.2018.12.002.
112. Kaji R, Osako Y, Suyama K, et al. Botulinum toxin type A in post-stroke upper limb spasticity. Curr Med Res Opin. 2010;26:1983–92. https://doi.org/10.1185/03007995.2010.497103.
113. Kaji R, Osako Y, Suyama K, et al. Botulinum toxin type A in post-stroke lower limb spasticity: a multicenter, double-blind, placebo-controlled trial. J Neurol. 2010;257:1330–7. https://doi.org/10.1007/s00415-010-5526-3.
114. Kamel JT, Cordivari C, Catania S. Treatment of upper limb tremor with botulinum toxin: an individualized approach. Mov Disord Clin Pract. 2019;6:652–5. https://doi.org/10.1002/mdc3.12832.
115. Kaňovský P, Slawek J, Denes Z, et al. Efficacy and safety of botulinum neurotoxin NT 201 in poststroke upper limb spasticity. Clin Neuropharmacol. 2009;32:259–65. https://doi.org/10.1097/WNF.0b013e3181b13308.
116. Karp BI, Alter K. Botulinum toxin treatment of blepharospasm, orofacial/oromandibular dystonia, and hemifacial spasm. Semin Neurol. 2016;36:84–91. https://doi.org/10.1055/s-0036-1571952.
117. Kasyan G, Pushkar D. Randomized controlled trial for efficacy of botulinum toxin type A in treatment of patients suffering bladder pain syndrome/interstitial cystitis with hunners' lesions preliminary results. J Urol. 2012;187. https://doi.org/10.1016/j.juro.2012.02.912.
118. Kerzoncuf M, Viton J-M, Pellas F, et al. People post-stroke' postural sway improved by botulinum toxin: a multicenter randomized double-blind controlled trial. Arch Phys Med Rehabil. 2019. https://doi.org/10.1016/j.apmr.2019.04.024.
119. Krack P, Marion MH. "Apraxia of lid opening," a focal eyelid dystonia: clinical study of 32 patients. Mov Disord. 1994;9:610–5. https://doi.org/10.1002/mds.870090605.
120. Kuo H-C, Chancellor MB. Comparison of intravesical botulinum toxin type A injections plus hydrodistention with hydrodistention alone for the treatment of refractory interstitial cystitis/painful bladder syndrome. BJU Int. 2009;104:657–61. https://doi.org/10.1111/j.1464-410X.2009.08495.x.
121. Kuo H-C, Jiang Y-H, Tsai Y-C, Kuo Y-C. Intravesical botulinum toxin-A injections reduce bladder pain of interstitial cystitis/bladder pain syndrome refractory to conventional treatment – a prospective, multicenter, randomized, double-blind, placebo-controlled clinical trial. Neurourol Urodyn. 2016;35:609–14. https://doi.org/10.1002/nau.22760.
122. Kwak CH, Hanna PA, Jankovic J. Botulinum toxin in the treatment of tics. Arch Neurol. 2000;57:1190–3.
123. Lagalla G, Millevolte M, Capecci M, et al. Botulinum toxin type A for drooling in Parkinson's disease: a double-blind, randomized, placebo-controlled study. Mov Disord. 2006;21:704–7. https://doi.org/10.1002/mds.20793.
124. Lagalla G, Millevolte M, Capecci M, et al. Long-lasting benefits of botulinum toxin type B in Parkinson's disease-related drooling. J Neurol. 2009;256:563–7. https://doi.org/10.1007/s00415-009-0085-1.
125. Lam K, Lau KK, So KK, et al. Can botulinum toxin decrease carer burden in long term care residents with upper limb spasticity? A randomized controlled study. J Am Med Dir Assoc. 2012;13:477–84. https://doi.org/10.1016/j.jamda.2012.03.005.
126. Lepore V, Defazio G, Acquistapace D, et al. Botulinum a toxin for the so-called apraxia of lid opening. Mov Disord. 1995;10:525–6. https://doi.org/10.1002/mds.870100425.
127. Lew MF, Adornato BT, Duane DD, et al. Botulinum toxin type B: a double-blind, placebo-controlled, safety and efficacy study in cervical dystonia. Neurology. 1997;49:701–7. https://doi.org/10.1212/WNL.49.3.701.
128. Lew MF, Brashear A, Dashtipour K, et al. A 500 U/2 mL dilution of abobotulinumtoxinA vs. placebo: randomized study in cervical dystonia. Int J Neurosci. 2018;128:619–26. https://doi.org/10.1080/00207454.2017.1406935.
129. Liu H-B, Fan J-P, Lin S-Z, et al. Botox transient treatment of tinnitus due to stapedius myoclonus: case report. Clin Neurol Neurosurg. 2011;113:57–8. https://doi.org/10.1016/j.clineuro.2010.07.022.

130. Lotia M, Jankovic J. New and emerging medical therapies in Parkinson's disease. Expert Opin Pharmacother. 2016;19:1–15.
131. Lotia M, Jankovic J. Botulinum toxin for the treatment of tremor and tics. Semin Neurol. 2016;36:054–63. https://doi.org/10.1055/s-0035-1571217.
132. Louis ED, Rios E, Applegate LM, et al. Jaw tremor: prevalence and clinical correlates in three essential tremor case samples. Mov Disord. 2006;21:1872–8. https://doi.org/10.1002/mds.21069.
133. Lowe NJ, Yamauchi PS, Lask GP, et al. Efficacy and safety of botulinum toxin type A in the treatment of palmar hyperhidrosis: a double-blind, randomized, placebo-controlled study. Dermatol Surg. 2002;28:822–7. https://doi.org/10.1046/j.1524-4725.2002.02039.x.
134. Maanum G, Jahnsen R, Stanghelle JK, et al. Effects of botulinum toxin A in ambulant adults with spastic cerebral palsy: a randomized double-blind placebo controlled-trial. J Rehabil Med. 2011;43:338–47. https://doi.org/10.2340/16501977-0672.
135. Machado D, Martimbianco ALC, Bussadori SK, et al. Botulinum toxin type A for painful temporomandibular disorders: systematic review and meta-analysis. J Pain. 2019. https://doi.org/10.1016/j.jpain.2019.08.011.
136. Mancini F, Zangaglia R, Cristina S, et al. Double-blind, placebo-controlled study to evaluate the efficacy and safety of botulinum toxin type A in the treatment of drooling in parkinsonism. Mov Disord. 2003;18:685–8. https://doi.org/10.1002/mds.10420.
137. Manning J, Dwyer P, Rosamilia A, et al. A multicentre, prospective, randomised, double-blind study to measure the treatment effectiveness of abobotulinum A (AboBTXA) among women with refractory interstitial cystitis/bladder pain syndrome. Int Urogynecol J. 2014;25:593–9. https://doi.org/10.1007/s00192-013-2267-8.
138. Manrique D. Application of botulinum toxin to reduce the saliva in patients with amyotrophic lateral sclerosis. Braz J Otorhinolaryngol. 2005;71:566–9. S0034-72992005000500004.
139. Marchese MR, D'Alatri L, Bentivoglio AR, Paludetti G. OnabotulinumtoxinA for adductor spasmodic dysphonia (ADSD): functional results and the role of dosage. Toxicon. 2018;155:38–42. https://doi.org/10.1016/j.toxicon.2018.10.006.
140. Marciniak CM, Harvey RL, Gagnon CM, et al. Does botulinum toxin type A decrease pain and lessen disability in hemiplegic survivors of stroke with shoulder pain and spasticity?: a randomized, double-blind, placebo-controlled trial. Am J Phys Med Rehabil. 2012;91:1007–19. https://doi.org/10.1097/PHM.0b013e31826ecb02.
141. Marras C, Andrews D, Sime E, Lang AE. Botulinum toxin for simple motor tics: a randomized, double-blind, controlled clinical trial. Neurology. 2001;56:605–10. https://doi.org/10.1212/WNL.56.5.605.
142. Matak I, Bölcskei K, Bach-Rojecky L, Helyes Z. Mechanisms of botulinum toxin type A action on pain. Toxins (Basel). 2019;11:459. https://doi.org/10.3390/toxins11080459.
143. McCrory P, Turner-Stokes L, Baguley IJ, et al. Botulinum toxin A for treatment of upper limb spasticity following stroke: a multi-centre randomized placebo-controlled study of the effects on quality of life and other person-centred outcomes. J Rehabil Med. 2009;41:536–44. https://doi.org/10.2340/16501977-0366.
144. Mendes RA, Upton LG. Management of dystonia of the lateral pterygoid muscle with botulinum toxin A. Br J Oral Maxillofac Surg. 2009;47:481–3. https://doi.org/10.1016/j.bjoms.2008.08.010.
145. Mikaeli J, Bishehsari F, Montazeri G, et al. Injection of botulinum toxin before pneumatic dilatation in achalasia treatment: a randomized-controlled trial. Aliment Pharmacol Ther. 2006;24:983–9. https://doi.org/10.1111/j.1365-2036.2006.03083.x.
146. Mikaeli J, Fazel A, Montazeri G, et al. Randomized controlled trial comparing botulinum toxin injection to pneumatic dilatation for the treatment of achalasia. Aliment Pharmacol Ther. 2001;15:1389–96. https://doi.org/10.1046/j.1365-2036.2001.01065.x.
147. Miller LS, Szych GA, Kantor SB, et al. Treatment of idiopathic gastroparesis with injection of botulinum toxin into the pyloric sphincter muscle. Am J Gastroenterol. 2002;97:1653–60. https://doi.org/10.1111/j.1572-0241.2002.05823.x.

148. Mittal SO, Lenka A, Jankovic J. Botulinum toxin for the treatment of tremor. 2019. https://doi.org/10.1016/j.parkreldis.2019.01.023.
149. Mittal SO, Machado D, Richardson D, et al. Botulinum toxin in Parkinson disease tremor. Mayo Clin Proc. 2017;92:1359–67. https://doi.org/10.1016/j.mayocp.2017.06.010.
150. Mittal SO, Machado D, Richardson D, et al. Botulinum toxin in essential hand tremor – a randomized double-blind placebo-controlled study with customized injection approach. Parkinsonism Relat Disord. 2018;56:65–9. https://doi.org/10.1016/j.parkreldis.2018.06.019.
151. Møller E, Bakke M, Dalager T, Werdelin LM. Oromandibular dystonia involving the lateral pterygoid muscles: four cases with different complexity. Mov Disord. 2007;22:785–90. https://doi.org/10.1002/mds.21304.
152. Monini S, De Carlo A, Biagini M, et al. Combined protocol for treatment of secondary effects from facial nerve palsy. Acta Otolaryngol. 2011;131:882–6. https://doi.org/10.3109/0001648 9.2011.577447.
153. Namin AW, Christopher KM, Eisenbeis JF. Botulinum toxin dosing trends in spasmodic dysphonia over a 20-year period. J Voice. 2017;31:107–10. https://doi.org/10.1016/j.jvoice.2016.01.006.
154. Narayanaswami P, Geisbush T, Tarulli A, et al. Drooling in Parkinson's disease: a randomized controlled trial of incobotulinum toxin A and meta-analysis of botulinum toxins. Parkinsonism Relat Disord. 2016;30:73–7. https://doi.org/10.1016/j.parkreldis.2016.07.001.
155. Nastasi L, Mostile G, Nicoletti A, et al. Effect of botulinum toxin treatment on quality of life in patients with isolated lingual dystonia and oromandibular dystonia affecting the tongue. J Neurol. 2016;263:1702–8. https://doi.org/10.1007/s00415-016-8185-1.
156. Naumann M, Lowe NJ. Botulinum toxin type A in treatment of bilateral primary axillary hyperhidrosis: randomised, parallel group, double blind, placebo controlled trial. BMJ. 2001;323:596–9. https://doi.org/10.1136/bmj.323.7313.596.
157. Naumann M, So Y, Argoff CE, et al. Assessment: botulinum neurotoxin in the treatment of autonomic disorders and pain (an evidence-based review): report of the Therapeutics and Technology Assessment Subcommittee of the American Academy of Neurology. Neurology. 2008;70:1707–14. https://doi.org/10.1212/01.wnl.0000311390.87642.d8.
158. Neville C, Venables V, Aslet M, et al. An objective assessment of botulinum toxin type A injection in the treatment of post-facial palsy synkinesis and hyperkinesis using the synkinesis assessment questionnaire. J Plast Reconstr Aesthet Surg. 2017;70:1624–8. https://doi.org/10.1016/j.bjps.2017.05.048.
159. Niemann N, Jankovic J. Botulinum toxin for the treatment of hand tremor. Toxins (Basel). 2018;10:299. https://doi.org/10.3390/toxins10070299.
160. Niemann N, Jankovic J. Treatment of tardive dyskinesia: a general overview with focus on the vesicular monoamine transporter 2 inhibitors. Drugs. 2018;78:525–41. https://doi.org/10.1007/s40265-018-0874-x.
161. Nitti VW, Dmochowski R, Herschorn S, et al. OnabotulinumtoxinA for the treatment of patients with overactive bladder and urinary incontinence: results of a phase 3, randomized, placebo controlled trial. J Urol. 2017;197:S216–23. https://doi.org/10.1016/j.juro.2016.10.109.
162. Nüssgens Z, Roggenkämper P. Comparison of two botulinum-toxin preparations in the treatment of essential blepharospasm. Graefes Arch Clin Exp Ophthalmol. 1997;235:197–9.
163. Odergren T, Hjaltason H, Kaakkola S, et al. A double blind, randomised, parallel group study to investigate the dose equivalence of Dysport and Botox in the treatment of cervical dystonia. J Neurol Neurosurg Psychiatry. 1998;64:6–12. https://doi.org/10.1136/jnnp.64.1.6.
164. Okuzumi A, Kurosawa M, Hatano T, et al. Rapid dissemination of alpha-synuclein seeds through neural circuits in an in-vivo prion-like seeding experiment. Acta Neuropathol Commun. 2018;6:96. https://doi.org/10.1186/s40478-018-0587-0.
165. Ondo WG, Hunter C, Moore W. A double-blind placebo-controlled trial of botulinum toxin B for sialorrhea in Parkinson's disease. Neurology. 2004;62:37–40. https://doi.org/10.1212/01.wnl.0000101713.81253.4c.

166. Ondo WG, Simmons JH, Shahid MH, et al. Onabotulinum toxin-A injections for sleep bruxism. Neurology. 2018;90:e559–64. https://doi.org/10.1212/WNL.0000000000004951.
167. Pacchetti C, Mancini F, Bulgheroni M, et al. Botulinum toxin treatment for functional disability induced by essential tremor. Neurol Sci. 2000;21:349–53. https://doi.org/10.1007/s100720070049.
168. Pahwa R, Busenbark K, Swanson-Hyland EF, et al. Botulinum toxin treatment of essential head tremor. Neurology. 1995;45:822–4. https://doi.org/10.1212/WNL.45.4.822.
169. Pandey S, Sarma N. Tremor in dystonia. Parkinsonism Relat Disord. 2016;29:3–9. https://doi.org/10.1016/j.parkreldis.2016.03.024.
170. Pandey S, Srivanitchapoom P, Kirubakaran R, Berman BD. Botulinum toxin for motor and phonic tics in Tourette's syndrome. Cochrane Database Syst Rev. 2018;1:CD012285. https://doi.org/10.1002/14651858.CD012285.pub2.
171. Panicker J, DasGupta R, Amit B. Neurourology. In: Bradley's neurology in clinical practice. 7th ed. London: Elsevier; 2016.
172. Papapetropoulos S, Singer C. Treatment of primary writing tremor with botulinum toxin type A injections. Clin Neuropharmacol. 2006;29:364–7. https://doi.org/10.1097/01.WNF.0000236765.00785.9C.
173. Pappert EJ, Germanson T, Myobloc/Neurobloc European Cervical Dystonia Study Group. Botulinum toxin type B vs. type A in toxin-naïve patients with cervical dystonia: randomized, double-blind, noninferiority trial. Mov Disord. 2008;23:510–7. https://doi.org/10.1002/mds.21724.
174. Park J, Park H. Botulinum toxin for the treatment of neuropathic pain. Toxins (Basel). 2017;9:260. https://doi.org/10.3390/toxins9090260.
175. Park YC, Lim JK, Lee DK, Yi SD. Botulinum a toxin treatment of hemifacial spasm and blepharospasm. J Korean Med Sci. 1993;8:334–40. https://doi.org/10.3346/jkms.1993.8.5.334.
176. Patel PN, Owen SR, Norton CP, et al. Outcomes of buccinator treatment with botulinum toxin in facial synkinesis. JAMA Facial Plast Surg. 2018;20:196. https://doi.org/10.1001/jamafacial.2017.1385.
177. Pedrero-Escalas MF, García-López I, Santiago-Pérez S, et al. Experiencia clínica en pacientes con síndrome de Meige primario y disfonía espasmódica. Acta Otorrinolaringol Esp. 2019;70:1–5. https://doi.org/10.1016/j.otorri.2017.11.007.
178. Penney SE, Bruce IA, Saeed SR. Botulinum toxin is effective and safe for palatal tremor: a report of five cases and a review of the literature. J Neurol. 2006;253:857–60. https://doi.org/10.1007/s00415-006-0039-9.
179. Persaud R, Garas G, Silva S, et al. An evidence-based review of botulinum toxin (Botox) applications in non-cosmetic head and neck conditions. JRSM Short Rep. 2013;4:10. https://doi.org/10.1177/2042533312472115.
180. Piccione F, Mancini E, Tonin P, Bizzarini M. Botulinum toxin treatment of apraxia of eyelid opening in progressive supranuclear palsy: report of two cases. Arch Phys Med Rehabil. 1997;78:525–9. https://doi.org/10.1016/s0003-9993(97)90169-6.
181. Pinto RA, Costa D, Morgado A, et al. Intratrigonal OnabotulinumtoxinA improves bladder symptoms and quality of life in patients with bladder pain syndrome/interstitial cystitis: a pilot, single center, randomized, double-blind, placebo controlled trial. J Urol. 2018;199:998–1003. https://doi.org/10.1016/j.juro.2017.10.018.
182. Pittock SJ, Moore AP, Hardiman O, et al. A double-blind randomised placebo-controlled evaluation of three doses of botulinum toxin type A (Dysport) in the treatment of spastic equinovarus deformity after stroke. Cerebrovasc Dis. 2003;15:289–300. https://doi.org/10.1159/000069495.
183. Poewe W, Burbaud P, Castelnovo G, et al. Efficacy and safety of abobotulinumtoxinA liquid formulation in cervical dystonia: a randomized-controlled trial. Mov Disord. 2016;31:1649–57. https://doi.org/10.1002/mds.26760.
184. Poewe W, Deuschl G, Nebe A, et al. What is the optimal dose of botulinum toxin A in the treatment of cervical dystonia? Results of a double blind, placebo controlled, dose ranging

study using Dysport. J Neurol Neurosurg Psychiatry. 1998;64:13–7. https://doi.org/10.1136/jnnp.64.1.13.

185. Pullman SL. Approach to the treatment of limb disorders with botulinum toxin A. Arch Neurol. 1996;53:617. https://doi.org/10.1001/archneur.1996.00550070055012.

186. Rahimi F, Bee C, Debicki D, et al. Effectiveness of BoNT A in Parkinson's disease upper limb tremor management. Can J Neurol Sci/J Can des Sci Neurol. 2013;40:663–9. https://doi.org/10.1017/S031716710001489X.

187. Rahimi F, Samotus O, Lee J, Jog M. Effective management of upper limb Parkinsonian tremor by IncobotulinumtoxinA injections using sensor-based biomechanical patterns. Tremor Other Hyperkinet Mov (N Y). 2015;5:348. https://doi.org/10.7916/D8BP0270.

188. Raina GB, Cersosimo MG, Folgar SS, et al. Holmes tremor: clinical description, lesion localization, and treatment in a series of 29 cases. Neurology. 2016;86:931–8. https://doi.org/10.1212/WNL.0000000000002440.

189. Ramirez-Castaneda J, Jankovic J. Long-term efficacy, safety, and side effect profile of botulinum toxin in dystonia: a 20-year follow-up. Toxicon. 2014;90:344–8. https://doi.org/10.1016/j.toxicon.2014.07.009.

190. Ramzan Z, Nassri AB. The role of botulinum toxin injection in the management of achalasia. Curr Opin Gastroenterol. 2013;29:468–73. https://doi.org/10.1097/MOG.0b013e328362292a.

191. Richardson D, Sheean G, Werring D, et al. Evaluating the role of botulinum toxin in the management of focal hypertonia in adults. J Neurol Neurosurg Psychiatry. 2000;69:499–506. https://doi.org/10.1136/jnnp.69.4.499.

192. Roggenkämper P, Jost WH, Bihari K, et al. Efficacy and safety of a new botulinum toxin type A free of complexing proteins in the treatment of blepharospasm. J Neural Transm. 2006;113:303–12. https://doi.org/10.1007/s00702-005-0323-3.

193. Rogozhin AA, Pang KK, Bukharaeva E, et al. Recovery of mouse neuromuscular junctions from single and repeated injections of botulinum neurotoxin A. J Physiol. 2008;586:3163–82. https://doi.org/10.1113/jphysiol.2008.153569.

194. Rosales RL, Efendy F, Teleg ES, et al. Botulinum toxin as early intervention for spasticity after stroke or non-progressive brain lesion: a meta-analysis. J Neurol Sci. 2016;371:6–14. https://doi.org/10.1016/j.jns.2016.10.005.

195. Rosales RL, Kong KH, Goh KJ, et al. Botulinum toxin injection for hypertonicity of the upper extremity within 12 weeks after stroke: a randomized controlled trial. Neurorehabil Neural Repair. 2012;26:812–21. https://doi.org/10.1177/1545968311430824.

196. Rovner E, Kennelly M, Schulte-Baukloh H, et al. Urodynamic results and clinical outcomes with intradetrusor injections of onabotulinumtoxina in a randomized, placebo-controlled dose-finding study in idiopathic overactive bladder. Neurourol Urodyn. 2011;30:556–62. https://doi.org/10.1002/nau.21021.

197. Ruiz-de-León-Hernández G, Díaz-Sánchez R-M, Torres-Lagares D, et al. Botulinum toxin A for patients with orofacial dystonia: prospective, observational, single-centre study. Int J Oral Maxillofac Surg. 2018;47:386–91. https://doi.org/10.1016/j.ijom.2017.11.006.

198. Rumbach A, Aiken P, Novakovic D. Outcome measurement in the treatment of spasmodic dysphonia: a systematic review of the literature. J Voice. 2018. https://doi.org/10.1016/j.jvoice.2018.03.011.

199. Rystedt A, Zetterberg L, Burman J, et al. A comparison of Botox 100 U/mL and Dysport 100 U/mL using dose conversion ratio 1. Clin Neuropharmacol. 2015;38:170–6. https://doi.org/10.1097/WNF.0000000000000101.

200. Saad J, Gourdeau A. A direct comparison of OnabotulinumtoxinA (Botox) and IncobotulinumtoxinA (Xeomin) in the treatment of benign essential blepharospasm. J Neuro-Ophthalmol. 2014;34:233–6. https://doi.org/10.1097/WNO.0000000000000110.

201. Sahai A, Khan MS, Dasgupta P. Efficacy of botulinum toxin-A for treating idiopathic detrusor overactivity: results from a single center, randomized, double-blind, placebo controlled trial. J Urol. 2007;177:2231–6. https://doi.org/10.1016/j.juro.2007.01.130.

202. Sahebally SM, Meshkat B, Walsh SR, Beddy D. Botulinum toxin injection *vs* topical nitrates for chronic anal fissure: an updated systematic review and meta-analysis of randomized controlled trials. Color Dis. 2018;20:6–15. https://doi.org/10.1111/codi.13969.

203. Samotus O, Lee J, Jog M. Long-term tremor therapy for Parkinson and essential tremor with sensor-guided botulinum toxin type A injections. PLoS One. 2017;12:e0178670. https://doi.org/10.1371/journal.pone.0178670.

204. Samotus O, Rahimi F, Lee J, Jog M. Functional ability improved in essential tremor by IncobotulinumtoxinA injections using kinematically determined biomechanical patterns – a new future. PLoS One. 2016;11:e0153739. https://doi.org/10.1371/journal.pone.0153739.

205. Sampaio C, Ferreira JJ, Simões F, et al. DYSBOT: a single-blind, randomized parallel study to determine whether any differences can be detected in the efficacy and tolerability of two formulations of botulinum toxin type A--Dysport and Botox--assuming a ratio of 4:1. Mov Disord. 1997;12:1013–8. https://doi.org/10.1002/mds.870120627.

206. Schneider SA, Bhatia KP. The entity of jaw tremor and dystonia. Mov Disord. 2007;22:1491–5. https://doi.org/10.1002/mds.21531.

207. Schneider SA, Edwards MJ, Cordivari C, et al. Botulinum toxin A may be efficacious as treatment for jaw tremor in Parkinson's disease. Mov Disord. 2006;21:1722–4. https://doi.org/10.1002/mds.21019.

208. Schnider P, Binder M, Auff E, et al. Double-blind trial of botulinum A toxin for the treatment of focal hyperhidrosis of the palms. Br J Dermatol. 1997;136:548–52.

209. Schurch B, de Sèze M, Denys P, et al. Botulinum toxin type A is a safe and effective treatment for neurogenic urinary incontinence: results of a single treatment, randomized, placebo controlled 6-month study. J Urol. 2005;174:196–200. https://doi.org/10.1097/01.ju.0000162035.73977.1c.

210. Scott K, Shannon R, Roche-Green A. Management of sialorrhea in amyotrophic lateral sclerosis #299. J Palliat Med. 2016;19:110–1. https://doi.org/10.1089/jpm.2015.0360.

211. Shaw LC, Price CIM, van Wijck FMJ, et al. Botulinum toxin for the upper limb after stroke (BoTULS) trial. Stroke. 2011;42:1371–9. https://doi.org/10.1161/STROKEAHA.110.582197.

212. Shinn JR, Nwabueze NN, Du L, et al. Treatment patterns and outcomes in botulinum therapy for patients with facial synkinesis. JAMA Facial Plast Surg. 2019;21:244. https://doi.org/10.1001/jamafacial.2018.1962.

213. Shoffel-Havakuk H, Rosow DE, Lava CX, et al. Common practices in botulinum toxin injection for spasmodic dysphonia treatment: a national survey. Laryngoscope. 2019;129:1650–6. https://doi.org/10.1002/lary.27696.

214. Shogan AN, Rogers DJ, Hartnick CJ, Kerschner JE. Use of botulinum toxin in pediatric otolaryngology and laryngology. 2014. https://doi.org/10.1016/j.ijporl.2014.06.026.

215. Simpson DM, Blitzer A, Brashear A, et al. Assessment: botulinum neurotoxin for the treatment of movement disorders (an evidence-based review): report of the Therapeutics and Technology Assessment Subcommittee of the American Academy of Neurology. Neurology. 2008;70:1699–706. https://doi.org/10.1212/01.wnl.0000311389.26145.95.

216. Simpson DM, Gracies JM, Yablon SA, et al. Botulinum neurotoxin versus tizanidine in upper limb spasticity: a placebo-controlled study. J Neurol Neurosurg Psychiatry. 2008;80:380–5. https://doi.org/10.1136/jnnp.2008.159657.

217. Simpson DM, Hallett M, Ashman EJ, et al. Practice guideline update summary: botulinum neurotoxin for the treatment of blepharospasm, cervical dystonia, adult spasticity, and headache: report of the Guideline Development Subcommittee of the American Academy of Neurology. Neurology. 2016;86:1818–26. https://doi.org/10.1212/WNL.0000000000002560.

218. Singer C, Papapetropoulos S. A comparison of jaw-closing and jaw-opening idiopathic oromandibular dystonia. Parkinsonism Relat Disord. 2006;12:115–8. https://doi.org/10.1016/j.parkreldis.2005.07.007.

219. Singer C, Papapetropoulos S, Spielholz NI. Primary writing tremor: report of a case success-fully treated with botulinum toxin A injections and discussion of underlying mechanism. Mov Disord. 2005;20:1387–8. https://doi.org/10.1002/mds.20590.
220. Sterling JL, Schey R, Malik Z. The role of botulinum toxin injections for esophageal motil-ity disorders. Curr Treat Options Gastroenterol. 2018;16:528–40. https://doi.org/10.1007/s11938-018-0212-0.
221. Stone CA, O'Leary N. Systematic review of the effectiveness of botulinum toxin or radio-therapy for sialorrhea in patients with amyotrophic lateral sclerosis. J Pain Symptom Manag. 2009;37:246–58. https://doi.org/10.1016/j.jpainsymman.2008.02.006.
222. Sulica L, Louis ED. Clinical characteristics of essential voice tremor: a study of 34 cases. Laryngoscope. 2010;120:516–28. https://doi.org/10.1002/lary.20702.
223. Sun L-C, Chen R, Fu C, et al. Efficacy and safety of botulinum toxin type A for limb spasticity after stroke: a meta-analysis of randomized controlled trials. Biomed Res Int. 2019;2019:1–17. https://doi.org/10.1155/2019/8329306.
224. Syan R, Briggs MA, Olivas JC, et al. Transvaginal ultrasound guided trigone and bladder injection: a cadaveric feasibility study for a novel route of intradetrusor chemodenervation. Investig Clin Urol. 2019;60:40. https://doi.org/10.4111/icu.2019.60.1.40.
225. Taha RM, Farahat A, Bahnasy M, et al. A prospective randomized study of intravesical pen-tosan polysulfate and botulinum toxin-A for the treatment of painful bladder syndrome/inter-stitial cystitis. Eur Urol Suppl. 2010;2(9):213.
226. Tan E-K, Jankovic J. Botulinum toxin A in patients with oromandibular dystonia: long-term follow-up. Neurology. 1999;53:2102. https://doi.org/10.1212/WNL.53.9.2102.
227. Tao W, Yan D, Li J-H, Shi Z-H. Gait improvement by low-dose botulinum toxin A injection treatment of the lower limbs in subacute stroke patients. J Phys Ther Sci. 2015;27:759–62. https://doi.org/10.1589/jpts.27.759.
228. Tarsy D, Ro SI. Unusual position-sensitive jaw tremor responsive to botulinum toxin. Mov Disord. 2006;21:277–8. https://doi.org/10.1002/mds.20737.
229. Tassorelli C, De Icco R, Alfonsi E, et al. Botulinum toxin type A potentiates the effect of neuromotor rehabilitation of Pisa syndrome in Parkinson disease: a placebo con-trolled study. Parkinsonism Relat Disord. 2014;20:1140–4. https://doi.org/10.1016/j.parkreldis.2014.07.015.
230. Thenganatt MA, Jankovic J. Recent advances in understanding and managing Tourette syn-drome. F1000Research. 2016;5:152. https://doi.org/10.12688/f1000research.7424.1.
231. Thomas AJ, Larson MO, Braden S, et al. Effect of 3 commercially available botulinum toxin neuromodulators on facial synkinesis. JAMA Facial Plast Surg. 2018;20:141. https://doi.org/10.1001/jamafacial.2017.1393.
232. Tincello DG, Kenyon S, Abrams KR, et al. Botulinum toxin A versus placebo for refrac-tory detrusor overactivity in women: a randomised blinded placebo-controlled trial of 240 women (the RELAX study). Eur Urol. 2012;62:507–14. https://doi.org/10.1016/j.eururo.2011.12.056.
233. Tintner R, Gross R, Winzer UF, et al. Autonomic function after botulinum toxin type A or B: a double-blind, randomized trial. Neurology. 2005;65:765–7. https://doi.org/10.1212/01.wnl.0000174433.76707.8c.
234. Trosch RM, Pullman SL. Botulinum toxin A injections for the treatment of hand tremors. Mov Disord. 1994;9:601–9. https://doi.org/10.1002/mds.870090604.
235. Truong D, Comella C, Fernandez HH, et al. Efficacy and safety of purified botulinum toxin type A (Dysport®) for the treatment of benign essential blepharospasm: a randomized, placebo-controlled, phase II trial. Parkinsonism Relat Disord. 2008;14:407–14. https://doi.org/10.1016/j.parkreldis.2007.11.003.
236. Truong D, Duane DD, Jankovic J, et al. Efficacy and safety of botulinum type A toxin (Dysport) in cervical dystonia: results of the first US randomized, double-blind, placebo-controlled study. Mov Disord. 2005;20:783–91. https://doi.org/10.1002/mds.20403.

237. Truong DD, Gollomp SM, Jankovic J, et al. Sustained efficacy and safety of repeated incobot-ulinumtoxinA (Xeomin(®)) injections in blepharospasm. J Neural Transm. 2013;120:1345–53. https://doi.org/10.1007/s00702-013-0998-9.

238. Turner-Stokes L, Baguley I, De Graaff S, et al. Goal attainment scaling in the evaluation of treatment of upper limb spasticity with botulinum toxin: a secondary analysis from a double-blind placebo-controlled randomized clinical trial. J Rehabil Med. 2010;42:81–9. https://doi.org/10.2340/16501977-0474.

239. van Hoeij FB, Tack JF, Pandolfino JE, et al. Complications of botulinum toxin injections for treatment of esophageal motility disorders†. Dis Esophagus. 2016;30:1–5. https://doi.org/10.1111/dote.12491.

240. Vastik M, Hok P, Hlustik P, et al. Botulinum toxin treatment of freezing of gait in Parkinson's disease patients as reflected in functional magnetic resonance imaging of leg movement. Neuro Endocrinol Lett. 2016;37:147–53.

241. Verma A, Steele J. Botulinum toxin improves sialorrhea and quality of living in bulbar amyotrophic lateral sclerosis. Muscle Nerve. 2006;34:235–7. https://doi.org/10.1002/mus.20545.

242. Verplancke D, Snape S, Salisbury CF, et al. A randomized controlled trial of botulinum toxin on lower limb spasticity following acute acquired severe brain injury. Clin Rehabil. 2005;19:117–25. https://doi.org/10.1191/0269215505cr827oa.

243. Vielotte J. Effectiveness of intramuscular injections of botulinum toxin in the treatment of disabling cerebellar tremor of the hand. Ann Phys Rehabil Med. 2016;59:e142. https://doi.org/10.1016/J.REHAB.2016.07.319.

244. Vijayakumar D, Jankovic J. Drug-induced dyskinesia, part 1: treatment of levodopa-induced dyskinesia. Drugs. 2016;76:759–77. https://doi.org/10.1007/s40265-016-0566-3.

245. Vijayakumar D, Jankovic J. Medical treatment of blepharospasm. Expert Rev Ophthalmol. 2018;13:233–43. https://doi.org/10.1080/17469899.2018.1503535.

246. Vives-Rodriguez A, Kim CY, Louis ED. Primary writing tremor. Tremor Other Hyperkinet Mov (N Y). 2018;8:586. https://doi.org/10.7916/D8T740ZZ.

247. von Coelln R, Raible A, Gasser T, Asmus F. Ultrasound-guided injection of the iliopsoas muscle with botulinum toxin in camptocormia. Mov Disord. 2008;23:889–92. https://doi.org/10.1002/mds.21967.

248. Vurture G, Peyronnet B, Feigin A, et al. Outcomes of intradetrusor onabotulinum toxin A injection in patients with Parkinson's disease. Neurourol Urodyn. 2018;37:2669–77. https://doi.org/10.1002/nau.23717.

249. Wabbels B, Reichel G, Fulford-Smith A, et al. Double-blind, randomised, parallel group pilot study comparing two botulinum toxin type A products for the treatment of blepharospasm. J Neural Transm. 2011;118:233–9. https://doi.org/10.1007/s00702-010-0529-x.

250. Wagle Shukla A, Malaty I. Botulinum toxin therapy for Parkinson's disease. Semin Neurol. 2017;37:193–204. https://doi.org/10.1055/s-0037-1602246.

251. Wald A, Bharucha AE, Cosman BC, Whitehead WE. ACG clinical guideline: management of benign anorectal disorders. Am J Gastroenterol. 2014;109:1141–57; (Quiz) 1058. https://doi.org/10.1038/ajg.2014.190.

252. Wan TK, Chen JT, Wang PC. EMG-guided salpingopharyngeus Botox injection for palatal myoclonus. B-ENT. 2013;9:67–9.

253. Wang L, Li Y-M, Li L. Meta-analysis of randomized and controlled treatment trials for achalasia. Dig Dis Sci. 2009;54:2303–11. https://doi.org/10.1007/s10620-008-0637-8.

254. Ward A, Wissel J, Borg J, et al. Functional goal achievement in post-stroke spasticity patients: the BOTOXÂ® Economic Spasticity Trial (BEST). J Rehabil Med. 2014;46:504–13. https://doi.org/10.2340/16501977-1817.

255. Warrick P, Dromey C, Irish JC, et al. Botulinum toxin for essential tremor of the voice with multiple anatomical sites of tremor: a crossover design study of unilateral versus bilateral injection. Laryngoscope. 2000;110:1366–74. https://doi.org/10.1097/00005537-200008000-00028.

256. Wijemanne S, Jankovic J. Hand, foot, and spine deformities in parkinsonian disorders. J Neural Transm. 2019;126:253–64. https://doi.org/10.1007/s00702-019-01986-1.
257. Wijemanne S, Jimenez-Shahed J. Improvement in dystonic camptocormia following botulinum toxin injection to the external oblique muscle. Parkinsonism Relat Disord. 2014;20:1106–7. https://doi.org/10.1016/j.parkreldis.2014.06.002.
258. Winterholler MG, Erbguth FJ, Wolf S, Kat S. Botulinum toxin for the treatment of sialorrhoea in ALS: serious side effects of a transductal approach. J Neurol Neurosurg Psychiatry. 2001;70:417–8. https://doi.org/10.1136/jnnp.70.3.417.
259. Wissel J, Masuhr F, Schelosky L, et al. Quantitative assessment of botulinum toxin treatment in 43 patients with head tremor. Mov Disord. 1997;12:722–6. https://doi.org/10.1002/mds.870120516.
260. Wu C-J, Lian Y-J, Zheng Y-K, et al. Botulinum toxin type A for the treatment of trigeminal neuralgia: results from a randomized, double-blind, placebo-controlled trial. Cephalalgia. 2012;32:443–50. https://doi.org/10.1177/0333102412441721.
261. Xiao L, Mackey S, Hui H, et al. Subcutaneous injection of botulinum toxin A is beneficial in postherpetic neuralgia. Pain Med. 2010;11:1827–33. https://doi.org/10.1111/j.1526-4637.2010.01003.x.
262. Yaltho TC, Jankovic J. The many faces of hemifacial spasm: differential diagnosis of unilateral facial spasms. Mov Disord. 2011;26:1582–92. https://doi.org/10.1002/mds.23692.
263. Yao G, Lam K, Perry K, et al. Crystal structure of the receptor-binding domain of botulinum neurotoxin type HA, also known as type FA or H. Toxins (Basel). 2017;9:93. https://doi.org/10.3390/toxins9030093.
264. Yi Y, Kim K, Yi Y, et al. Botulinum toxin type A injection for cervical dystonia in adults with dyskinetic cerebral palsy. Toxins (Basel). 2018;10:203. https://doi.org/10.3390/toxins10050203.
265. Yoshimura DM, Aminoff MJ, Tami TA, Scott AB. Treatment of hemifacial spasm with botulinum toxin. Muscle Nerve. 1992;15:1045–9. https://doi.org/10.1002/mus.880150909.
266. Yuan RY, Sheu JJ, Yu JM, et al. Botulinum toxin for diabetic neuropathic pain: a randomized double-blind crossover trial. Neurology. 2009;72:1473–8. https://doi.org/10.1212/01.wnl.0000345968.05959.cf.
267. Yun JY, Kim JW, Kim H-T, et al. Dysport and Botox at a ratio of 2.5:1 units in cervical dystonia: a double-blind, randomized study. Mov Disord. 2015;30:206–13. https://doi.org/10.1002/mds.26085.
268. Zakin E, Simpson D. Botulinum toxin in management of limb tremor. Toxins (Basel). 2017;9:365. https://doi.org/10.3390/toxins9110365.
269. Zaninotto G, Annese V, Costantini M, et al. Randomized controlled trial of botulinum toxin versus laparoscopic heller myotomy for esophageal achalasia. Ann Surg. 2004;239:364–70. https://doi.org/10.1097/01.sla.0000114217.52941.c5.
270. Zhang H, Lian Y, Ma Y, et al. Two doses of botulinum toxin type A for the treatment of trigeminal neuralgia: observation of therapeutic effect from a randomized, double-blind, placebo-controlled trial. J Headache Pain. 2014;15:65. https://doi.org/10.1186/1129-2377-15-65.
271. Zhang L-L, Canning SD, Wang X-P. Freezing of gait in Parkinsonism and its potential drug treatment. Curr Neuropharmacol. 2016;14:302–6.
272. Zúñiga C, Piedimonte F, Díaz S, Micheli F. Acute treatment of trigeminal neuralgia with onabotulinum toxin A. Clin Neuropharmacol. 2013;36:146–50. https://doi.org/10.1097/WNF.0b013e31829cb60e.

Chapter 5
Basic Science of Pain and Botulinum Toxin

Zdravko Lacković, Ivica Matak, and Lidija Bach-Rojecky

Abstract The use of botulinum toxin type A (BoNT-A) in pain conditions is continuously growing largely because of its long-lasting effect after local application and safety profile. These unique features distinguish BoNT-A from other conventional and adjuvant analgesic drugs. Furthermore, BoNT-A diminishes only the pathological pain, without affecting the normal pain threshold. Preclinical data from several complex pain models suggested the central site of its action on pain after retrograde axonal transport from the peripheral site of application. Further investigations of the mechanism of BoNT-A antinociceptive action are ongoing as well as experiments on new recombinant BoNTs with higher selectivity for nociceptive neurons.

Keywords Botulinum toxins · Pain · CNS · Experimental models of pain · Recombinant toxins

> Clinicians… loathe chronic pain, perhaps the symptom that brings more patients into our practices than any other but also the symptom most likely to make us feel helpless as healers.
>   Crofford LJ (2015). Chronic Pain: Where the Body Meets the Brain. Trans Am Clin Climatol Assoc. 126:167–83 [1]

Over the last decades, our understanding of botulinum toxin mechanism of action has changed. Intensive research has shown that peripherally administered botulinum toxin type A (BoNT-A) reaches the central nervous system (CNS) by axonal transport. Major molecular mechanism is prevention of neurotransmitter release: synaptic silencing. Such effect is long-lasting but reversible. This action might

Z. Lacković (✉) · I. Matak
Laboratory of Molecular Neuropharmacology, Department of Pharmacology, University of Zagreb School of Medicine, Zagreb, Croatia
e-mail: zdravko.lackovic@mef.hr

L. Bach-Rojecky
Department of Pharmacology, University of Zagreb Faculty of Pharmacy and Biochemistry, Zagreb, Croatia

© Springer Nature Switzerland AG 2020
B. Jabbari (ed.), *Botulinum Toxin Treatment in Surgery, Dentistry, and Veterinary Medicine*, https://doi.org/10.1007/978-3-030-50691-9_5

occur at central synapse of the first sensory neuron. Whether there is occurrence of transcytosis is not yet known. Events after first sensory neuron are just at the beginning of intensive research. There are influences on other neurons and glial cells in the CNS. Unique characteristic of BoNT-A is lack of analgesic action on acute nociceptive pain that has important warning function; in humans, analgesic activity usually is monthslong. In spite of some still missing pieces of the puzzle, there is increasing evidence that botulinum toxin, especially type A (BoNT-A), is preventing pain in a growing range of disorders. In the absence of unexpected findings, or an increase in the uncontrolled use of illicit preparations by uneducated persons, BoNT-A is emerging as a new long-lasting and relatively safe analgesic. BoNT-A is not devoid of side effect – even fatalities occurred; however, in the usage of registered product by well-trained professionals, side effects are mild and rare.

Basic Science of Pain

Pain is defined by the International Association for the Study of Pain (IASP) as "an unpleasant sensory and emotional experience associated with actual or potential tissue damage, or described in terms of such damage" [2].

Classification of pain is complex and a matter of debate [3, 4]. Classification could be based on localization (somatic or visceral; organ or body part) and cause (nociception, inflammation, tumors, neurogenic, psychogenic). According to mechanism, pain can be divided into nociceptive (peripheral and central), reflexive and nonreflexive, neuropathic (also peripheral and central), and psychogenic; according to duration, pain is commonly divided into acute and chronic. There is no unified definition of chronic pain. Chronicity depends on disease, for example, migraine is considered chronic if there are more than 15 days of attack per month, while in some other disorders chronic pain should last more longer, usually 3 months. Pain that is caused by the presence of a painful stimulus on nociceptors is called nociceptive pain. Nociceptive pain in its acute form usually serves an important biological (or evolutionary) function as it warns the organism of impending danger and informs the organism of tissue damage or injury.

Neuropathic pain as experimental prototype of chronic pain is caused by a primary lesion or dysfunction in the nervous system and could be peripheral or central. However, the pain is projected into the region supplied by the nerve ("projected pain"). Some of the most baffling types of chronic pain, such as diabetic neuropathy, phantom limb pain, and postherpetic neuralgia, are neuropathic in origin. A significant proportion of patients suffering from chronic low back pain or cancer pain have, in addition to a nociceptive part, also a neuropathic component.

Psychogenic pain is caused by the mental processes of the sufferer rather than by immediate physiological causes. Purely psychogenic pain is rare, and its incidence is often overestimated. Nevertheless, chronic pain frequently has a secondary psychological component resulting in a mixed presentation (e.g., psychosomatic pain) (Fig. 5.1).

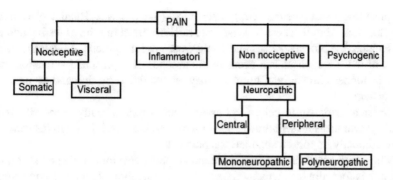

Fig. 5.1 Compilation of attempts to present classification of pain

Anatomy of Pain Classical anatomy of pain is well known: Shortly painful information travels from peripheral pain receptors (nociceptors) to the spinal cord through primary afferent neurons or "first-order" sensory neurons consisting of A-delta and C fibers. Pain transmitted by A-delta fibers is described as sharp and is felt first. This is followed by a duller pain carried by the C fibers. Cell bodies of unipolar neurons in sensory dorsal root ganglia have central projections that reach dorsal column of the spinal cord. Besides different interneurons, A-delta and C fibers innervate "second-order" nerve fibers in laminae II and III of the dorsal horns. They form spinothalamic tract and reach thalamus and finally somatosensory cortex. In cranial nerves (i.e., *n. trigeminus*, n. *facialis*, etc.), first-order neurons innervate second-order neurons in their nuclei in the brainstem.

In addition to the described ascendant system, there is also a complex descending pain modulatory system that influences nociceptive input from the spinal cord or the brainstem sensory nuclei. This descendant system is under influence of cortical, subcortical, and brainstem structures that can modulate perception of pain. Accordingly, perception of pain in humans is influenced by experience, emotions, cultural social factors, etc. Such influence in a more simple way exists in experimental animals as well and can influence results of pharmacological research in rodents [5]. It is a common knowledge that different individuals, humans but some higher animals as well, have very different reactions to pain. Consequently, measurement of pain can be considered as a prototype for the quantitative study of subjective responses [6].

In vitro experiments are basis to elucidate molecular mechanism of physiological functions including sensory system and pain. The hope of in vitro experiments is that they reflect the biology of the intact organism. Investigators doing in vitro work must be careful to avoid overinterpretation of their results, which can lead to erroneous conclusions [7].

Measuring pain and analgesia in experimental animals in vivo is the mainstream of study of pain and analgesic drug assessment and development. There are a number of tests developed to measure reflexive pain and evaluate behavioral, withdrawal responses after the application of painful stimuli like heat (like tail flick or hot plate test), cold (acetone, etc.), mechanical (like pinprick, Randall-Selitto test), and electrical stimuli. These tests activate nociceptors at the site of testing and trigger localized, motor responses and could exist even in animals without the pain as many of these responses can occur in the absence of supraspinal activation; however, in higher animals and humans, they are modified by descending pain control system.

Classical criticism to behavioral assessment of pain, usually in rodents, is that most of them measure withdrawal responses to evoked painful stimuli instead of the more clinically important spontaneous pain [8].

Nonreflexive pain tests record spontaneous pain behavior [9]. The most common example is formalin test, which refers to the quantification of pain behavior, such as time spent licking chemically injured part of the body (usually paw pad or vibrissal pad in the face). Additional pain behavior could include, for example, paw elevation and smoothing. Application of other irritant substances (capsaicin, mustard oil, carrageenan, etc.) can also be used. Similarly, quantification of writhing behaviors after an intraperitoneal injection of acetic acid can be useful to quantify visceral pain.

Ultrasonic vocalization was used to measure pain intensity in chronic cancer pain and neuropathic pain models in mice. Mice and rats communicate by ultrasound; thus, distinguishing pain and normal ultrasound communication might not be easy [10].

Grimace scale is the most recent test that records and measures pain-induced facial expression. It is described both, in mice [11] and rats [10]. Based on orbital tightening, nose bulge, cheek bulge, ear position, and whisker change, a score on a 0–2 scale for their prominence in still photographs allows quantification of spontaneous pain (Fig. 5.2). There are reports that facial grimace scale in rats and mice

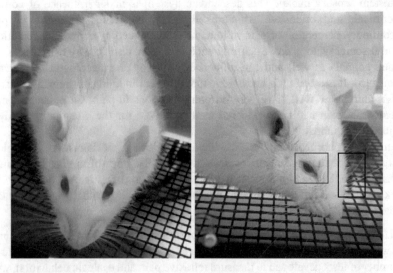

Fig. 5.2 Rat grimace in normal rat (left) and a rat feeling modest pain (right). Nose/cheek flattening and ear changes are not visible

after infraorbital nerve constriction injury remains high for 10 days or more [12]. Fentanyl reversed the changes in rat grimace scale scores, suggesting that these scores reflect pain perception [12].

In animals with chronic pain, usually behavioral responses to additional painful stimuli (mechanical or thermal) reflect hypersensitivity to pain and allodynia using additional pain test, often von Frey filaments. Thus, what is measured is not "basic," "tonic" spontaneous chronic pain but rather a reaction to the additional stimulation. Therefore, instead of spontaneous pain, supersensitivity to pain and allodynia are measured.

A review of tests to measure pain in experimental animals shows that they are all movement-related. They are based on avoidance or the reduction of painful stimuli, that is, the movements of the experimental animals. Because BoNT-A reduces movement due to its effect on muscles, this can significantly affect the results of behavioral experiments. This is probably why in behavioral tests no one has so far shown an acceptable relationship between BoNT-A dose and effect. A detailed analysis shows that such research often yields yes/no results. In conclusion, by investigating the effect of botulinum toxin on pain, we obtain a response that represents a balance between the analgesic and paralytic effects of BoNT-A.

The Studies of Pain in Humans In assessment of pain in patients, some mechanical tests are sometimes applied like pinprick, von Frey filaments, but most common assessments are based on subjective feeling by a particular patient. To standardize patient rating of pain feeling, numerous rating scales have been developed.

Haefeli and Elfering describe and discuss most commonly used pain measurement scales [13]. All of them are subjective and based on patient assessment of intensity of pain, for example, on the scale of 1–10. Best known are the visual analogue scale, numerical rating scale, verbal rating scale, pain drawing, etc.

Besides rating scales, clinical drug testing on a larger group of patients have many methodological requirements to make results more reliable. Those requirements are described in many documents on Good Clinical Practice and are also a part of the American Academy of Neurology (AAN) criteria for evaluation of new drugs.

Structural and functional neuroimaging clearly demonstrated central nervous system contributors to chronic pain in humans. There is a belief that brain imaging could provide objective biomarkers of chronic pain and guide treatment for personalized pain management; however, before that, there is a need for standardization and validation [14].

Synaptic Silencing: The Main Molecular Effect of BoNT-A

As described many times, BoNTs are produced primarily by bacteria of the genus *Clostridium* and have been classified as eight distinct types (A–G and X) [15], while over 40 subtypes are known, five for BoNT-A (BoNT-A1–5). BoNT-A1 is only one commercially available in the USA and Europe (Botox® and Botox Cosmetic® *ona-botulinumtoxinA* by Allergan; Dysport® *abobotulinumtoxinA* by Ipsen; Xeomin® *incobotulinumtoxinA* by Merz; and only one BoNT-B1 preparation Myobloc® *rimabotulinumtoxinB*, by Solstice Neurosciences) [16]. BoNTs contain two core subunits responsible for toxic and therapeutic activity: light chain (50 kDa) and heavy chain (100 kDa), linked by disulfide bond. The light chain is Zn^{2+} metallopro-tease that represents the actual toxic domain of the holoprotein [17]. This enzyme specifically cleaves the particular proteins responsible for the fusion of synaptic vesicles with the plasma membrane: synaptosomal N-ethylmaleimide-sensitive attachment protein receptors (SNAREs) containing several different proteins: syn-taxin, synaptobrevin (VAMP), and synaptosomal-associated protein 25 (SNAP-25). BoNT-A, BoNT-E, and BoNT-C cleave SNAP-25, and BoNT-B, BoNT-D, BoNT-F, and BoNT-G cleave VAMP, while BoNT-C cleaves both SNAP-25 and syntaxin [17, 18]. Consequently, function of synaptic vesicles is prevented, and the result is neu-ronal silencing. Silencing of neuromuscular junction causes flaccid paralysis as a main sign of botulism. As could be expected, heterozygous missense mutation in the SNAP-25 gene causes *congenital myasthenic syndrome-18* with myasthenia, cortical hyperexcitability, ataxia, and intellectual disability [19]. Less predictable is association of SNAP-25 polymorphisms with *attention-deficit disorder* [20].

Molecular action of BoNTs consists of several steps [21–23]:

(a) Binding of BoNTs to the presynaptic membrane, mediated with gangliosides (polysialogangliosides, PSG) and synaptic vesicle protein 2 (SV2)
(b) Internalization of BoNTs, via endocytosis of the BoNTs-acceptor complex (PSG and SV2) inside the neurons
(c) Translocation of BoNTs' light chain from the endocytosed vesicle to the neuro-nal cytosol and release of the light chain in the cytosol by reduction of the interchain disulfide bond.
(d) Cleavage of protein target by Zn^{2+}-endopeptidase blocking the activity of spe-cific SNARE proteins (Fig. 5.3)
(e) Axonal transport (retrograde and anterograde) to the place of enzymatic action [24, 25]
(f) Cell-to-cell, transsynaptic transport to remote place of action [24, 26].

The high potency and neurospecificity of the BoNTs is associated with binding two acceptors ganglioside and SV2 [23]. Dual acceptor binding is probably respon-sible for high neurospecificity of BoNT, including higher affinity to block the release of acetylcholine and then the release of other neurotransmitters. As could be expected, transgenic mice and cell lines devoid of PSG are largely resistant to BoNTs [27]. Interestingly, BoNT-s is not toxic for insects that are devoid of PSG. This makes insects an excellent vector to spread botulism among birds and fishes [28].

Pharmacologically unique characteristic of BoNT-A is long-lasting effect. Following i.m. injection of radioiodinated BoNT-A, the radioactivity returned to control value within 12 h. In vitro in neuronal culture, enzymatic activity of BoNT-A persists for up to 1 year; in humans, the effect can last 3–6 months and in

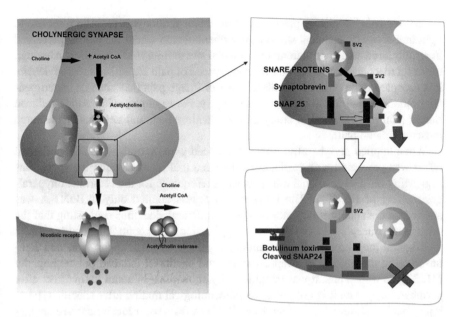

Fig. 5.3 Synapse silencing by BoNT-A

experimental animals usually up to 30 days. Turnover of SNARE proteins is estimated to be 4–5 days. However, BoNT-A duration of action is much longer than
turnover rate of SNARE. There are several theories that attempt to explain the length
of the BoNT-A effect, but a definitive answer is still to be expected.

Fifteen Years' Debate: Controversies About Botulinum Toxin A Site of Analgesic Action

The question whether BoNT-A affects only peripheral nerve endings or is it axonally transported to the CNS was a matter of debate lasting over 15 years. BoNT-A
and even BoNT-B have a remarkable similarity to tetanus toxin (TeNT). Molecular
structure is similar, molecular target in both cases is SNARE protein complex, and
final results of BoNTs and tetanus toxin are neuronal silencing. Difference is in
central target(s) that are known for TeNT. Clinical difference is remarkable as well:
spastic vs. flaccid paralysis occurs. This makes the debate if BoNTs are axonally
transported or not from periphery toward CNS fundamentally important. Most
important arguments demonstrated the existence of axonal transport, and central
effects of peripherally applied BoNT-A are shortly discussed in the following text.

Out of many behavioral experiments (review Matak and Lackovic [29]), most
convincing arguments showing central effects of peripherally applied BoNT-A are
obtained in studies of mirror pain.

"Mirror pain," typically presented as mechanical allodynia (pain in response to light innocuous mechanical stimuli), is a phenomenon where the pain is perceived in an uninjured area contralateral to the actual site of injury/inflammation. Although the exact mechanisms for the contralateral spread of pain are still a matter of debate, it is accepted to be centrally mediated. Mirror image pain (MP) can be experimentally induced by different types of tissue injury. For example, acidic saline-induced mirror pain is developed to study chronic, widespread, and neuronally mediated musculoskeletal pain.

When applied peripherally, BoNT-A reduced pain on both sides. This bilateral effect was prevented with ipsilateral colchicine that blocks axonal transport, thus suggesting retrograde axonal transport as a prerequisite for the central antihyperalgesic effect of BoNT-A. The bilateral effect was elicited only if BoNT-A was applied on the side of injury, not on the contralateral side, thus suggesting that the toxin is not transported from the site of application to the contralateral side [30].

Bilateral long-lasting effect of unilateral peripheral toxin application was demonstrated in the models of streptozotocin- and paclitaxel-induced polyneuropathy [31, 32], as well. Thus, it was unequivocally shown that bilateral toxin effect after peripheral application is not just a phenomenological finding after specific type of injury but is a feature that distinguishes BoNT-A from other locally applied analgesic drugs.

The quantities of BoNT-A that might come into the CNS structure are extremely low, and up to now it was not possible to detect functionally active toxin in the spinal cord or the brain. However, light chain of BoNT-A is a Zn^{2+} endopeptidase cleaving SNAP-25. In series of immunohistochemical experiments using specific antibody against cleaved SNAP-25, Matak et al. were able to identify the presence of cleaved SNAP-25, clear footstep of the enzymatic activity of BoNT-A (Fig. 5.4), in dorsal horn of the spinal cord and trigeminal nuclei in the brainstem [25, 33, 34]. It is important that those immunohistochemical experiments were performed at the end of behavioral experiments showing antinociceptive action of peripherally applied BoNT-A.

All mentioned experiments clearly demonstrate the existence of axonal transport of peripherally applied BoNT-A and enzymatic action within CNS. Some experiments like those on bilateral and mirror pain cannot be explained differently other by central action of BoNT-A. However, this does not exclude the participation of peripheral endings of sensory neurons in some actions of BoNT-A.

Botulinum Toxin Beyond First Sensory Neuron: Mechanism of Analgesic Effect

The exact mechanism of BoNT-A action on pain in the dorsal horn of the spinal cord or brain nuclei is not completely elucidated. There are two general possibilities for the central action of BoNT-A:

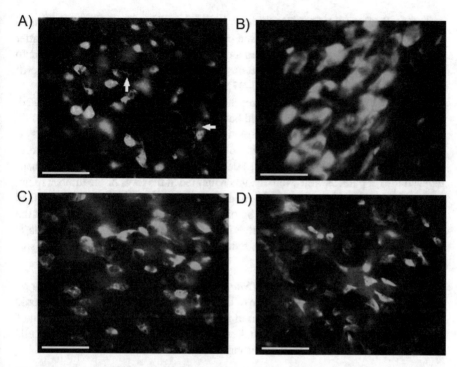

Fig. 5.4 Presence of BoNT-A-cleaved SNAP-25 occurrence in the trigeminal nucleus caudalis (TNC) and the lack of detectable action in sensory regions upstream from TNC. Cleaved SNAP-25 was examined 6 days after peripheral BoNT-A injection into the rat whisker pad (5 U/kg). SNAP-25 immunoreactivity (red) was visible in TNC (**a**). Cleaved SNAP-25 (red) was not visible in ipsilateral locus coeruleus (**b**), periaqueductal gray (**c**), or contralateral ventral posteromedial nucleus of thalamus (**d**). NeuN (green) represents neuronal counterstaining. Scale bar = 100 μm. (From Matak I. PhD thesis)

1. The activity ends by silencing primary sensory neuron, thereby stopping the pain information further in the CNS.
2. Or thereafter, indirectly or transsynaptically, BoNT-A modulates smaller or larger neural loops which participate in the forming of memory of pain in the CNS that could explain bilateral effects after unilateral peripheral administration, similar effect in mirror image allodynia, and the like.

Investigation of pain in the area of trigeminal innervation provided additional important insights into the central mechanisms of BoNT-A action on pain. BoNT-A unilateral peripheral application significantly reduced bilateral mechanical allodynia induced after unilateral infraorbital nerve injury and temporomandibular joint inflammation. After intraganglionic application, colchicine also prevented BoNT-A bilateral effect on pain. Additionally, it was shown that peripherally injected BoNT-A reaches trigeminal nucleus caudalis where it inhibits the expression of TRPA1, TRPV1, and TRPV2 that was induced after infraorbital nerve injury. Furthermore, enzymatic activity of BoNT-A (cl-SNAP-25) in ipsilateral dura mater and colocalization with CGRP in intracranial dural nerve endings was demonstrated after peripheral toxin application. Based on these results, it was suggested that after entering extracranial trigeminal afferents and upon retrograde axonal transport to the trigeminal ganglion, BoNT-A is transcytosed to meningeal afferents and anterogradely transported to dura mater [35–37].

Neuronal events after BoNT-A reaches CNS are only partially investigated. Other neurons and also glial cell could be affected.

Experimental data propose the interaction with opioid and GABA inhibitory systems that have a role in the attenuation of sensory input to the spinal dorsal horn. Involvement of these two systems was demonstrated in the model of carrageenan-induced mirror pain, as well. Namely, when applied at the level of the lumbar spinal cord, opioid antagonist naloxonazine and GABA antagonist bicuculline abolished toxin's bilateral effect on pain. Since opioid and GABA antagonists didn't affect the BoNT-A action on pain if injected either in cisterna magna or cerebral ventricles, it was logical to conclude that BoNT-A reduces pain primarily at the level of the spinal cord [38–40].

Effects on Astroglia and Microglia (Neuroinflammation) While searching for an explanation for the central mechanism of the long-term effect of BoNT-A on chronic pain, investigation of the involvement of glial cells in the antinociceptive action of BoNT-A seemed the logical next step, keeping in mind important role of glial cells in the induction and persistence of chronic pain.

In 2011, Mika et al. showed that a single intraplantar administration of BoNT-A, after chronic constriction nerve injury in rat, diminished the injury-induced ipsilateral spinal and dorsal root ganglia upregulation of microglial C1q mRNA (measured by RT-PCR). These results suggested that reduction in neuroimmune interactions between microglia and neurons is connected and according to authors could be the key to the long-lasting BoNT-A effect on neuropathic pain [41]. Furthermore, in the same model in mice, it was demonstrated that intraplantar BoNT-A (15 pg/paw) injection reduced microglia activation but also astrocyte number and the percentage of activated astrocytes in both the dorsal and ventral horns of the spinal cord [42]. Similarly, Finocchiaro et al. when investigating the analgesic effect of BoNT-B found reduced abundance and activation of astrocytes in the ipsilateral dorsal but not ventral horn of the spinal cord after the constriction injury of the mice sciatic nerve. In contrast to BoNT-A, BoNT-B did not change the expression of activated microglia, thus suggesting different effects of BoNT-A and BoNT-B in neuropathic pain [43].

Using colocalization experiments of cl-SNAP-25 (a marker of enzymatic activity of BoNT-A) with markers of either microglia or astrocyte, it was shown that after peripheral injection of BoNT-A, its enzymatic product cl-SNAP-25 colocalized with glial fibrillary acidic protein (GFAP), a protein marker expressed in non-myelinating Schwann cells, and in spinal cord astrocytes, but not with the marker of microglial activation [44]. This was an indication that BoNT-A may be transcytosed from nociceptive fibers in spinal cord and may enter into glial cells. The absence of cl-SNAP-25 in microglia can be explained with predominant expression of SNAP-23 in these cells, in contrast to astrocyte which expresses both proteins.

Additionally, in satellite glial cells (SGCs) of rat trigeminal ganglion expressing both SNAP-23 and SNAP-25, BoNT-A in a concentration of 100 pM blocked ionomycin-stimulated glutamate release. These findings demonstrate the existence of vesicular glutamate release from SGCs, which could potentially play a role in the trigeminal sensory transmission and additionally suggested interaction of BoNTA with non-neuronal cells at the level of TG [45].

Except in the models of neuropathic pain, mostly induced by nerve injury, glial cell activation was demonstrated in models of chronic inflammation. Specific glial cell populations become activated in both the trigeminal ganglia and the CNS following induction of temporomandibular joint inflammation using complete Freund's adjuvant (CFA) intra-articular injection. Seventy-two hours after CFA injection, activated microglial cells can be observed in the ipsilateral trigeminal subnucleus caudalis and the cervical dorsal horn, with a significant upregulation of ionized calcium binding adaptor molecule (Iba1) immunoreactivity but with no signs of reactive astrogliosis in the same areas [46].

In the CFA-induced monoarthritis model, significant elevation of microglial activation markers Iba-1 and phosphorylation of P38MAPK (P-p38MAPK) was detected in the lumbar spinal cord even 21 days after induction of ankle joint inflammation, thus suggesting the role of microglia not just in induction but in maintenance of chronic hyperalgesia as well, at least in this chronic pain model. The intra-articular administration of a single effective dose of BoNT-A (5 U/ankle) on day 21 after CFA injection significantly decreased protein overexpression and immunoreactivity for Iba-1 and P-p38MAPK in CFA-induced rat. It additionally inhibited the increase in TNF-α mRNA and P2X4R mRNA expression induced by CFA injection. These results suggested that BoNT-A can modulate neuroinflammation in chronic inflammatory pain by reducing the activation of microglial cells and the release of microglia-derived TNF-α, possibly by inhibiting the activation of the P2X4R-P38MAPK signaling pathways in spinal microglial cells [47].

The emerging results provide novel insights into the potential mechanism of BoNT-A action on chronic pain at the level of the spinal cord, with the reduction of neuroinflammation in its center.

Antinociceptive Effects of Other BoNT Serotypes

In humans, naturally occurring botulism is caused by serotypes A, B, E, and F, while intoxication with other serotypes is also possible. Thus, theoretically other BoNT serotypes could be employed for the treatment of neurological disorders, particularly in case of a developed immune resistance to BoNT-A. Apart from BoNT-A, BoNT-B (rimabotulinumtoxinA) is the only clinically used serotype registered for treatment of cervical dystonia. BoNT-B cleaves synaptotagmin part of SNARE proteins and also prevents neurotransmitter release the same as BoNT-A. BoNT-B reduces pain associated with cervical dystonia [48]. Case reports or retrospective studies have reported possible efficacy in the treatment of migraine headache [49, 50], but there are no placebo-controlled clinical studies.

In the formalin test, BoNT-B injected intrathecally (0.5 U) or intraplantarly (1 U) reduced nocifensive behavior, c-Fos activation, and neurokinin-1 (NK1) receptor internalization (indicative of substance P release) in intraplantar formalin-evoked pain. Intrathecally or intraplantarly injected BoNT-B reduces the experimental mononeuropathic pain evoked by spinal nerve ligation or constriction of sciatic nerve and polyneuropathic pain evoked by cisplatin [43, 51–53]. Interestingly, BoNT-B did not induce a regenerative effect upon sciatic nerve injury comparable to BoNT-A [43].

The effect of peripherally injected BoNT-B was associated with lowered VAMP-1 expression in dorsal root or trigeminal ganglia, a possible indication of toxin's retrograde axonal transport and cleavage of the synaptic protein. In addition, unilateral reduction of otherwise bilateral increase of NK1 receptor internalization induced by intrathecal injection of TRPV1 activator capsaicin suggests the BoNT-B action at the level of central afferent terminals. Blockade of c-Fos expression after intrathecal substance P injection was interpreted as a possible transsynaptic cell-to-cell traffic of the toxin within the dorsal horn [52]; however, this has not been definitively confirmed. Antinociceptive effect upon dural stimulation with capsaicin and reduction of VAMP-1 expression in trigeminovascular neurons innervating the dura after facial BoNT-B injection suggest the toxin transcytosis within trigeminal neurons innervating different intracranial and extracranial targets [54].

Up to now, other toxin serotypes have not been investigated for analgesic efficacy in humans or preclinically in pain models; however, some insights into their actions have been obtained by employing cultured sensory neurons. BoNT-E was shown not to affect the evoked CGRP release, due to the possibility that BoNT-E heavy chain lacks acceptor binding activity on rat sensory neurons [55]. BoNT-B, on the other hand, did not prevent the evoked neurotransmitter release most likely due to the mutated VAMP-1 which is resistant to the proteolytic activity of the toxin, which was also reported in vivo [51]. Unlike BoNT-B, BoNT-D was able to cleave VAMP isoforms and prevent the neurotransmitter release [56]. BoNT-C1 prevents the capsaicin-evoked CGRP release most likely due to its effect on both, SNAP-25 and syntaxin1, compared to BoNT-A which cleaves SNAP-25 only and has no effect on CGRP release in vitro [56, 57].

Antinociceptive Effects of Recombinant BoNT-A-Based Molecules

Considerable efforts have been made in designing new recombinant BoNT-A-based toxins with higher selectivity for nociceptive neurons and, supposedly, reduced risk for potential side effects mediated by native holotoxin's nonspecific action in other types of neurons. One of the common strategies has been to develop a chimeric molecule which retains the enzymatic light chain (L) and heavy chain (HC) translocation domains of the native toxin molecule and to exchange the acceptor binding domain of HC for another domain that targets primarily first-order or second-order sensory nociceptive neurons [58].

First of the studies employing these strategies used a plant-derived lectin that recognizes sensory neurons by binding to the glycoproteins residing on their neuronal surface. Duggan et al. reported that such construct reduces the glutamate and substance P release from embryonic dorsal root ganglion neurons [59]. Despite being successfully retargeted to block the neurotransmitter release from sensory neurons and shown to have improved toxicity profiles, lectin containing construct exhibited much lower in vitro potency on substance P release.

A more recent study (Maiarù et al. 2018) reported the use of L-HN construct linked to substance P or endogenous opioid dermorphin, applying the so-called "protein stapling" technique [60]. Stapling technique employed for connection of L-HN to native HC of BoNT-A produces a recombinant toxin termed BiTOX with larger size and lowered paralytic potency, supposedly due to a larger size compared to native toxin. In rats, BiTOX injected intraplantarly reduces CFA, capsaicin, or neuropathic pain-evoked mechanical hyperalgesia [61]. Mentioned results suggest reduced spectrum of antinociceptive effects of BiTOX compared to native holotoxin.

One of the major hurdles in employing such high doses of recombinant retargeted toxins could be the development of immunological resistance upon repeated use, already considered a major problem even at low doses of BoNT-A native toxin-based preparations used. In line with that possibility, it was reported that recombinant BoNT-A with lower potency compared to native toxin, already after second injection (200 ng dose), exhibits lower reduction of toe spreading reflex – indicative of reduced response to BoNT-A suggested to be due to immune response [62].

Dolly and collaborators conducted a series of studies by combining the BoNT-A with light chains of other serotypes into functional chimeras. Based on findings that, unlike BoNT-A itself, BoNT-E light chain coupled with BoNT-A heavy chain prevents capsaicin-evoked CGRP release under certain experimental conditions, it was hypothesized that BoNT-E protease could be more efficacious sensory neurotransmitter release blocker [55, 63]. More recent studies employing a similar chimera demonstrated a prolonged activity in neuropathic pain models [64]. Moreover, repeated injection of the recombinant toxin reproduced the unchanged analgesic efficacy, suggesting the lack of immune response. The overall efficacy of L(E)-BoNT-A against neuropathic pain was higher compared to native BoNT-A, which is, thus, the first observation of a recombinant molecule with improved efficacy compared to BoNT-A holotoxin. This could be of clinical benefit since, due to the lack of dose-response relation within the safe non-paralytic range, employing higher BoNT-A doses does not lead to improved antinociceptive efficacy.

References

1. Crofford LJ (2015). Chronic Pain: Where the Body Meets the Brain. Trans Am Clin Climatol Assoc. 126:167–83.
2. Loeser JD, Treede RD. The Kyoto protocol of IASP basic pain terminology. Pain. 2008;137(3):473–7. https://doi.org/10.1016/j.pain.2008.04.025.
3. Kosek E, Cohen M, Baron R, Gebhart GF, Mico JA, Rice AS, Rief W, Sluka AK. Do we need a third mechanistic descriptor for chronic pain states? Pain. 2016;157(7):1382–6. https://doi.org/10.1097/j.pain.0000000000000507.
4. Granan LP. We do not need a third mechanistic descriptor for chronic pain states! Not yet. Pain. 2017;158(1):179. https://doi.org/10.1097/j.pain.0000000000000735.
5. Heinricher MM, Tavares I, Leith JL, Lumb BM. Descending control of nociception: specificity, recruitment and plasticity. Brain Res Rev. 2008;60(1):214–25. https://doi.org/10.1016/j.brainresrev.2008.12.009.
6. Beecher HK. The measurement of pain: prototype for the quantitative study of subjective responses. Pharmacol Rev. 1957;9(1):59–209.
7. Rothman SS. Lessons from the living cell: the culture of science and the limits of reductionism. New York: McGraw-Hill; 2002. ISBN 0-07-137820-0.
8. Chapman CR, Casey KL, Dubner R, Foley KM, Gracely RH, Reading AE. Pain measurement: an overview. Pain. 1985;22:1–31. https://doi.org/10.1016/0304-3959(85)90145-9.
9. Gregory N, Harris AL, Robinson CR, Dougherty PM, Fuchs PN, Sluka KA. An overview of animal models of pain: disease models and outcome measures. J Pain. 2013;14(11):1255–69. https://doi.org/10.1016/j.jpain.2013.06.008.
10. Kurejova M, Nattenmüller U, Hildebrandt U, Selvaraj D, Stösser S, Kuner R. An improved behavioural assay demonstrates that ultrasound vocalizations constitute a reliable indicator of chronic cancer pain and neuropathic pain. Mol Pain. 2010;6:18. https://doi.org/10.1186/1744-8069-6-18.
11. Langford DJ, Bailey AL, Chanda ML, Clarke SE, Drummond TE, Echols S, Glick S, Ingrao J, Klassen-Ross T, Lacroix-Fralish ML, Matsumiya L, Sorge RE, Sotocinal SG, Tabaka JM, Wong D, van den Maagdenberg AM, Ferrari MD, Craig KD, Mogil JS. Coding of facial expressions of pain in the laboratory mouse. Nat Methods. 2010;7(6):447–9. https://doi.org/10.1038/nmeth.1455.
12. Akintola T, Raver C, Studlack P, Uddin O, Masri R, Keller A. The grimace scale reliably assesses chronic pain in a rodent model of trigeminal neuropathic pain. Neurobiol Pain. 2017;2:13–7. https://doi.org/10.1016/j.ynpai.2017.10.001.
13. Haefeli M, Elfering A. Pain assessment. Eur Spine J. 2006;15(Suppl 1):S17–24. https://doi.org/10.1007/s00586-005-1044-x.
14. Martucci KT, Mackey SC. Neuroimaging of pain: human evidence and clinical relevance of central nervous system processes and modulation. Anesthesiology. 2018;128(6):1241–54. https://doi.org/10.1097/ALN.0000000000002137.
15. Zhang S, Masuyer G, Zhang J, Shen Y, Lundin D, Henriksson L, Miyashita SI, Martínez-Carranza M, Dong M, Stenmark P. Identification and characterization of a novel botulinum neurotoxin. Nat Commun. 2017;8:14130. https://doi.org/10.1038/ncomms14130.
16. Pier CL, Chen C, Tepp WH, Lin G, Janda KD, Barbieri JT, Pellett S, Johnson EA. Botulinum neurotoxin subtype A2 enters neuronal cells faster than subtype A1. FEBS Lett. 2011;585(1):199–206. https://doi.org/10.1016/j.febslet.2010.11.045.
17. Blasi J, Chapman ER, Link E, Binz T, Yamasaki S, De Camilli P, Südhof TC, Niemann H, Jahn R. Botulinum neurotoxin A selectively cleaves the synaptic protein SNAP-25. Nature. 1993;365(6442):160–3. https://doi.org/10.1038/365160a0.
18. Schiavo G, Santuci A, Dasgupta BR, Mehta PP, Jontes J, Benfenati F, Wilson M, Montecucco C. Botulinum neurotoxins serotypes A and E cleave SNAP-25 at distinct COOH-terminal peptide bonds. FEBS Lett. 1993;335(1):99–103a. https://doi.org/10.1016/0014-5793(93)80448-4.

19. Shen XM, Selcen D, Brengman J, Engel AG. Mutant SNAP25B causes myasthenia, cortical hyperexcitability, ataxia, and intellectual disability. Neurology. 2014;83(24):2247–55. https://doi.org/10.1212/WNL.0000000000001079.
20. Feng Y, Crosbie J, Wigg K, Pathare T, Ickowicz A, Schachar R, Tannock R, Roberts W, Malone M, Swanson J, Kennedy JL, Barr C. The SNAP25 gene as a susceptibility gene contributing to attention-deficit hyperactivity disorder. Mol Psychiatry. 2005;10:998–1005. https://doi.org/10.1038/sj.mp.4001722.
21. Dolly JO, Black J, Williams RS, Melling J. Acceptors for botulinum neurotoxin reside on motor nerve terminals and mediate its internalization. Nature. 1984;307(5950):457–60. https://doi.org/10.1038/307457a0.
22. Montecucco C. How do tetanus and botulinum toxins bind to neuronal membranes? Trends Biochem Sci. 1986;11:314–7.
23. Rummel A. Double receptor anchorage of botulinum neurotoxins accounts for their exquisite neurospecificity. Curr Top Microbiol Immunol. 2013;364:61–90. https://doi.org/10.1007/978-3-642-33570-9_4.
24. Antonucci F, Rossi C, Gianfranceschi L, Rossetto O, Caleo M. Long-distance retrograde effects of botulinum neurotoxin A. J Neurosci. 2008;2;28(14):3689–96. https://doi.org/10.1523/JNEUROSCI.0375-08.2008.
25. Matak I, Bach-Rojecky L, Filipović B, Lacković Z. Behavioral and immunohistochemical evidence for central antinociceptive activity of botulinum toxin A. Neuroscience. 2011;186:201–7. https://doi.org/10.1016/j.neuroscience.2011.04.026.
26. Caleo M, Spinelli M, Colosimo F, Matak I, Rossetto O, Lackovic Z, Restani L. Transsynaptic action of botulinum neurotoxin type A at central cholinergic boutons. J Neurosci. 2018;38(48):10329–37. https://doi.org/10.1523/JNEUROSCI.0294-18.2018.
27. Kitamura M, Igimi S, Furukawa K, Furukawa K. Different response of the knockout mice lacking b-series gangliosides against botulinum and tetanus toxins. Biochim Biophys Acta. 2005;1741(1–2):1–3. https://doi.org/10.1016/j.bbadis.2005.04.005.
28. Montecucco C, Rasotto MB. On botulinum neurotoxin variability. mBio. 2015;6(1):e02131–14. https://doi.org/10.1128/mBio.02131-14.
29. Matak I, Lacković Z. Botulinum toxin A, brain and pain. Prog Neurobiol. 2014;119–120:39–59. https://doi.org/10.1016/j.pneurobio.2014.06.001.
30. Bach-Rojecky L, Lacković Z. Central origin of the antinociceptive action of botulinum toxin type A. Pharmacol Biochem Behav. 2009;94(2):234–8. https://doi.org/10.1016/j.pbb.2009.08.012pain.
31. Bach-Rojecky L, Salković-Petrišić M, Lacković Z. Botulinum toxin type A reduces pain supersensitivity in experimental diabetic neuropathy: bilateral effect after unilateral injection. Eur J Pharmacol. 2010;633(1–3):10–4. https://doi.org/10.1016/j.ejphar.2010.01.020.
32. Favre-Guilmard C, Auguet M, Chabrier PE. Different antinociceptive effects of botulinum toxin type A in inflammatory and peripheral polyneuropathic rat models. Eur J Pharmacol. 2009;617(1–3):48–53. https://doi.org/10.1016/j.ejphar.2009.06.047.
33. Matak I, Riederer P, Lacković Z. Botulinum toxin's axonal transport from periphery to the spinal cord. Neurochem Int. 2012;61(2):236–9. https://doi.org/10.1016/j.neuint.2012.05.001.
34. Matak I, Rossetto O, Lacković Z. Botulinum toxin type A selectivity for certain types of pain is associated with capsaicin-sensitive neurons. Pain. 2014;155(8):1516–26. https://doi.org/10.1016/j.pain.2014.04.027.
35. Filipović B, Matak I, Bach-Rojecky L, Lacković Z. Central action of peripherally applied botulinum toxin type A on pain and dural protein extravasation in rat model of trigeminal neuropathy. PLoS One. 2012;7(1):e29803. https://doi.org/10.1371/journal.pone.0029803.
36. Wu C, Xie N, Lian Y, Xu H, Chen C, Zheng Y, Chen Y, Zhang H. Central antinociceptive activity of peripherally applied botulinum toxin type A in lab rat model of trigeminal neuralgia. Springerplus. 2016;5:431. https://doi.org/10.1186/s40064-016-2071-2.
37. Lacković Z, Filipović B, Matak I, Helyes Z. Activity of botulinum toxin type A in cranial dura: implications for treatment of migraine and other headaches. Br J Pharmacol. 2016;173(2):279–91. https://doi.org/10.1111/bph.13366.

38. Drinovac Vlah V, Filipović B, Bach-Rojecky L, Lacković Z. Role of central versus peripheral opioid system in antinociceptive and anti-inflammatory effect of botulinum toxin type A in trigeminal region. Eur J Pain. 2018;22(3):583–91. https://doi.org/10.1002/ejp.1146.

39. Drinovac V, Bach-Rojecky L, Lacković Z. Association of antinociceptive action of botulinum toxin type A with GABA-A receptor. J Neural Transm (Vienna). 2014;121(6):665–9. https://doi.org/10.1007/s00702-013-1150-6.

40. Drinovac V, Bach-Rojecky L, Matak I, Lacković Z. Involvement of µ-opioid receptors in antinociceptive action of botulinum toxin type A. Neuropharmacology. 2013;270:331–7. https://doi.org/10.1016/j.neuropharm.2013.02.011.

41. Mika J, Rojewska E, Makuch W, Korostynski M, Luvisetto S, Marinelli S, Pavone F, Przewlocka B. The effect of botulinum neurotoxin A on sciatic nerve injury-induced neuroimmunological changes in rat dorsal root ganglia and spinal cord. Neuroscience. 2011;175:358–66. https://doi.org/10.1016/j.neuroscience.2010.11.040.

42. Vacca V, Marinelli S, Luvisetto S, Pavone F. Botulinum toxin A increases analgesic effects of morphine, counters development of morphine tolerance and modulates glia activation and µ opioid receptor expression in neuropathic mice. Brain Behav Immun. 2013;32:40–50. https://doi.org/10.1016/j.bbi.2013.01.088.

43. Finocchiaro A, Marinelli S, De Angelis F, Vacca V, Luvisetto S, Pavone F. Botulinum toxin B affects neuropathic pain but not functional recovery after peripheral nerve injury in a mouse model. Toxins. 2018;10(3):128. https://doi.org/10.3390/toxins10030128.

44. Marinelli S, Vacca V, Ricordy R, Uggenti C, Tata AM, Luvisetto S, Pavone F. The analgesic effect on neuropathic pain of retrogradely transported botulinum neurotoxin A involves Schwann cells and astrocytes. PLoS One. 2012;7(10):e47977. https://doi.org/10.1371/journal.pone.0047977.

45. da Silva LB, Poulsen JN, Arendt-Nielsen L, Gazerani P. Botulinum neurotoxin type A modulates vesicular release of glutamate from satellite glial cells. J Cell Mol Med. 2015;19(8):1900–9. https://doi.org/10.1111/jcmm.12562.

46. Villa G, Ceruti S, Zanardelli M, Magni G, Jasmin L, Ohara PT, Abbracchio MP. Temporomandibular joint inflammation activates glial and immune cells in both the trigeminal ganglia and in the spinal trigeminal nucleus. Mol Pain. 2010;6:89. https://doi.org/10.1186/1744-8069-6-89.

47. Shi X, Gao C, Wang L, Chu X, Shi Q, Yang H, Li T. Botulinum toxin type A ameliorates adjuvant-arthritis pain by inhibiting microglial activation-mediated neuroinflammation and intracellular molecular signaling. Toxicon. 2019;178:33–40. https://doi.org/10.1016/j.toxicon.2019.12.153.

48. Lew MF, Chinnapongse R, Zhang Y, Corliss M. RimabotulinumtoxinB effects on pain associated with cervical dystonia: results of placebo and comparator-controlled studies. Int J Neurosci. 2010;120(4):298–300. https://doi.org/10.3109/00207451003668408.

49. Fadeyi MO, Adams QM. Use of botulinum toxin type B for migraine and tension headaches. Am J Health Syst Pharm. 2002;59(19):1860–2. https://doi.org/10.1093/ajhp/59.19.1860.

50. Grogan PM, Alvarez MV, Jones L. Headache direction and aura predict migraine responsiveness to rimabotulinumtoxinB. Headache. 2013;53(1):126–36. https://doi.org/10.1111/j.1526-4610.2012.02288.x.

51. Huang PP, Khan I, Suhail MS, Malkmus S, Yaksh TL. Spinal botulinum neurotoxin B: effects on afferent transmitter release and nociceptive processing. PLoS One. 2011;6(4):e19126. https://doi.org/10.1371/journal.pone.0019126.

52. Marino MJ, Terashima T, Steinauer JJ, Eddinger KA, Yaksh TL, Xu Q. Botulinum toxin B in the sensory afferent: transmitter release, spinal activation, and pain behavior. Pain. 2014;155(4):674–84. https://doi.org/10.1016/j.pain.2013.12.009.

53. Park HJ, Marino MJ, Rondon ES, Xu Q, Yaksh TL. The effects of intraplantar and intrathecal botulinum toxin type B on tactile allodynia in mono and polyneuropathy in the mouse. Anesth Analg. 2015;121(1):229–38. https://doi.org/10.1213/ANE.0000000000000777.

54. Ramachandran R, Lam C, Yaksh TL. Botulinum toxin in migraine: role of transport in trigemino-somatic and trigemino-vascular afferents. Neurobiol Dis. 2015;79:111–22. https://doi.org/10.1016/j.nbd.2015.04.011.
55. Meng J, Ovsepian SV, Wang J, Pickering M, Sasse A, Aoki KR, Lawrence GW, Dolly JO. Activation of TRPV1 mediates calcitonin gene-related peptide release, which excites trigeminal sensory neurons and is attenuated by a retargeted botulinum toxin with anti-nociceptive potential. J Neurosci. 2009;29(15):4981–92. https://doi.org/10.1523/JNEUROSCI.5490-08.2009.
56. Meng J, Wang J, Lawrence G, Dolly JO. Synaptobrevin I mediates exocytosis of CGRP from sensory neurons and inhibition by botulinum toxins reflects their anti-nociceptive potential. J Cell Sci. 2007;120(Pt 16):2864–74. https://doi.org/10.1242/jcs.012211.
57. Meng J, Dolly JO, Wang J. Selective cleavage of SNAREs in sensory neurons unveils protein complexes mediating peptide exocytosis triggered by different stimuli. Mol Neurobiol. 2014;50(2):574–88. https://doi.org/10.1007/s12035-014-8665-1.
58. Foster KA. A new wrinkle on pain relief: re-engineering clostridial neurotoxins for analgesics. Drug Discov Today. 2005;10(8):563–9. https://doi.org/10.1016/S1359-6446(05)03389-1.
59. Duggan MJ, Quinn CP, Chaddock JA, Purkiss JR, Alexander FC, Doward S, Fooks SJ, Friis LM, Hall YH, Kirby ER, Leeds N, Moulsdale HJ, Dickenson A, Green GM, Rahman W, Suzuki R, Shone CC, Foster K. Inhibition of release of neurotransmitters from rat dorsal root ganglia by a novel conjugate of a Clostridium botulinum toxin A endopeptidase fragment and Erythrina cristagalli lectin. J Biol Chem. 2002;277(38):34846–52. https://doi.org/10.1074/jbc.M202902200.
60. Maiarù M, Leese C, Certo M, Echeverria-Altuna I, Mangione AS, Arsenault J, Davletov B, Hunt SP. Selective neuronal silencing using synthetic botulinum molecules alleviates chronic pain in mice. Sci Transl Med. 2018;10(450):eaar7384. https://doi.org/10.1126/scitranslmed.aar7384.
61. Mangione AS, Obara I, Maiarú M, Geranton SM, Tassorelli C, Ferrari E, Leese C, Davletov B, Hunt SP. Nonparalytic botulinum molecules for the control of pain. Pain. 2016;157(5):1045–55. https://doi.org/10.1097/j.pain.0000000000000478.
62. Vazquez-Cintron E, Tenezaca L, Angeles C, Syngkon A, Liublinska V, Ichtchenko K, Band P. Pre-clinical study of a novel recombinant botulinum neurotoxin derivative engineered for improved safety. Sci Rep. 2016;6:30429. https://doi.org/10.1038/srep30429.
63. Wang J, Zurawski TH, Meng J, Lawrence G, Olango WM, Finn DP, Wheeler L, Dolly JO. A dileucine in the protease of botulinum toxin A underlies its long-lived neuroparalysis: transfer of longevity to a novel potential therapeutic. J Biol Chem. 2011;286(8):6375–85. https://doi.org/10.1074/jbc.M110.181784.
64. Wang J, Casals-Diaz L, Zurawski T, Meng J, Moriarty O, Nealon J, Edupuganti OP, Dolly O. A novel therapeutic with two SNAP-25 inactivating proteases shows long-lasting anti-hyperalgesic activity in a rat model of neuropathic pain. Neuropharmacology. 2017;118:223–32. https://doi.org/10.1016/j.neuropharm.2017.03.026.

Chapter 6
Botulinum Toxin Therapy in Medical Pain Disorders

Delaram Safarpour and Bahman Jabbari

Abstract Animal studies have shown that local injection of botulinum neurotoxins (BoNTs) reduces neuropathic pain. This effect is exerted via interfering with the function of pain transmitters and modulators at peripheral and central levels. Recent studies in humans have demonstrated an analgesic effect in several pain disorders. In this chapter, the effect of BoNT therapy in different medical, human pain syndromes is reviewed. The level of efficacy in each pain syndrome is determined according to the guidelines of the Assessment Subcommittee of the American Academy of Neurology.

Keywords Botulinum toxin · Botulinum neurotoxin · Pain · Neuropathic pain · Pain disorder

Introduction

Over the past 30 years, treatment with botulinum neurotoxins (BoNTs) has established a firm role in many fields of medicine and, most notably, in the treatment of hyperkinetic movement disorders (mainly dystonias), focal spasms, spasticity, autonomic dysfunctions (sialorrhea; hyperhidrosis), and migraine [1]. During the past 15 years, with emergence of data from animal studies, clinical researchers expressed interest in investigating the role of BoNT therapy in human pain disorders. Recent publication of high-quality studies in this field indicates that, in addition to migraine, many pain syndromes are amenable to BoNT therapy.

In this chapter, we describe the current status of BoNT therapy in different human medical pain disorders. In each category, the efficacy of BoNT therapy is defined according to the criteria set forward by the Guideline and Assessment

D. Safarpour
Department of Neurology, Oregon Health &Science University, Portland, OR, USA

B. Jabbari (✉)
Department of Neurology, Yale University School of Medicine, New Haven, CT, USA
e-mail: bahman.jabbari@yale.edu

© Springer Nature Switzerland AG 2020   131
B. Jabbari (ed.), *Botulinum Toxin Treatment in Surgery, Dentistry,
and Veterinary Medicine*, https://doi.org/10.1007/978-3-030-50691-9_6

Table 6.1 Injection paradigm recommended by the PREEMPT study: injected muscles, muscle location, muscle function, and the dose of onaA (Botox) administered per site(s)

Muscle	Location	Function of muscle	Number of injection sites per muscle	Dose per site
Corrugator	Above the medial edge of eyebrow	Draws the eye brows together and downward	One on each side	5 units
Procerus	Helps to pull the skin between eyebrows downward	Pulling eyebrows together	Single muscle One injection at midline	5 units
Frontalis	Whole forehead	Pulling eyebrows up	Two on each side, total 4	5 units
Temporal	Temple	Closes the mouth	Four on each side, total 8	5 units
Occipitalis	Back of the head	Moves the scalp back	Three on each side, total 6	5 units
Splenius	Upper neck	Turns and tilts the head to the same side	Two on each side, total 4	5 units
Trapezius	Shoulder	Moves the shoulders up and head back	Three on each site, total 6	5 units

From Jabbari [70]

Subcommittee of the American Academy of Neurology [2, 3]. The efficacy levels A, B, C, and U reflect established, probable, possible, and undetermined efficacy, respectively. The level of efficacy depends on the number of certain class of studies available, designated as A, B, C, and D (see Table 6.1 for definition). These levels reflect the strength of available studies. For instance, a level A efficacy requires at least two published class A studies. A level A study is a well-designed, double-blind, placebo-controlled clinical trial that meets all five criteria [2, 3]. This information may be considered complementary to the data that will be presented in the succeeding chapters of this book on the effect of BoNTs on surgical and dental pain as well as pain disorders encountered in veterinary medicine. Detailed information regarding our current knowledge of mechanisms through which BoNTs alleviate pain is described by Lacovik and colleagues in Chap. 4 of this book.

Pain Disorders with Level A efficacy

This category includes five pain disorders in which the efficacy of BoNT injections is considered established (level A) based on two or more class I studies (see Table 6.1 for definition). These disorders are chronic migraine, postherpetic neuralgia, post-traumatic neuralgia, trigeminal neuralgia, and diabetic neuropathy. Among these, only chronic migraine is currently approved by FDA for BoNT therapy.

Level A, FDA-Approved Pain Disorder: Chronic Migraine

Migraine affects over a billion people per year worldwide and is the second cause of workday loss due to disability [4]. It affects 17% of women and 6% of men [5]. Migraine headaches are usually moderate to severe in intensity and last 4–72 hours. The term episodic migraine applies to migraine with headache days of less than 15/month. The term chronic migraine indicates that headache frequency equals or exceeds 15 days per month with at least in 8 of those headache days; headache has characteristics of migraine [6]. High-quality (blinded and placebo-controlled) studies of botulinum toxin therapy in episodic migraine have failed to show positive results. With chronic migraine however, the efficacy has been established via two large-scale, well-designed, high-quality clinical trials (PREEMPT studies) [7, 8]. Each study includes close to 700 patients (total 1384). Each study had a blind arm (24 weeks) followed by an open label arm of 32 weeks. During the blind period, patients were injected either with onabotulinumtoxinA (onaA) or placebo every 3 months. The pooled data of the two PREEEMPT studies showed significant reduction of pain days in the onaA group (8.4 days) compared to the placebo group ($P < 0.001$) [9]. Migraine severity, frequency of migraine days, and migraine duration were also significantly reduced in the onaA injected group ($P < 0.001$). Subsequent studies of PREEMPT patients have shown onaA efficacy in subgroup of patients with medication overuse, improvement of quality of life with onaA therapy, and sustained improvement after five cycles (every three to 4 months) of onaA therapy in migraine [10–12].

Technique and Dosage

A total dose of 165 units is recommended in PREEMPT studies which is distributed over several muscles, each receiving injections at multiple sites (Table 6.1, Fig. 6.1) [13]. The total dose may be increased to 195 units at the discretion of the treating physician. The total number of injections is 31.

Since the publication of PREEMPT studies in 2010, several investigators have attempted to find a technique that provides similar results with fewer sites of injections. Jabbari and his colleagues at Yale University provided evidence that a technique with 21 injection sites can produce comparable results to PREEMPT studies of onaA therapy in chronic migraine. The logic for the Yale technique is based on the following four principles:

1. In the PREEMPT injection scheme, the lower site of injection into temporalis muscle is probably into the tendon and not into the muscle itself. The tendon of temporalis muscle can be quite large and can extend a considerable distance upward [14]. The Yale protocol recommends injections into two sites with 15 units per site (30 units per site) eliminating inferior and superior temporal injections. Such a dose does not cause appreciable weakness of the powerful temporalis muscle.

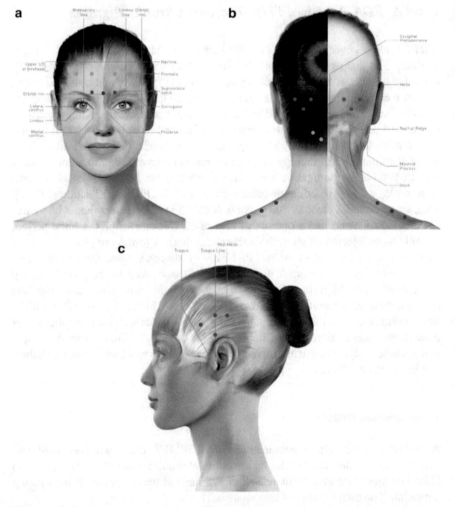

Fig. 6.1 (a) Corrugator, as depicted by purple dots; procerus, as depicted by the red dot; frontalis, as depicted by orange dots. (b) Occipitalis area, as depicted by purple dots; cervical paraspinal area, as depicted by orange dots; trapezius, as depicted by red dots. (c) Temporalis, as depicted by purple dots. Sites of injections in PREEMPT technique. (From Blumenfeld et al. [13]. Printed with permission from Wiley and Sons)

2. The six injections (three on each side) into trapezius muscles are eliminated in the Yale technique as it is unlikely that trapezius muscles contribute significantly to migraine headaches.
3. Occipital injection is reduced from three injections at each side to one injection per site using a larger dose of 10 units. Occipitalis muscle is a small muscle, and a larger dose delivered in one injection is likely to cover the muscle.

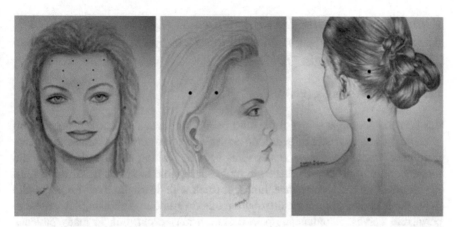

Fig. 6.2 The sites of injection in the Yale technique. (From Jabbari [71]. Drawing courtesy of Drs. Tahere Mousavi and Damoun Safarpour)

4. Injection sites into the cervical region are increased from two to three sites (Fig. 6.2) with a larger dose of 15 units per site (10 units/site for small necks). Splenius capitis is also a powerful muscle, and the vast experience of past 30 years with injection into this muscle has shown no appreciable weakness with such doses. In the PREEMPT technique, the medial high cervical site of injection is most likely into semispinalis cervicis. In Yale protocol, the three cervical injections into splenius capitis are not too close to midline.

In an open label study of 50 patients with chronic migraine when using the Yale technique, 72% of the patients after first injection and 85% after third injection reported their experience after onaA injection as "very satisfactory" using Patient Global Impression of Change (PGIC) [15]. No serious side effects were reported over 2–8 years of observation. After the first year of treatment, 73% of the patients reported no more emergency department visit for additional therapy. By 12 months of treatment, 50% of the patients discontinued their daily preventive medications, and 61% had no longer any need for abortive medicine. In a subsequent double-blind, placebo-controlled study of 25 patients [16], injections of onaA, using the Yale technique, reduced the headache days significantly compared to the placebo at 4 and 8 weeks ($P = 0.0031$). Using PGIC, 9 of 11 patients in the onaA group and 3 of 10 patients in the placebo group described their experience very satisfactory ($P = 0.030$). In the open arm of the study, 58.8% of the patients reported 50% or more reduction of pain days at 4 weeks postinjection, and 88.2% demonstrated reduction of HIT scores compared to baseline. Larger blinded and placebo-controlled studies are necessary to establish the Yale technique as an alternative to the technique of PREEMPT.

Pain Disorders with Level A Efficacy (Effective), Not FDA Approved: Postherpetic Neuralgia, Post-traumatic Neuralgia, Trigeminal Neuralgia (Table 6.2)

Postherpetic Neuralgia (PN)

Postherpetic neuralgia is one of the most painful human pain disorders. It is a complication of herpes zoster infection. In adults, herpes zoster infection is due to reactivation of inactive varicella zoster virus acquired during childhood. Elderly and immunocompromised individuals are more susceptible to zoster reactivation [23]. Zoster infection can involve face, limbs, or trunk with distribution of vesicles, while in the latter regions follow the distribution of skin eruptions following the course of peripheral nerves. Spontaneous pain cessation may occur, but, in many patients, continued pain (for months even years) despite antiviral and analgesic therapy handicaps the patient. Two double-blind and placebo-controlled class I studies [17, 18] have reported significant improvement of pain in PN after administration of local botulinum toxin injections (Table 6.2). In one study [17], pain improvement was associated with significant reduction of opioid use when BoNT treatment was compared to lidocaine and placebo groups (toxin, 78%; lidocaine, 48%; placebo, 34%).

Post-traumatic Neuralgia

Ranoux et al. [19] studied the effect effects of onabotulinumtoxinA on post-traumatic neuralgia. Twenty patients were investigated via a double-blind, placebo-controlled clinical trial. Injections were given into the areas of skin affected by pain and allodynia. The injections were administered intradermally, 1.5 centimeters apart. The dose varied from 20 to 190 units based on the area involvement. The magnitude of pain was measured by VAS using a 0 to10 scale. The authors found significant reduction of pain intensity during the second week following injection ($P = 0.02$), and this positive effect lasted 14 weeks ($P = 0.03$). In the area of involvement, allodynia to brush was also improved significantly. Authors reported no side effects.

More recently, Attal et al. [20] described similar responses to BoNT therapy in a double-blind, placebo-controlled clinical trial conducted on 46 patients with post-traumatic neuralgia. The percentage of pain relief, their primary outcome, was significantly higher in the toxin group (26.4 versus 10.6 for the placebo) ($P = 0.008$). The two secondary outcome measures, reduction of pain frequency and improvement of sleep, also significantly improved in the toxin-treated group ($P = 0.001$ and $P = 0.02$).

Trigeminal Neuralgia

Trigeminal neuralgia (TN) has an estimated lifetime prevalence of 0.3% and usually affects individuals over age 50 years of age [24]. Secondary TN can be seen in patients with multiple sclerosis and has an earlier age of onset. TN is characterized by severe, brief bouts of pain, usually lasting a few seconds. Patient may experience

Table 6.2 Pain syndromes with level A efficacy (effective) based on two or more class I randomized double-blind, placebo-controlled clinical trials

Authors	Pain syndrome	AAN class	Number of Patients in Study	Type of toxin	Total dose units	Injection site	Primary outcome (PO)	Secondary outcome (SO)	Results
Xiao et al. (2010) [17]	Postherpetic neuralgia	I	60	Prosigne	100 U	Subcutaneous Multiple sites Grid-like	Pain intensity (VAS), days 7 and 90	Sleep hours	Both PO and SO were met (P < 0.01)
Apalla et al. (2013) [18]	Postherpetic neuralgia	I	30	onaA	100 U	Subcutaneous Administered in five sites	50% reduction in pain intensity (VAS)	Quality of sleep on 5-point scale	Pain intensity and quality of sleep improved (P < 0.0001)
Ranoux et al. (2008) [19]	Post-traumatic neuralgia	I	24	onaA	20 to 190 U	Intradermal 1.5 cm apart Number based on extent of skin involvement	Pain intensity (VAS)	Allodynia to brush	Significant improvement of VAS – week 2 (P = 0.02), week 14 (P = 0.03)
Attal et al. (2016) [20]	Post-traumatic neuralgia	I	46	onaA	20–190 U	Intradermal 1.5 cm apart Number based on extent of skin involvement	Percentage of pain intensity relief	Pain frequency and sleep	Pain intensity improved (P = 0.008). SOs (P = 0.001) and (P = 0.01), respectively
Wu et al. (2012) [21]	Trigeminal neuralgia	I	40	Prosigne	75 U	Subcutaneous/ epidermal 16 sites on the face	50% reduction in pain intensity (VAS)	Patient Global Impression of Change (PGIC)	Both PO and SO improved (P < 000.1)
Zhang et al. (2014) [22]	Trigeminal neuralgia	I	84	Prosigne	25 versus 75 U group	Subcutaneous/ epidermal 16 sites on the face	50% reduction in pain intensity (VAS)	Patient Global Impression of Change (PGIC)	Both PO and SO improved (P < 0.05) No difference between two dose groups

onabA onabotulinumtoxinA(Botox), *Prosigne* Chinese type A toxin from Lanzhou Institute, *PO* primary outcome, *SO* secondary outcome, *PGIC* Patient Global Impression of Change, *VAS* Visual Analogue Scale many (tens to hundreds) of pain bouts per day. Medical treatment consisting of treatment with anticonvulsants (carbamazepine, phenytoin, and valproic acid) provides limited relief. Patients with advanced age often poorly tolerate high doses of such medications which may be required for satisfactory pain relief. Microvascular surgery and the Gamma Knife procedure offer relief in some patients, but recurrence of pain is not uncommon after these interventions.

Two class I, randomized, double-blind, placebo-controlled clinical trials evaluated the efficacy of BoNT therapy in trigeminal neuralgia [21, 22] (the last two studies listed in Table 6.2). Both studies reported that intradermal and subcutaneous injections of BoNT-A into the area of the face affected by pain improves pain of TN significantly. Injections were carried out using a grid-like pattern (8–16 sites) (Fig. 6.3). The toxin used in these studies was Prosigne. Prosigne is a Chinese type A toxin with suggested unit comparability to onabotulinumtoxinA (Botox). One of the two abovementioned studies compared 25 and 75 units of Prosigne in TN and found the low dose of the toxin to be equally effective as the high dose [22]. In this study, seven patients developed mild facial asymmetry, and three developed mild facial swelling after injections; all side effects disappeared within a week.

A prospective study on 88 patients with TN demonstrated that repeated injections of onabotulinumA over 14 months sustained pain relief efficacy and continued to reduce anxiety and depression along with improving the patients' sleep and the quality of life [25].

In our experience, more than 50% of the patients with refractory TN respond to BoNT injections. Injections are done subcutaneously in a grid-like pattern covering the region(s) of pain. With onabotulinumtoxinA (Botox), we use 2.5 units/site (Fig. 6.3).

Fig. 6.3 Subcutaneous grid-like BoNT injections in trigeminal neuralgia covering the distribution of pain. (Drawing courtesy of Tahere Mousavi M.D.)

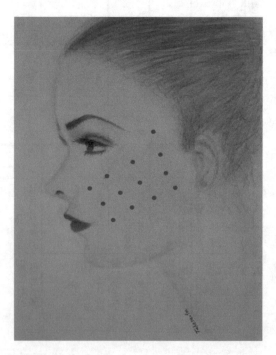

Level B Efficacy (Probably Effective) Based on Availability of Class I and II Studies: Diabetic Neuropathy, Chronic Low Back Pain, Plantar Fasciitis, Piriformis Syndrome, Lateral Epicondylitis, Neuropathic Pain After Spinal Cord Injury, and Male Pelvic Pain (Table 6.3)

Diabetic Neuropathy

Peripheral neuropathy is a common finding in diabetic patients. Painful diabetic neuropathy is more common in type 2 diabetes and often seen in older individuals (25–26% in type 2 versus 16% in type 1) [50, 51]. The type of pain is usually neuropathic, characterized by burning, tingling, pricking, and sometimes electric-shock sensation. Affected regions of skin (usually feet) demonstrate allodynia (touch perceived as pain). The second type of pain is muscle cramps which are often associated with the neuropathic pain. There is now strong evidence from randomized clinical trials that local injection of botulinum toxins can alleviate both neuropathic pain and muscle cramps in diabetic neuropathy.

Yuan et al. [26], in a double-blind, placebo-controlled study, investigated the effect of onabotulinumtoxinA (Botox) in 20 patients with painful diabetic neuropathy. The study had a crossover design. A total dose of 50 units was used. Injections were administered on the dorsum of the foot at 12 sites. Outcomes were measures by Visual Analogue Scale (VAS), depicting pain intensity at a 0–10 scale and by CPSQI, a Chinese version of the Pittsburgh Sleep Quality Index. There was significant improvement of VAS in the toxin group compared to the placebo group at weeks 1, 4, 8, and 12 ($P < 0.05$). CPSQI, measured at week 4, also demonstrated significant improvement compared to the placebo ($P < 0.05$). One patient in the toxin group developed mild local skin infection at the site of injection that cleared up within days.

Ghasemi et al. [27] studied 40 patients with painful diabetic neuropathy. Twenty patients were assigned to aboA toxin group (100 units) and 20 to saline (placebo) group. The study was blinded and had a parallel design. The outcomes were evaluated 3 weeks after injections. In the toxin group, 30% experienced no pain after treatment, while 0% reported no pain in the placebo group ($P = 0.01$). After treatment, diabetic neuropathy scores (DPN4) in the toxin group were significantly reduced for electric shocks, burning, pins and needles, and brushing ($P < 0.005$). In neuropathic pain scale (NPS), all items, except cold sensation, improved ($P = 0.05$). No side effects were reported.

Salehi et al. [29] also studied the effect of aboA toxin injections (100 units) on pain relief in diabetic painful neuropathy. The protocol studied 32 patients and had a parallel, placebo-controlled, double-blind design. The injection pattern was similar to the two abovementioned studies. Outcome measures included VAS for pain, PSQI for sleep, and SF-36 for quality of life. At 12 weeks, all measures improved for the toxin group: VAS and PSQI, $P < 0.001$, and SF-32, $P = 0.050$. The duration of study was 3 months. No side effects were reported.

Table 6.3 Pain disorders with level B efficacy (probably effective) based on one class I or two class II studies. All studies are double-blind and placebo-controlled

Authors	Diagnosis	Class	Number of Patients in Study	BoNT type	Total dose in units	Site(s) of injection	Outcome measure	Results
Yuan et al. (2009) [26]	Diabetic neuropathy Neuropathic pain	II Crossover	20	onaA	50 U	Intradermal – dorsum of the foot 12 sites	Pain intensity (VAS), sleep CPSQI	VAS improved at 1, 4, 8, 12 wks ($P < 0.05$); CPSQI improved ($P < 0.05$)
Ghasemi et al. (2014) [27]	Diabetic neuropathy Neuropathic pain	I Parallel	40	aboA	100 U	Intradermal – dorsum of the foot 12 sites	Pain intensity (VAS); NPS	Both VAS and NPS improved ($P < 0.05$)
Restivo et al. (2018) [28]	Diabetic neuropathy Painful cramps	I Parallel	50	incoA	100 U 30 U	Gastrocnemius small flexor of the foot	PO: pain intensity (VAS); SO: QoL	VAS and cramp frequency improved: ($P = 0.037$) and ($P = 0.004$)
Salehi et al. (2019) [29]	Diabetic neuropathy Neuropathic pain	II Parallel	32	aboA	100 U	Foot surface, 12 points	Pain (VAS) Sleep (PSQI) Quality of life (SF-36)	VAS improved at 12 wks ($P < 0.001$) PSQI ($P < 0.001$) SF-36 psychological Scale ($P = 0.050$)
Foster et al. (2001) [30]	Low back pain	II Parallel	31	onaA	200 U	Unilateral Erector spinae at all five lumbar levels (40 U/level)	Pain (VAS); ADL (Oswestry)	VAS improved 3 wks:($P = 0.012$ 8 wks: ($P = 0.009$) Oswestry improved 8 wks: P (0.011)
Machado et al. (2016) [31]	Low back pain	II Parallel	37	aboA	500 U 1000 U	Unilateral bilateral Erector spinae at all five lumbar levels (40 U/level)	Pain (VAS); Oswestry; PGIC	VAS improved 8 weeks: (0.048) Oswestry improved 8 weeks: (0.040) PGIC improved 8 weeks: (0.029)

Study	Condition	Phase	N	Toxin	Dose	Injection site	Measures	Results
De Andres et al. (2010) [32]	Low back pain	II	27	onaA	50 U	Quadratus lumborum Psoas major	Pain (VAS)	More patients showed VAS improvement in the aboA group but statistically not significant
Cogne et al. (2017) [33]	Low back pain	II Crossover	17	onaA	200 U	Bilateral Erector spinae lumbar region (20 U/level)	PO: pain (VAS) SO: Quebec Back Pain Disability Scale, QoL scale	No significant difference between toxin and placebo in either PO or SO
Babcock et al. (2005) [34]	Plantar fasciitis	II Parallel	27	onaA	70 U	Medial heal Midfoot into plantar fascia	Pain (VAS) MFS Pressure algometry (PA)	All improved significantly VAS: $P < 0.0005$ MFS: $P = 0.001$ PA: $P = 0.003$
Huang et al. (2010) [35]	Plantar fasciitis	II Parallel	50	onaA	50 U	Below calcaneus into plantar fascia	Pain (VAS) Thickness of fascia	VAS improved Thickness of fascia reduced ($P < 0.001$)
Peterlein et al. (2012) [36]	Plantar fasciitis	II Parallel	40	aboA	200 U	Fan shape from the origin of PF	Pain (VAS) proportion of responders	AboA 25% versus saline 5% Statistically not significant
Rodriguez et al. (2013) [37]	Plantar fasciitis	II[a] Parallel	40	aboA	250 U	Gastrocnemius Soleus	Pain (VAS) MFS FADI	More improvement of VAS, MFS, and FADI in aboA group compared to steroid group ($P < 0.05$)
Ahmad et al. (2017) [38]	Plantar fasciitis	II Parallel	50	incoA	100 U	Single injection into plantar – medial aspect of calcaneus	Pain (VAS) Foot and Ankle Ability Measure (FAAM)	Both VAS and FAAM improved $P = 0.01$

(continued)

Table 6.3 (continued)

Authors	Diagnosis	Class	Number of Patients in Study	BoNT type	Total dose in units	Site(s) of injection	Outcome measure	Results
Abbasian et al. (2020) [39]	Plantar fasciitis	II Parallel	32	BoNT-A?	70 U	Medial gastrocnemius	Pain (VAS) AOFAS score Patient satisfaction	Improvement of VAS and AOFAS significant compared to placebo $P < 0.01$
Fishman et al. (2002) [40]	Piriformis syndrome	II Parallel	36	onaA	200 U	Into piriformis muscle	Pain (VAS)	65% of onaA and 6% of placebo improved in VAS ($P = 0.001$)
Childers et al. (2002) [41]	Piriformis syndrome	II Crossover	9	onaA	100 U	Into piriformis muscle	Pain (VAS)	Significant improvement of VAS and daily activity ($P < 0.05$)
Fishman et al. (2017) [42]	Piriformis syndrome	II Parallel	56	incoA	300 U	Into piriformis muscle	Pain (VAS) FAIR physical score	VAS improved $P < 0001$; FAIR: improvement varied from $P = 0.003$ to $P = 0.046$
Wong et al. (2005) [43]	Lateral epicondylitis	II Parallel	60	aboA	60 U	Deep into SC tissue and muscle, 1 cm from lateral epicondyle (LE)	Pain (VAS) Grip strength	VAS improved, Wk 4: $P < 0.01$ Wk 12: $P < 0.006$ Finger strength (ns)
Hyton et al. (2005) [44]	Lateral epicondylitis	II Parallel	40	aboA	50 U	Into muscle, 5 cm distal to the tender epicondyle	Pain (VAS) SF-12 Hand grip	No significant difference between aboA and placebo in those measures

Placzek et al. (2007) [45]	Lateral epicondylitis	I	Parallel	130	aboA	60 U	3–4 cm distal to the tender epicondyle, at two points	Pain (VAS) Patient and physician satisfaction	VAS improved ($P < 0.05$) Physician satisfied
Espandar et al. (2012) [46]	Lateral epicondylitis	II	Parallel	48	aboA	60 U	33% of arm's length, below epicondyle	Pain (VAS) Maximum pinch pain	VAS improved $P = 0.01$ Maximum pinch $P = 0.004$
Han et al. (2016) [47]	Neuropathic pain after spinal cord surgery	I	Parallel	40	Meditox	200 U	Subcutaneous Multiple sites	Pain (VAS) WHO-QoL	VAS improved ($P < 005$) WHO-QoL: trend $P = 0.052$
Gottsch et al. (2011) [48]	Male pelvic pain – prostatitis	II	Parallel	13	onaA	100 U	Into bulbospongiosus muscle	Pain (VAS) Chronic pain syndrome index (CPSI)	VAS improvement 30% (toxin) versus 13% (placebo) $P < 0.0002$ CPSI pain subset also improved ($P = 0.05$)
Falahatkar et al. (2015) [49]	Male pelvic pain – prostatitis	I	Parallel	60	aboA	100 U 200 U	Into lateral lobe of prostate, three sites	Pain (VAS) NIH-CPSI	Significantly improved pain (VAS) and quality of life (CPSI)

Prosigne, Chinese type A toxin from Lanzhou Institute, *PGIC* Patient Global Impression of Change, *VAS* Visual Analogue Scale, *PSQI* Pittsburgh Sleep Quality Index, *CPSQI* Chinese version of Pittsburgh Sleep Quality Index, *onaA* onabotulinumtoxinA (Botox), *incoA* incobotulinumtoxinA (Xeomin), *aboA* abobotulinumtoxin (Dysport), *NPS* neuropathic pain scale, *MFS* Maryland Foot Score, *aboA* abobotulinumtoxin/A (Dysport), *FADI* Foot and Ankle Disability Index, *FAAM* Foot and Ankle Ability Measure, *CPSI* Chronic Prostatitis Symptom Index
[a]Comparator study (toxin versus steroid)

Restivo et al. [28] assessed the efficacy of intramuscular injections of onaA on painful cramps associated with diabetic neuropathy. Fifty patients were studied in a clinical trial with a parallel, double-blind, placebo-controlled design. Injections of either 30 or 100 units of onaA into medial gastrocnemius or small foot flexors muscles were compared with placebo (saline) injections. A decrease of 50% or more of cramp frequency and cramp intensity was taken as primary outcome which was met in the toxin group after one week and lasted for 14 weeks (*P* values 0.037 and 0.04, respectively). The maximum effect was at week 6. Mild pain at the site of injection occurred in 25 patients in the toxin group which disappeared within 2–3 days.

Comment
The level of evidence for analgesic effect of BoNT therapy in neuropathic pain of diabetic neuropathy is B (probably effective) based on one class I and two class II studies. The level of efficacy is also B for BoNT therapy for muscle cramps in diabetic neuropathy. All three type A toxins (ona, abo, and inco) have demonstrated analgesic effects. Larger controlled studies are needed to support these encouraging findings. No serious side effects were reported in these studies with the applied doses of BoNTs.

Chronic Low Back Pain

"Chronic back pain is defined as pain that persists for 12 weeks or longer, even after an initial injury or underlying cause of acute low back pain has been treated." Approximately 20 percent of people affected by acute low back pain develop chronic low back pain [52]. The anatomic basis of low back pain is complex; hence, the pain can originate from malfunction of several structures among the low back muscles, vertebral column, facet joints, and nerve roots. Potent analgesics such as narcotics can provide pain relieve in chronic low back pain, but their use is associated with side effects, and there is always a potential for addition. Spinal stimulation, a relatively new treatment modality for low back pain, is often more effective than conventional therapy but has higher risk of complications.

Botulinum Toxin Treatment

BoNT therapy aims to alleviate low back pain through several mechanisms:

1. Relaxing tense and contracted muscles via blocking the release of acetylcholine from presynaptic vesicles in neuromuscular junction.
2. Reducing arrival of pain signals to the spinal cord by influencing peripheral pain neurotransmitters.
3. A central analgesic effect due to retrograde transfer of the toxin from periphery to the spinal cord [53]. This would reduce the phenomenon of central sensitization which is a part of pathophysiology of any chronic pain disorders.

4. By reducing the activity of muscle spindles after intramuscular injection [54] cuts down a powerful excitatory input to the spinal cord.
5. When a tight compartment in the back is playing a role in the pathophysiology of low back pain (tight compartment syndrome [55]), injection of BoNT into the tight muscles may alleviate pain by causing reversible atrophy tense back muscles.

Botulinum Toxin Studies of Low Back Pain Targeting Erector Spinae (ES) Muscles

This category includes three controlled clinical trials. Two of these trials reported significant improvement of low back pain in patients with no history of prior surgery using an identical technique of injection and dosage. In one study [30], conducted at Walter Reed Army Medical Center, authors studied 31 patients with predominately unilateral chronic low back pain comparing the effects of onaA injections blindly with placebo. In the onaA group, each patient received 40 units injected into ES muscle at each of the five lumbar levels ipsilateral to the side of pain. The outcome measures included VAS for pain and Oswestry Low Back Pain Questionnaire (OLBPQ) for the activities of daily living. Three weeks following injection, 11 of 15 patients (73.8%) in the onaA group and 4 of 16 (25%) patients in the placebo group had 50% or more reduction of pain intensity ($P = 0.012$) which remained reduced at 8 weeks only in the onaA group ($P = 0.0009$). At 8 weeks, OLBPQ demonstrated significant improvement of activities of daily living in 10 of 15 patients in the onaA group and 3 of 16 in the saline group, respectively ($P = 0.011$). No patient reported any side effects. In the second study [32], investigators at Yale University blindly studied the effects of aboA injection into ES muscles in 37 patients with unilateral and bilateral chronic low back pain (no history of surgery). The technique was identical to that of the first study – injection into ES muscle at four lumbar levels. A total dose of 500 units was used for unilateral and 1000 units for bilateral injections. Although the units of different toxins are not truly interchangeable, a conversion ratio of 1:2.5 is used between onaA and aboA often in clinical trials which makes the dose of the two studies comparable. The second study found significant improvements by VAS (proportion of responders), activities of daily living, and Patient Global Impression of Change in the aboA group compared to the placebo group (P values of 0.008, 0.048, and 0.0930, respectively). Three patients in the toxin group and two patients in the placebo group developed local pain at the site of injection lasting a few days. In contrast to the two abovementioned studies, another study which used the same technique and onaA toxin did not find a significant difference between the toxin and placebo group in any of the outcome measures (VAS, Quebec Back Pain Disability Scale) [33]. The authors stated that the response failure might have been related to the lower dose of the toxin used in their study (half compared the other two studies).

Botulinum Toxin Study Targeting Quadratus Lumborum and Iliopsoas Muscles

De Andres et al. [32] compared the effect of a single injection of 100 units of onaA with placebo and lidocaine in a blinded study of 27 patients with myofascial pain at lumbar area.

The onaA was injected into quadratus lumborum and iliopsoas major muscles at one side (27 patients) and compared with the effect of saline (14 patients) and lidocaine (13 patients) injected into the same muscles on the other side. The pain outcome was measured by VAS. Patient activities of daily living were assessed through five different questionnaires including OLBPQ. At the end of the study, a trend for significant VAS improvement was noted only on the side that patients had received onaA injection.

Comment

Injection of botulinum toxin A (ona or inco) into the erector spinae muscles using Walter Reed-Yale protocol (injecting 40 units of abo or inco A per each lumbar level) significantly improves low back pain in patients with no surgical history. The level of efficacy for this protocol in chronic low back pain is B (probably effective) based on publication of two class II (placebo-controlled and blinded) studies. The failure of another study that was conducted under a very similar protocol [33] most likely reflects using a much lower dose (half of that of prior studies) as suggested by authors. The short-term positive results of the Walter Reed-Yale protocol in chronic low back pain need to be confirmed in clinical trials with larger number of patients and conducted over longer periods of time.

Plantar Fasciitis (Plantar Fasciopathy)

Plantar fasciitis (PF) is a common pain problem that affects 10% of runners [56]. Plantar fascia is a layer of fibrous tissue that connects the base of the toes to the medial part of the calcaneum. It is believed that repeated trauma to plantar fascia during running, playing football, or jobs that require heavy labor causes microtears in the PF. In some patients, the pathology also involves local inflammation. The main symptom of PF is pain that is often felt at or close to the heel. Patients with mild symptoms respond to stretching, night splint, orthosis, and nonsteroidal, anti-inflammatory medications. Injection of steroids into the plantar fascia, acupuncture, ultrasound therapy, cryosurgery, and application of shock waves is often used to achieve pain relief in more severe cases. These remedies, however, are not without complications; steroid injections may cause rupture of plantar fascia, and application of shock waves may be hard to tolerate due to its painful nature. Because of these issues, many patients with severe PF are unsatisfied with their management.

BoNT Therapy in Plantar Fasciitis

The senior author of this chapter and his colleagues first studied the effect of local BoNT injection in patients with PF under a double-blind, placebo-controlled proto-col [34]. Twenty-seven patients were randomized into toxin and placebo groups. In the toxin group, onabotulinumtoxinA (Botox) was injected into the medial aspect of the heel (40 units) and into the plantar fascia between the anterior part of the heel and midfoot (30 units). A thin needle, gauge 27.5, was used for injections to avoid injury to PF. Treatment outcome was assessed by VAS, Maryland Foot Score (MFS), and pressure algometry at 3 and 8 weeks after injection. All measures were signifi-cantly improved at 3 and 8 weeks (P values at week 3: < 0.005, < 0.0005, $P = 0.003$, respectively). Except for mild local pain at the site of injection for a few minutes, no other side effects were reported. A later blinded study conducted in 50 patients with PF [35] also reported significant improvement of VAS in the toxin group compared to placebo ($P = 0.001$). The toxin group also demonstrated significant reduced thickness of plantar fascia. The authors injected 50 units of onaA into the plantar fascia via posterior calcaneal approach under ultrasound guidance. No side effects were reported. Two other blinded, placebo-controlled studies have shown similar results using different techniques [38, 39]. In one of the two studies [38] which included 50 patients, a single injection with 100 units of incoA or saline was admin-istered into the most tender part of plantar fascia at the distal aspect of plantar-medial aspect of calcaneus where the plantar fascia is adjacent to flexor digitorum brevis. Pain (VAS) and function (ankle ability measure – FAAM) outcomes were measured at 6 and 12 months. Both VAS and FAAM improved in the toxin group at 6 and 12 months ($P = 0.01$ and <0.005, respectively). Three patients in the saline group, but none in the toxin group, required surgery after 12 months. No side effects were reported. In a very recent publication [39], authors have provided evidence from a controlled clinical trial that a single injection of 70 units of onaA into the medial gastrocnemius under ultrasound guidance can significantly improve the symptoms of PF. Improvement of pain (measured by VAS) and the improved score from the American Orthopedic Foot and Ankle Society Scale (AOFAS) were both statistically significant compared to the placebo at 12 months ($P < 0.01$). Two patients in the toxin group and one in the placebo group reported mild, transient "local inflammation" at the site of injection. Elizondo-Rodriguez et al. [37] blindly compared the effect of abobotulinumA (aboA) injection with steroid and lidocaine injections in 40 patients with PF. BoNT injection was superior to steroid in terms of long-term pain relief and foot function (Table 6.3).

Comment
Five controlled clinical trials (blinded and placebo-controlled) have shown injection of BoNT-A improves pain and foot function in plantar fasciitis both short term and up to at least 12 months. All three marketed types of type A toxin (onaA, incoA, and aboA) have demonstrated a positive effect. Side effects are mild, infrequent, and transient. These studies (all class II) provide a B level of evidence (probably effec-tive) for efficacy of BoNT-As in PF. The optimal location of injection (into the

plantar fascia or gastrocnemius/soleus muscles) remains to be determined by future studies. Larger clinical trials are needed in order to raise the level of significance for this indication from B to A (see chapter supplement).

Piriformis Syndrome (PS)

Piriformis syndrome is caused by a tense and overactive piriformis muscle and its pressure against the adjacent sciatic nerve. Pain is the major symptom of PS, often felt deep in the buttock; it occasionally radiates to the thigh. Pain of PS is mainly felt during sitting and squatting. Piriformis muscle is a deep triangular muscle, located behind gluteus maximus with attachments to the sacrum and the greater trochanter. The true incidence of PS is not known, but one investigator reported that 6% of patients diagnosed with sciatica represent piriformis syndrome [57].

Treatment of Piriformis Syndrome

Treatment begins with physical therapy alone or combined with oral analgesics. A special stretching technique which lengthens the piriformis muscle is sometimes helpful [58]. Heat application and ultrasound therapy may promote the positive effects of physical therapy [59]. One retrospective study in 500 patients over a 10-year period reported that injection of 1.5–2% lidocaine mixed with 20 mg of triamcinolone into the piriformis muscle improves pain in 70% of patients [60]. Sustained pain relief using current medical managements is uncommon in many PS patients.

BoNT Therapy in Piriformis Syndrome

In 2002, two groups of investigators reported the results of blinded, placebo-controlled studies that have assessed the efficacy of onabotulinumtoxinA (Botox) in piriformis syndrome. Childers et al. [41] in a crossover study of nine patients reported that injection of 100 units of onaA into the piriformis muscle (PM) relieved pain significantly (measured by VAS) ($P < 0.05$). In a larger parallel study of 36 patients, 25 patients were injected with 200 U of onaA, and 15 patients were injected with the same volume of saline into PM [42]. In blinded assessments of the results, 65% of the patients in the onaA group and 6% of the patients in the saline group demonstrated >50% decrease in pain intensity as measured by VAS ($P = 0.001$). Furthermore, flexion, adduction, and internal rotation of the affected leg (FAIR test) produced less pain in the onaA group compared to the placebo group. In both studies, piriformis muscle injection was performed under electromyogrphic guidance using a long needle (3.5 cm or longer) in order to reach the deep piriformis muscle located behind gluteus maximus. In 2017, 15 years later, the same senior investigator published a controlled study [44] in which the results of incobotulinumtoxinA (Xeomin) injection were blindly compared with that of placebo injections into the piriformis muscle in patients with PS. Following injection of 200 units, pain (measured by VAS) was significantly reduced in the incoA group at 2, 4, 8, 10, and 12 postinjection weeks ($P < 0.0001$). The FAIR test also significantly improved in the incoA group compared to placebo over 2, 4, 6, and 8 postinjection weeks ($P < 0.05$). In addition to clinical features of pain, the authors have used specific abnormalities of H-reflex, elicited from posterior tibialis muscle to support the diagnosis of piriformis syndrome. Side effects were reported to be mild and transient in the toxin group consisted of pain at the site of injection (2), flue-like symptoms (1), neck pain (1), and wobbly neck (1). Similar side effects were reported in the placebo group.

Comment
Although piriformis syndrome as the cause of sciatic pain remains controversial [61], three class II studies have provided evidence that injection of BoNT into piriformis muscle can reduce sciatic pain in the affected patients. The larger studies used an injection dose of 200 units of BoNT-A (onaA or inco-A) which did not cause any serious side effects. The data indicates that injection of BoNT-A into the piriformis muscle is probably effective (level B evidence, two class II studies) in relieving sciatic pain in piriformis syndrome.

Chronic Lateral Epicondylitis (CLE)

Chronic lateral epicondylitis is a common pain disorder affecting 1–3% of general population each year [62]. It is an overuse injury that is caused by repeated wrist extension against resistance. Heavy works requiring elbow extension and sports, particularly tennis, that often requires overextension of the elbow commonly cause CLE. Up to 50% of tennis players, especially those with poor or heavy swings, may develop this complication [62]. Although most acute cases improve with time if repeated elbow overextension is avoided, close to 20% develop CLE a year after the onset of their symptoms [63]. The lateral epicondyle is often tender to touch, and extension of the elbow generates pain. The pathology consists of degeneration of extensor tendons which is demonstrated well on in ultrasound examination, sometimes associated with inflammation [64]. Physical therapy avoiding elbow overuse and bracing helps in mild cases. Pharmacotherapy with nonsteroidal analgesics and GABAergic drugs such as pregabalin and gabapentin offers help. Local injection of steroids and anesthetic agents is reserved for more severe cases.

BoNT Therapy for Chronic Lateral Epicondylitis (CLE)

Four groups of investigators [43–46] conducted double-blind, placebo-controlled studies assessing the efficacy of BoNT injections in CLE (Table 6.3). All studies used abobotulinumtoxinA (Dysport) injections. The injection site was along the course of the extensor muscles. The dose varied from 50 to 60 units. Different investigators chose different distances from lateral epicondyle as the site of BoNT injection. One group injected into extensors 1 cm below the tender epicondyle [43], two groups injected between 3 and 5 cm below the epicondyle [44, 45], and one group injected 33% of the arm's length below the epicondyle [46]. Three studies [43, 45, 46] with larger group of patients and employing a larger dose of toxin (60 units) reported improvement of pain ($P < 0.05$, measured by VAS) and physician satisfaction scale, whereas one study with smaller number of patients, injected close to epicondyle (cm) and employing a smaller dose of the toxin (50 units), did not report significant difference between the toxin and placebo groups [44]. Unfortunately, up to one-third of the patients after BoNT injection developed weakness of finger extensors that in some patients lasted up to 3 months.

Comment

Injection of abobotulinumtoxinA (Dysport) below the tender lateral epicondyle into elbow extensors is probably effective in CLE (level B: one class I and two class II studies). Development of finger weakness is a bothersome side effect. Hopefully, future studies may reduce the frequency of this complication via refinement of injection technique and BoNT dose adjustment.

Neuropathic Pain After Spinal Cord Injury

Han and coworkers [47] evaluated the analgesic effect of botulinum toxin type A (BTX-A) in 40 patients who experienced neuropathic pain after spinal cord injury. The study was randomized, double-blind, placebo-controlled, and parallel in design. In the toxin group, each patient received 200 units of Meditox (Korean toxin) injected subcutaneously into the area of skin affected by the neuropathic pain. The total dose of 200 U was distributed into several injection sites. The outcome measures consisted of Visual Analogue Scale for pain assessment (VAS), the Korean version of the short-form McGill Pain Questionnaire, and the World Health Organization WHOQOL-BREF quality of life. The patients' response to the injected toxin or placebo was evaluated at 4 and 8 weeks postinjection. At 4 and 8 weeks following injection, the VAS score was significantly reduced in the toxin group (18.6 ± 16.8 and 21.3 ± 26.8, respectively) compared to the placebo group (2.6 ± 14.6 and 0.3 ± 19.5, respectively) ($P < 0.05$). There was a trend toward significance in WHOQOL-BREF for the BONT-A group at 4 weeks ($P = 0.0521$). No side effects were reported.

Comment

This class I study provides a level B evidence (probably effective) for efficacy of subcutaneous injection of Meditoxin (type A, Korean BoNT) in neuropathic pain incurred in patients with spinal cord injury.

Chronic Pelvic Pain (CPP)

Chronic pelvic pain is defined as a noncyclic pain in the pelvic region of more than 6 months' duration. It is a common disorder in both genders. In one prospective study of a large number of women (n = >5000), 14.7% met the criteria for chronic pelvic pain [65]. There is evidence from blinded, placebo-controlled studies that both male and female pelvic pain may benefit from BoNT treatment. For male pelvic pain, these studies, one class I and one class II, provide a level B efficacy (probably effective), whereas for female pelvic pain, availability of one class II study denotes a possible level of efficacy (C level).

Gottsch el al. [48] have studied 11 male patients with CPP related to prostatitis in a randomized, placebo-controlled, double-blind protocol. A total of 100 units of BoNT-A was injected into the bulbospongiosus muscle. One month following treatment, the response measured by Global Response Assessment (GRA) was significantly better in the BoNT-A group compared to the placebo group (30% vs. 13%, p = 0.0002). The NIH-CPSI pain subdomain of NIH-CPSI score also significantly improved in the BoNT group. Another group of investigators injected 100 and 200 units of abobotulinumtoxinA (Dysport) into the lateral lobe of the prostate (at three sites) of 60 patients with prostatitis and CPP [49]. Pain was evaluated by VAS, American Urological Symptom Score (AUA-SS), NIH-CPSI, and frequency of diurnal and nocturnal urination. Injections and assessments were performed under a double-blind, placebo-controlled protocol. All measures improved following BoNT treatment. NIH-CPSI pain subdomain and the VAS scores showed the most significant improvements (scores were decreased by 79.9% and 82.1% at 6-month follow-up, respectively).

Recently, the beneficial effect of BoNT therapy in male chronic pelvic pain was supported by a class III study in that the effect of transurethral injection of 200 units of onaA into prostate was compared in 43 patients with no treatment over 12 months [66]. All patients had chronic pelvic pain due to chronic prostatitis (mean duration of 7 years). The outcome measures consisted of VAS for pain and NIH-CPSI total score. The toxin-injected group demonstrated a significant reduction of VAS (P < 0.0001 and significant improvement of NIH-CPSI score (P < 0.0001) at 3 months.

There are several other pain disorders in which efficacy of botulinum toxins for pain relief is suggested based on limited (one class II study) and small double-blind, placebo-controlled clinical trials. These conditions which by AAN guidelines will currently have a C level evidence (possibly effective) include female pelvic pain syndrome, painful knee osteoarthritis, pain in children with cerebral palsy after adductor release surgery, and vastus lateralis imbalance syndrome [67].

The level of efficacy of BoNT therapy in myofascial pain syndrome (MFPS) has been designated as U (undetermined) by AAN's assessment and guideline committee due to contradicting results from two large, class I clinical trials. However, the two studies employed different injection techniques: Gobel et al. [68] who reported statistically significant pain relief used a flexible injection pattern and injected 10 trigger points, whereas Ferrante et al. [69] who reported failure of BoNT to relieve pain in MPS injected less than five trigger points (in many patients one trigger point). The authors of this chapter feel that MFPS with Gobel et al.'s method should have a level B efficacy (probably effective) based on one well-designed and conducted class I study.

References

1. Jankovic J. Botulinum toxin: state of the art. Mov Disord. 2017;32(8):1131–8. https://doi. org/10.1002/mds.27072.
2. Gronseth G, French J. Practice parameters and technology assessments: what they are, what they are not, and why you should care. Neurology. 2008;71(20):1639–43. https://doi. org/10.1212/01.wnl.0000336535.27773.c0.
3. French J, Gronseth G. Lost in a jungle of evidence: we need a compass. Neurology. 2008;71(20):1634–8. https://doi.org/10.1212/01.wnl.0000336533.19610.1b.
4. Lipton RB, Bigal ME, Diamond M, et al. Migraine prevalence, disease burden, and the need for preventive therapy. Neurology. 2007;68(5):343–9. https://doi.org/10.1212/01. wnl.0000252808.97649.21.
5. Eller M, Goadsby PJ. Migraine: a brain state amenable to therapy. Med J Aust. 2020;212(1):32– 9. https://doi.org/10.5694/mja2.50435.
6. Parikh SK, Silberstein SD. Preventive treatment for episodic migraine. Neurol Clin. 2019;37(4):753–70. https://doi.org/10.1016/j.ncl.2019.07.004.
7. Aurora SK, Dodick DW, Turkel CC, et al. OnabotulinumtoxinA for treatment of chronic migraine: results from the double-blind, randomized, placebo-controlled phase of the PREEMPT 1 trial. Cephalalgia. 2010;30(7):793–803. https://doi.org/ 10.1177/0333102410364676.
8. Diener HC, Dodick DW, Aurora SK, et al. OnabotulinumtoxinA for treatment of chronic migraine: results from the double-blind, randomized, placebo-controlled phase of the PREEMPT 2 trial. Cephalalgia. 2010;30(7):804–14. https://doi.org/10.1177/0333102410364677.
9. Dodick DW, Turkel CC, DeGryse RE, et al. OnabotulinumtoxinA for treatment of chronic migraine: pooled results from the double-blind, randomized, placebo-controlled phases of the PREEMPT clinical program. Headache. 2010;50(6):921–36. https://doi. org/10.1111/j.1526-4610.2010.01678.x.
10. Silberstein SD, Blumenfeld AM, Cady RK, et al. OnabotulinumtoxinA for treatment of chronic migraine: PREEMPT 24-week pooled subgroup analysis of patients who had acute headache medication overuse at baseline. J Neurol Sci. 2013;331(1–2):48–56. https://doi.org/10.1016/j. jns.2013.05.003.
11. Lipton RB, Varon SF, Grosberg B, et al. OnabotulinumtoxinA improves quality of life and reduces impact of chronic migraine. Neurology. 2011;77(15):1465–72. https://doi.org/10.1212/ WNL.0b013e318232ab65.
12. Aurora SK, Dodick DW, Diener HC, et al. OnabotulinumtoxinA for chronic migraine: efficacy, safety, and tolerability in patients who received all five treatment cycles in the PREEMPT clinical program. Acta Neurol Scand. 2014;129(1):61–70. https://doi.org/10.1111/ane.12171.
13. Blumenfeld AM, Silberstein SD, Dodick DW, Aurora SK, Brin MF, Binder WJ. Insights into the functional anatomy behind the PREEMPT injection paradigm: guidance on achieving optimal outcomes. Headache. 2017;57(5):766–77. https://doi.org/10.1111/head.13074.
14. Choi YJ, Lee WJ, Lee HJ, Lee KW, Kim HJ, Hu KS. Effective botulinum toxin injection guide for treatment of temporal headache. Toxins (Basel). 2016;8(9):265. Published 2016 Sep 8. https://doi.org/10.3390/toxins8090265.

15. Schaefer SM, Gottschalk CH, Jabbari B. Treatment of chronic migraine with focus on botulinum neurotoxins. Toxins (Basel). 2015;7(7):2615–28. Published 2015 Jul 14. https://doi.org/10.3390/toxins7072615.

16. Richardson D, Jabbari B. Botulinum treatment of chronic migraine. A double- blind study with a novel technique employing fewer injections. Poster 124- American Academy of Neurology annual meeting, Vancouver, Canada, April 19, 2016.

17. Xiao L, Mackey S, Hui H, Xong D, Zhang Q, Zhang D. Subcutaneous injection of botulinum toxin a is beneficial in postherpetic neuralgia. Pain Med. 2010;11(12):1827–33. https://doi.org/10.1111/j.1526-4637.2010.01003.x.

18. Apalla Z, Sotiriou E, Lallas A, Lazaridou E, Ioannides D. Botulinum toxin A in postherpetic neuralgia: a parallel, randomized, double-blind, single-dose, placebo-controlled trial. Clin J Pain. 2013;29(10):857–64. https://doi.org/10.1097/AJP.0b013e31827a72d2.

19. Ranoux D, Attal N, Morain F, Bouhassira D. Botulinum toxin type A induces direct analgesic effects in chronic neuropathic pain [published correction appears in Ann Neurol. 2009;65(3):359]. Ann Neurol. 2008;64(3):274–83. https://doi.org/10.1002/ana.21427.

20. Attal N, de Andrade DC, Adam F, et al. Safety and efficacy of repeated injections of botulinum toxin A in peripheral neuropathic pain (BOTNEP): a randomised, double-blind, placebo-controlled trial. Lancet Neurol. 2016;15(6):555–65. https://doi.org/10.1016/S1474-4422(16)00017-X.

21. Wu CJ, Lian YJ, Zheng YK, et al. Botulinum toxin type A for the treatment of trigeminal neuralgia: results from a randomized, double-blind, placebo-controlled trial. Cephalalgia. 2012;32(6):443–50. https://doi.org/10.1177/0333102412441721.

22. Zhang H, Lian Y, Ma Y, et al. Two doses of botulinum toxin type A for the treatment of trigeminal neuralgia: observation of therapeutic effect from a randomized, double-blind, placebo-controlled trial. J Headache Pain. 2014;15(1):65. Published 2014 Sep 27. https://doi.org/10.1186/1129-2377-15-65.

23. Yawn BP, Saddier P, Wollan PC, St Sauver JL, Kurland MJ, Sy LS. A population-based study of the incidence and complication rates of herpes zoster before zoster vaccine introduction [published correction appears in Mayo Clin Proc. 2008;83(2):255]. Mayo Clin Proc. 2007;82(11):1341–9. https://doi.org/10.4065/82.11.1341.

24. Mueller D, Obermann M, Yoon MS, et al. Prevalence of trigeminal neuralgia and persistent idiopathic facial pain: a population-based study. Cephalalgia. 2011;31(15):1542–8. https://doi.org/10.1177/0333102411424619.

25. Li S, Lian YJ, Chen Y, et al. Therapeutic effect of botulinum toxin-A in 88 patients with trigeminal neuralgia with 14-month follow-up. J Headache Pain. 2014;15(1):43. Published 2014 Jun 22. https://doi.org/10.1186/1129-2377-15-43.

26. Yuan RY, Sheu JJ, Yu JM, et al. Botulinum toxin for diabetic neuropathic pain: a randomized double-blind crossover trial. Neurology. 2009;72(17):1473–8. https://doi.org/10.1212/01.wnl.0000345968.05959.cf.

27. Ghasemi M, Ansari M, Basiri K, Shaigannejad V. The effects of intradermal botulinum toxin type A injections on pain symptoms of patients with diabetic neuropathy. J Res Med Sci. 2014;19(2):106–11.

28. Restivo DA, Casabona A, Frittitta L, et al. Efficacy of botulinum toxin A for treating cramps in diabetic neuropathy. Ann Neurol. 2018;84(5):674–82. https://doi.org/10.1002/ana.25340.

29. Salehi H, Moussaei M, Kamiab Z, Vakilian A. The effects of botulinum toxin type A injection on pain symptoms, quality of life, and sleep quality of patients with diabetic neuropathy: a randomized double-blind clinical trial. Iran J Neurol. 2019;18(3):99–107.

30. Foster L, Clapp L, Erickson M, Jabbari B. Botulinum toxin A and chronic low back pain: a randomized, double-blind study. Neurology. 2001;56(10):1290–3. https://doi.org/10.1212/wnl.56.10.1290.

31. Machado D, Kumar A, Jabbari B. Abobotulinum toxin A in the treatment of chronic low back pain. Toxins (Basel). 2016;8(12):374. Published 2016 Dec 15. https://doi.org/10.3390/toxins8120374.

32. De Andrés J, Adsuara VM, Palmisani S, Villanueva V, López-Alarcón MD. A double-blind, controlled, randomized trial to evaluate the efficacy of botulinum toxin for the treatment of lumbar myofascial pain in humans. Reg Anesth Pain Med. 2010;35(3):255–60. https://doi.org/10.1097/AAP.0b013e3181d23241.

33. Cogné M, Petit H, Creuzé A, Liguoro D, de Seze M. Are paraspinous intramuscular injections of botulinum toxin a (BoNT-A) efficient in the treatment of chronic low-back pain? A randomised, double-blinded crossover trial. BMC Musculoskelet Disord. 2017;18(1):454. Published 2017 Nov 15. https://doi.org/10.1186/s12891-017-1816-6.

34. Babcock MS, Foster L, Pasquina P, Jabbari B. Treatment of pain attributed to plantar fasciitis with botulinum toxin a: a short-term, randomized, placebo-controlled, double-blind study. Am J Phys Med Rehabil. 2005;84(9):649–54. https://doi.org/10.1097/01.phm.0000176339.73591.d7.

35. Huang YC, Wei SH, Wang HK, Lieu FK. Ultrasonographic guided botulinum toxin type A treatment for plantar fasciitis: an outcome-based investigation for treating pain and gait changes. J Rehabil Med. 2010;42(2):136–40. https://doi.org/10.2340/16501977-0491.

36. Peterlein CD, Funk JF, Hölscher A, Schuh A, Placzek R. Is botulinum toxin A effective for the treatment of plantar fasciitis? Clin J Pain. 2012;28(6):527–33. https://doi.org/10.1097/AJP.0b013e31823ae65a.

37. Elizondo-Rodriguez J, Araujo-Lopez Y, Moreno-Gonzalez JA, Cardenas-Estrada E, Mendoza-Lemus O, Acosta-Olivo C. A comparison of botulinum toxin A and intralesional steroids for the treatment of plantar fasciitis: a randomized, double-blinded study. Foot Ankle Int. 2013;34(1):8–14. https://doi.org/10.1177/1071100712460215.

38. Ahmad J, Ahmad SH, Jones K. Treatment of plantar fasciitis with botulinum toxin. Foot Ankle Int. 2017;38(1):1–7. https://doi.org/10.1177/1071100716666364.

39. Abbasian M, Baghbani S, Barangi S, et al. Outcomes of ultrasound-guided gastrocnemius injection with botulinum toxin for chronic plantar fasciitis. Foot Ankle Int. 2020;41(1):63–8. https://doi.org/10.1177/1071100719875220.

40. Fishman LM, Anderson C, Rosner B. BOTOX and physical therapy in the treatment of piriformis syndrome. Am J Phys Med Rehabil. 2002;81(12):936–42. https://doi.org/10.1097/00002060-200212000-00009.

41. Childers MK, Wilson DJ, Gnatz SM, Conway RR, Sherman AK. Botulinum toxin type A use in piriformis muscle syndrome: a pilot study. Am J Phys Med Rehabil. 2002;81(10):751–9. https://doi.org/10.1097/00002060-200210000-00006.

42. Fishman LM, Wilkins AN, Rosner B. Electrophysiologically identified piriformis syndrome is successfully treated with incobotulinum toxin a and physical therapy. Muscle Nerve. 2017;56(2):258–63. https://doi.org/10.1002/mus.25504.

43. Wong SM, Hui AC, Tong PY, Poon DW, Yu E, Wong LK. Treatment of lateral epicondylitis with botulinum toxin: a randomized, double-blind, placebo-controlled trial. Ann Intern Med. 2005;143(11):793–7. https://doi.org/10.7326/0003-4819-143-11-200512060-00007.

44. Hayton MJ, Santini AJ, Hughes PJ, Frostick SP, Trail IA, Stanley JK. Botulinum toxin injection in the treatment of tennis elbow. A double-blind, randomized, controlled, pilot study. J Bone Joint Surg Am. 2005;87(3):503–7. https://doi.org/10.2106/JBJS.D.01896.

45. Placzek R, Drescher W, Deuretzbacher G, Hempfing A, Meiss AL. Treatment of chronic radial epicondylitis with botulinum toxin A: a double-blind, placebo-controlled, randomized multicenter study. J Bone Joint Surg Am. 2007;89(2):255–60. https://doi.org/10.2106/JBJS.F.00401.

46. Espandar R, Heidari P, Rasouli MR, et al. Use of anatomic measurement to guide injection of botulinum toxin for the management of chronic lateral epicondylitis: a randomized controlled trial. CMAJ. 2010;182(8):768–73. https://doi.org/10.1503/cmaj.090906.

47. Han ZA, Song DH, Oh HM, Chung ME. Botulinum toxin type A for neuropathic pain in patients with spinal cord injury. Ann Neurol. 2016;79(4):569–78. https://doi.org/10.1002/ana.24605.

48. Gottsch HP, Yang CC, Berger RE. A pilot study of botulinum toxin A for male chronic pelvic pain syndrome. Scand J Urol Nephrol. 2011;45(1):72–6. https://doi.org/10.3109/00365599.2010.529820.

49. Falahatkar S, Shahab E, Gholamjani Moghaddam K, Kazemnezhad E. Transurethral intraprostatic injection of botulinum neurotoxin type A for the treatment of chronic prostatitis/chronic pelvic pain syndrome: results of a prospective pilot double-blind and randomized placebo-controlled study. BJU Int. 2015;116(4):641–9. https://doi.org/10.1111/bju.12951.

50. Barrett AM, Lucero MA, Le T, Robinson RL, Dworkin RH, Chappell AS. Epidemiology, public health burden, and treatment of diabetic peripheral neuropathic pain: a review. Pain Med. 2007;8(Suppl 2):S50–62. https://doi.org/10.1111/j.1526-4637.2006.00179.x.

51. Boulton AJ. Diabetic neuropathy: classification, measurement and treatment. Curr Opin Endocrinol Diabetes Obes. 2007;14(2):141–5. https://doi.org/10.1097/MED.0b013e328014979e.

52. National Institute of Health (NIH) fact sheet 8-2019. Back Pain Fact Sheet, NINDS, Publication date March 2020. NIH Publication No. 20-NS-5161.

53. Matak I, Bölcskei K, Bach-Rojecky L, Helyes Z. Mechanisms of botulinum toxin type A action on pain. Toxins (Basel). 2019;11(8):459. Published 2019 Aug 5. https://doi.org/10.3390/toxins11080459.

54. Filippi GM, Errico P, Santarelli R, Bagolini B, Manni E. Botulinum A toxin effects on rat jaw muscle spindles. Acta Otolaryngol. 1993;113(3):400–4. https://doi.org/10.3109/00016489309135834.

55. Nathan ST, Roberts CS, Deliberato D. Lumbar paraspinal compartment syndrome. Int Orthop. 2012;36(6):1221–7. https://doi.org/10.1007/s00264-011-1386-4.

56. Chandler TJ, Kibler WB. A biomechanical approach to the prevention, treatment and rehabilitation of plantar fasciitis. Sports Med. 1993;15(5):344–52. https://doi.org/10.2165/00007256-199315050-00006.

57. Hallin RP. Sciatic pain and the piriformis muscle. Postgrad Med. 1983;74(2):69–72. https://doi.org/10.1080/00325481.1983.11698378.

58. Gulledge BM, Marcellin-Little DJ, Levine D, et al. Comparison of two stretching methods and optimization of stretching protocol for the piriformis muscle. Med Eng Phys. 2014;36(2):212–8. https://doi.org/10.1016/j.medengphy.2013.10.016.

59. Kirschner JS, Foye PM, Cole JL. Piriformis syndrome, diagnosis and treatment. Muscle Nerve. 2009;40(1):10–8. https://doi.org/10.1002/mus.21318.

60. Fishman LM, Dombi GW, Michaelsen C, et al. Piriformis syndrome: diagnosis, treatment, and outcome--a 10-year study. Arch Phys Med Rehabil. 2002;83(3):295–301. https://doi.org/10.1053/apmr.2002.30622.

61. Jankovic D, Peng P, van Zundert A. Brief review: piriformis syndrome: etiology, diagnosis, and management. Can J Anaesth. 2013;60(10):1003–12. https://doi.org/10.1007/s12630-013-0009-5.

62. Cutts S, Gangoo S, Modi N, Pasapula C. Tennis elbow: a clinical review article. J Orthop. 2019;17:203–7. Published 2019 Aug 10. https://doi.org/10.1016/j.jor.2019.08.005.

63. Smidt N, van der Windt DA, Assendelft WJ, Devillé WL, Korthals-de Bos IB, Bouter LM. Corticosteroid injections, physiotherapy, or a wait-and-see policy for lateral epicondylitis: a randomised controlled trial. Lancet. 2002;359(9307):657–62. https://doi.org/10.1016/S0140-6736(02)07811-X.

64. Connell D, Burke F, Coombes P, et al. Sonographic examination of lateral epicondylitis. AJR Am J Roentgenol. 2001;176(3):777–82. https://doi.org/10.2214/ajr.176.3.1760777.

65. Mathias SD, Kuppermann M, Liberman RF, Lipschutz RC, Steege JF. Chronic pelvic pain: prevalence, health-related quality of life, and economic correlates. Obstet Gynecol. 1996;87(3):321–7. https://doi.org/10.1016/0029-7844(95)00458-0.

66. Abdel-Meguid TA, Mosli HA, Farsi H, Alsayyad A, Tayib A, Sait M, Abdelsalam A. Treatment of refractory category III nonbacterial chronic prostatitis/chronic pelvic pain syndrome with intraprostatic injection of onabotulinumtoxinA: a prospective controlled study. Can J Urol. 2018;25:9273–80.

67. Safarpour Y, Jabbari B. Botulinum toxin treatment of pain syndromes -an evidence- based review. Toxicon. 2018;147:120–8. https://doi.org/10.1016/j.toxicon.2018.01.017.

68. Göbel H, Heinze A, Reichel G, Hefter H, Benecke R, Dysport myofascial pain study group. Efficacy and safety of a single botulinum type A toxin complex treatment (Dysport) for the relief of upper back myofascial pain syndrome: results from a randomized double-blind placebo-controlled multicentre study. Pain. 2006;125(1–2):82–8. https://doi.org/10.1016/j.pain.2006.05.001.
69. Ferrante FM, Bearn L, Rothrock R, King L. Evidence against trigger point injection technique for the treatment of cervicothoracic myofascial pain with botulinum toxin type A. Anesthesiology. 2005;103(2):377–83. https://doi.org/10.1097/00000542-200508000-00021.
70. Jabbari B. Botulinum toxin Treatment- what everybody should know. New York: Springer; 2018.
71. Jabbari B. Botulinum toxin treatment in clinical medicine – a disease-oriented approach. New York: Springer Publisher; 2018.

Chapter 7
Botulinum Toxin Treatment in Cardiovascular Surgery

Omer Tanyeli and Mehmet Isik

Abstract Although the use of Botulinum Toxin (BTX) is a common practice especially in cosmetics, plastic and ophthalmic surgery over the last four decades, cardiac and vascular use is relatively new. The new articles published and ongoing studies for cardiovascular use are promising. Although the basic data and researches performed so far are rather limited, cardiac use can be sampled as suppression of postoperative rhythm, especially atrial fibrillation. Vascular use of BTX is mainly investigated for prevention of arterial spasm, mainly in graft patencies, or native arteries. BTX-A might be considered as an alternative topical agent for prevention of arterial graft spasms (Internal mammarian and radial artery) in coronary artery bypass graft surgery. Its effectiveness was also documented in different studies, involving the functional popliteal artery entrapment syndrome and vasospastic disorders, including Raynaud's phenomenon. With the highlights of recent articles gathered and our experience, this chapter briefly identifies the experimental and clinical use of BTX in cardiovascular area.

Keywords Botulinum toxin · Atrial fibrillation · Vasospasm · Radial artery ·
Internal mammarian artery · Raynaud's phenomenon

Introduction

Botulinum toxin (BTX) is a potent neurotoxin, which causes relaxation of striated muscles by blocking the release of acetylcholine at the neuromuscular junction. BTXs are produced by *Clostridium botulinum* and cause the clinical syndrome of botulism, causing flaccid paralysis of the skeletal muscles. Seven different subtypes are described so far, which are known to be the most potent toxins. The basic mechanism of action of the BTX subtypes (A–G) has been extensively studied, and their mechanisms of action can be found in previous chapters in detail.

O. Tanyeli (✉) · M. Isik
Necmettin Erbakan University, Meram Medicine Faculty,
Department of Cardiovascular Surgery, Konya, Turkey

© Springer Nature Switzerland AG 2020   157
B. Jabbari (ed.), *Botulinum Toxin Treatment in Surgery, Dentistry,
and Veterinary Medicine*, https://doi.org/10.1007/978-3-030-50691-9_7

BTXs have been increasingly used worldwide in clinical practice since the 1980s. The clinical use of BTX has dramatically increased in the last two decades, predominantly in cosmetics, hyperkinetic movement disorders, spasticity, and migraine. The clinical use of BTX in cardiovascular diseases is rather limited when compared to other fields of medicine where BTX has been in common use for over 30 years. Among researchers, there has been an increased interest in the use of BTXs for vascular and cardiac conditions based on both experimental and clinical studies. The long duration of action and relatively irreversible but potent effects make BTX subtypes valuable in clinical use, especially in vascular surgery.

The main use of BTX subtypes can be categorized into either cardiac use or vascular use in cardiovascular disorders. The basic data and research performed in this area so far is rather limited. Cardiac use has focused on suppression of post-operative rhythm, especially atrial fibrillation (AF). Vascular use of BTX (mainly BTX-A and BTX-B) is mainly investigated for prevention of arterial spasm, either in graft patencies or native arteries as in Raynaud's phenomenon. This chapter will briefly review the experimental data and clinical use of BTX in cardiovascular disorders, highlighting recent published articles and our experience; new perspectives for potential use of BTX will be addressed as well.

Cardiac Use of BTX for Rhythm Disturbances

The concept of using BTX in management of cardiac disorders began in the late 1980s by Lamanna et al. [1]. They injected BTX into the coronary artery of experimental animals and reported direct cardiac effects. In their study, crystalline-type BTX-A caused temporary bradycardia and electrocardiographic changes in mice, rats, rabbits, and dogs. Cardiac contractile force was found to be depressed in dogs. What's more, electrocardiographic changes were indicative of conduction defects. The cardiac effects were spontaneously reversible in the intact animal without removal of the toxin, whereas in vitro studies of the isolated rat heart showed recovery of the cardiac effects of BTX-A only after washing out the toxin, denoting a physical rather than a chemical mechanism for the reversibility of its effects on the heart.

Physiologically, heart rate is regulated by parasympathetic ganglia in the heart. Acetylcholine released from the parasympathetic nerve terminals decreases heart rate. In humans, almost all parasympathetic inputs that influence the heart rate pass through the ganglionic cells in the sinoatrial (SA) fat pad, which overlies the right atrial junction of the right pulmonary veins [2]. This is also true for the dogs, and stimulation of parasympathetic neural elements in the SA fat pad decreases atrial rate, which may cause sinus arrest in dogs [3]. Tsuibo et al. tested whether BTX inhibits the parasympathetic ganglionic neurotransmission in the heart by selective injection of BTX-A into the SA fat pad in the anesthetized dog heart [4]. They demonstrated that BTX-A inhibited a decrease in sinus rate in response to cervical vagus nerve stimulation, when BTX had been injected into the SA fat pad before the vagus nerve stimulation. As a result, they suggested that BTX could inhibit the parasympathetic ganglionic neurotransmission in the dog heart in situ as it did in the neuromuscular junction in humans. Interestingly, BTX injected into the SA fat pad showed negative chronotropic responses to both stimulation of the cervical vagus nerves and to stimulation of the SA fat pad's parasympathetic neural elements but did not affect atrioventricular conduction time. They speculated that, by injection of BTX, they could regulate bradycardia at the ganglionic neurotransmission site in the heart. This idea would theoretically prevent the patients with certain ventricular arrhythmias from sudden death by reducing the sympathetic nerve stimulation of the heart.

After the suggestion that BTX injection into the epicardial fat pads could suppress AF inducibility, the idea was also tested in humans to determine if it could be effective in prevention of atrial tachyarrhythmias. As a cardiovascular surgeon, the most common arrhythmia we see after open heart surgery is AF. It is commonly seen 2–5 days after surgery, with an incidence of 10–50% [5]. Postoperative AF may lead to serious complications including impaired heart contractility leading to hemodynamic instability, cardiac failure, stroke, and even death [6]. To prevent AF in the postoperative period, beta-blocking agents are strongly recommended by the guidelines [7, 8]. If AF develops in the postoperative period, anticoagulation for a certain period of time is mandatory to prevent embolic attacks which may lead to postoperative bleeding, in conjunction with the use of antiarrhythmic drugs (e.g., amiodarone), or cardioversion in the early phase. Any of the medications suggested above have both beneficial and adverse effects on hemodynamic stability.

Experimentally and clinically, it is well known that autonomic nervous system plays a critical role in the initiation and maintenance of AF and activation of both the sympathetic and the parasympathetic nervous systems often precedes the onset of AF [9]. Since BTX blocks the exocytotic release of acetylcholine stored in the synaptic vesicles and thus interferes with cholinergic neurotransmission, it may have an effective role in regulating the SA node's electrical activity and signal transmission. Pokushalov et al. were the first to randomly compare the efficacy and safety of BTX injection into epicardial fat pads for preventing atrial tachyarrhythmias; the patients were followed for a period of 1 year [10]. In this study, patients with history of paroxysmal AF and indication for coronary artery bypass graft surgery were randomized to BTX or placebo groups. Fifty units of BTX-A was injected at four major epicardial fat pads during open heart surgery. There were no procedural complications. The incidence of early postoperative AF within 30 days after coronary artery bypass operation was 2 among the 30 patients (7%) in the BTX group and 9 among the 30 patients in the placebo group, which was statistically significant. The most important finding was observed in later follow-up of patients. In examinations between 30 days and up to 12 months after surgery, 7 of the 30 patients in the placebo group (27%) had recurrent AF, but none (0%) of the BTX patients developed AF, which was also statistically significant. Although the blocking effect of BTX is temporary and usually limited to 3–6 months, the longevity of the effects was more than predicted. Since the patients are more susceptible to postoperative AF and other tachyarrhythmias in the early postoperative period, tempo-

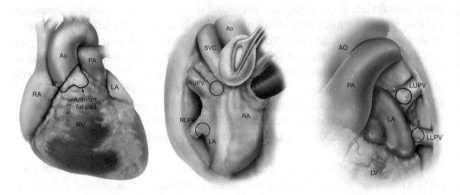

Fig. 7.1 Injection sites of BTX, as viewed from the perspective of the operating surgeon. (Figure is derived from the article Waldron et al. [12], with permission of the publisher)

rary (3–6 months) effect of BTX might lead to more AF-free periods after the operations. One of the major advantages of BTX injection is suppression of AF without any destruction of the anatomic structures, or conduction pathways, in contrast to surgical management of arrhythmia (e.g., Maze operations). This study also showed that BTX injection did not delay timing of discharge from the intensive care unit, increase hospital length of stay, or cause any other identifiable postoperative complications.

The same group also extended the follow-up of the patients to 3 years and published their data in 2018 [11]. The main findings of this report were that during the completed 3-year follow-up period, the incidence of any atrial tachyarrhythmia as well as AF burden was significantly lower in patients who received BTX injections during coronary artery bypass graft operation than those who received placebo. Also, the number of hospitalizations, mainly due to arrhythmia recurrences, was significantly lower in the BTX group.

Recently, a new randomized study was published by Waldron et al., with epicardial injection of BTX-A [12]. In this study, a broader spectrum of patients was studied including not only coronary artery bypass graft but also valvular procedures and patients with higher median age. A total of 130 patients were enrolled in this study and were assigned to receive either BTX-A or saline injection in five epicardial pads containing ganglionic plexi. In terms of methodology, the trial targeted left atrial ganglionic plexus as well as the anterior fat pad, which differs from the previously tested methodology (Fig. 7.1). Although the overall incidence of postoperative AF was reduced (36.5% and 47.8%, respectively), this difference was not statistically significant. Also, no significant differences were seen between length of hospital stay and occurrence of adverse effects in patients who received BTX injection or placebo. As a result, this study failed to show prevention of postoperative AF after BTX injection.

The left atrial sizes, as a marker of atrial structural remodeling, which commonly is associated with increased risk for AF, were considerably different between the studies of Pokushalov and Waldron. Not only the standard patients but also the inclusion of valvular diseases with increased left atrial sizes might be the possible explanations for the inconsistent results between studies [13]. To better identify the role of BTX in prevention of postoperative AF, larger controlled studies to identify the best injection points in the epicardial fat are needed.

Vascular Use of BTX in Cardiac Surgery for Vessel Preparation and Anastomosis

Coronary artery bypass graft surgery is the most common cardiac surgery worldwide, since it is the most effective method of revascularization. In order to supply blood flow distal to the occluded/stenotic coronary arteries, vascular grafts are used. Among the vascular grafts used, arterial grafts (internal mammary artery, radial artery) are known to have better patency rates when compared to venous grafts (e.g., great saphenous vein). The most common problem for arterial graft use in bypass surgery is graft spasm, which may lead to failure of the graft patency as a result of occlusion. Various surgical techniques and pharmacological agents have been proposed to overcome this problem. Unfortunately, there is no perfect vasodilator agent since vasospasm can have multiple causes. Generally, calcium channel blocking agents, sodium nitroprusside, and papaverine are the most commonly used agents to prevent spasm. In coronary artery bypass graft surgery, papaverine is used topically (1 mg/mL, 2.7 mmol/L) to prevent spasm of internal mammary artery. However, slow onset of action and acidity of the material, which may harm the endothelium if used intraluminally, are potential side effects. Sodium nitroprusside (1.7 mmol/L, 0.5 mg/mL) is very potent but may cause hypotension if it enters into systemic circulation [14]. The ideal vasodilator agent should have long-lasting effects with minimal, if any, systemic side effects and should not be toxic to the grafts. Unfortunately, currently, there is no ideal vasodilator agent readily available for this procedure.

The idea of using BTX for inhibition of muscle contraction to assess whether it might be effective in preventing arterial graft spasm was investigated by Murakami et al. [15]. Samples of abdominal aorta from male Wistar rats were cut into 2 mm rings and treated with various doses of BTX (type C solution) or papaverine for 30 min. In the presence of KCl and noradrenaline, almost all concentrations of BTX completely inhibited arterial contraction when compared with controls. Spasm prevention was lost after 60 min in rings with papaverine but persisted for 120 min in rings with BTX. Histologically, there was no arterial wall deformity with BTX. A positive change in blood flow of the femoral arteries was also observed after direct injection of BTX-A in rats [16].

As cardiovascular surgeons, we routinely use internal mammary and radial arteries as conduits during bypass surgery. The concept of using radial artery was almost abandoned after its improper use in the 1990s but became popular again after the concept of "full arterial revascularization" in the 2010s. Better preservation of the graft and choosing target vessels improved the patency of radial arteries. Although the prevention of vasospasm is overcome by the use of vasodilator agents, such as papaverine, the idea of finding nontoxic and long-lasting agents is still a common problem for surgeons. For this reason, we conducted a study using human radial artery in vitro and compared the vasodilatory effects of papaverine and BTX-A [17]. This study is the first in the literature using human radial arteries in isolated organ baths to test for prevention of vasospasm by BTX-A. Contraction responses for different doses of serotonin and endothelin-1 were evaluated as a percent of maximum contraction response elicited by 80 mM KCl. The inhibitory effects of BTX-A and papaverine on contraction responses taken at the beginning were compared with the 1st and 2nd hour responses. Inhibitory effects of BTX-A and papaverine against the contractile agent were evaluated by comparing the results of the first and the last (0th and 2nd hour) application.

Results of this in vitro study showed that pretreatment with both papaverine and BTX-A prevents vasospasm of human radial artery rings. In low concentrations (BTX-A, 10^{-8} M, and papaverine, 10^{-6} M), papaverine was found to be more effective on serotonin, both at 0th and 2nd hours. Both BTX-A and papaverine inhibited the maximum contractile effect of endothelin-1 to the same extent at the 0th hour, but the inhibitory effect of BTX-A was significantly stronger at the 2nd hour.

In high concentrations (BTX-A, 10^{-6} M, and papaverine, 10^{-4} M), papaverine showed stronger inhibition on serotonin, whereas both agents had similar action of inhibition on endothelin-1-mediated maximum contraction responses.

The most important point of this study was to show the long-lasting action of BTX-A, which is crucial for ideal vasodilatory agents, since most of the occlusions of the conduits are seen during the first 24 hours or within early postoperative periods (30 days), which are mainly due to anastomotic problems, graft vasospasm and thrombosis, or hemodynamic instability of the patients. This study successfully proved that BTX-A inhibited both endothelin-1 and serotonin-induced contractions, and its effectiveness did not decrease over time in contrast to what was observed with papaverine. The histological examination also revealed that all of the vascular layers (intima, media, and adventitia) kept their integrity without any signs of fibrosis, inflammation, mitosis, or necrosis, which is the desired and the optimal outcome expected of a vasodilatory agent.

In another study, we studied the effects of BTX-A and papaverine on human saphenous vein and internal mammary artery grafts in the same manner, and the preliminary results are presented here [18]. This study showed, for the first time, that incubation with BTX-A effectively relaxed both internal mammary artery and saphenous vein rings contracted with serotonin and endothelin-1. Duration of the vasodilatory effect of BTX-A was longer than papaverine. This inhibition of contraction and vasodilatory effect varied according to vasoconstrictor agent, dose, and vessel type, and contrary to papaverine did not decrease with time. As seen in the radial artery study, no vascular damage was seen after incubation with BTX-A. The details of this study will be published later.

These two studies performed in human radial and internal mammary arteries may open new perspectives in clinical use; for example, BTX-A might be considered as an alternative topical agent for prevention of arterial graft spasms in coronary artery bypass graft surgery. Positive in vitro results might not be seen in in vivo conditions; to be able to give definitive recommendations about its clinical use, in vivo randomized clinical trials should be designed.

Another issue in preservation of graft patency is thrombosis. Usually, thrombosis is prevented by the use of anti-aggregating agents, such as acetyl salicylic acid or clopidogrel. Not only cardiovascular surgeons but also plastic surgeons and orthopedic surgeons deal with vascular anastomosis for tissue transfer for reconstruction of complex defects throughout the body. The most common cause of free flap failure is vascular anastomotic problems and thrombosis. Its prevalence is evenly distributed among isolated arterial and venous structures or simultaneous arterial and venous failure [19]. Factors contributing to a difficult anastomosis include vasospasm, traumatized recipient vessels within the zone of injury, scar, infection, and radiation. In an animal model where free tissue transfer was performed, Clemens et al. used BTX-A in Sprague-Dawley rats [20]. Rats were pretreated with BTX-A subcutaneously injected into a randomly selected femoral vessel. The contralateral limb in each animal was similarly injected with saline and served as a control. After 5 days, femoral vessels were measured to determine the effect of neuromuscular blockade on diameter. Vessels were then divided and reanastomosed and subjected to systemic peripheral vasoconstrictor, phenylephrine, and lower extremity thermal effect of ice bath. Vessel patency was recorded before cold challenge and 1 hour thereafter. In this experimental model, the diameter was larger in all neuromuscularly blocked vessels. The BTX-A-treated arterial average was larger than the matched control, and also the venous average was significantly larger. As a result, anastomosis difficulty and time spent on the procedure were significantly less in BTX-A-pretreated group. Patency was 100% in BTX group, whereas it was 44% in the saline control group 1 hour after vasospastic challenge.

Similarly, Janz et al. transected and immediately repaired bilateral femoral arteries and veins of 25 rats via microscopic techniques [21]. Each rat had one leg randomly assigned to receive BTX-B; the contralateral side received normal saline. The rats were divided into five different groups, and each group was exposed to different vasospastic stresses, including systemic phenylephrine, and lower extremity cold temperature challenge at different time points (12, 24, 48, 72, and 120 hours). Then the wounds were reopened for evaluation of vessel diameter and thrombosis. Vessel thrombosis rate was significantly lower in BTX-B-treated group, and the average increase in diameter was significantly greater than that of control, regardless of patency.

This demonstration of both arterial and venous diameter increase and resistance to contraction in animal studies was consistent with our findings in the human radial artery, internal mammary artery, and great saphenous vein. As a future perspective, these findings may lead to the use of BTX-A in coronary artery anastomosis for enlargement of vessels, avoiding excessive contraction, and prevention of thrombosis. Also, they may be used for below-the-knee bypass surgery in patients with peripheral artery disease, where the vessel diameter is pretty small and subject to thrombosis due to poor runoff. Since BTX-A affects both arterial and venous systems, it might have beneficial effects on early maturation of arteriovenous fistula in end-stage renal failure patients. Of course, these are just theoretically derived possible effects and need to be objectively confirmed by well-designed, randomized, prospective studies.

Use of BTX in the Treatment of Functional Popliteal Artery Entrapment Syndrome

Popliteal artery entrapment syndrome (PAES) is a rare cause of exertional leg pain, caused by compression of neurovascular structures situated in the popliteal fossa by hypertrophic muscles. PAES is classified into two groups: anatomical and functional [22]. In the anatomical type, there is a clearly defined anatomical lesion which causes direct occlusion of the artery. According to the course of the popliteal artery, the anatomical variants were classified into types I–IV, with type V involving the popliteal vein in any of these types. These patients are typically older with sedentary lifestyle and present a relatively small group (0.6–3.4%) among PAES patients [23]. Usually the treatment is surgical in order to overcome symptoms.

Functional PAES is a more common form of the disease, with normal anatomy. Embryological development of the medial head of gastrocnemius muscle is more lateralized and responsible for the arterial compression of popliteal artery between it and the lateral condyle, lateral head of gastrocnemius, or plantaris [24]. Functional PAES patients are typically more active patients, younger, and with female predominance [23].

For management of functional PAES, surgical approach with myotomy is the treatment of choice. Surgical management often consists of lysis of fascial attachments and release of tendons (i.e., plantaris) and/or myotomy of the gastrocnemius, plantaris, and/or soleus muscles [25]. Unlike the management of anatomical PAES, most of the patients with functional PAES do not require vascular reconstruction; that's why myotomy is often enough and, hence, is the gold standard therapeutic option. Turnipseed reported 0% rate of recurrence among 43 patients treated by myotomy with a follow-up period of 8–84 months [26].

BTX injection for paralysis of muscles to manage various medical conditions is well established in the literature. BTX is commonly used for treatment of muscle spasticity, especially in cerebral palsy patients. Since functional PAES is caused predominantly by muscular factors affecting the flow of popliteal artery and the treatment of choice is mainly myotomy, the idea of a less invasive approach using BTX injections has been proposed. Theoretically, BTX injection might result in paralysis of muscular sliding, which may be responsible for the dynamic arterial occlusion; might provide localized muscle atrophy which may increase the space for vessel; and possibly might cause arterial smooth muscle relaxation of the popliteal artery resulting in vasodilation [27]. Gandor et al. were the first to apply BTX-A injections into the gastrocnemius and plantaris muscles in eight patients with functional popliteal entrapment syndrome [28]. In this study, 50 MU BTX-A was injected into the medial head of the gastrocnemius muscle, and 50 MU BTX-A into the plantaris muscle under EMG guidance. Clinical symptoms were reported to have improved in 81.3% of patients. A marked improvement was reported for ten legs (62.5%), a moderate improvement for two legs (12.5%), and a mild improvement for one leg (6.3%). Symptom improvement lasted for 4 months on average. As a result, they suggested BTX-A injection could be used as a noninvasive alternative to surgery.

In a series of two studies, Shahi et al. analyzed the use of BTX-A injection in 35 patients [25]. For the BTX treatment group, improvement of symptoms was achieved in 66% of patients at an average follow-up time of ten months.

In another study published by Hislop et al., functional PAES was treated with ultrasound-guided BTX-A injection [29]. In this study, 27 patients were included, with a mean age of 29 years (range of 16–65 years). All patients had symptoms for at least 3 months, and 18 patients (67%) had symptoms for longer than 2 years prior to diagnosis. After taking baseline treatment, all patients were given repeated "top-up" injections at 6–12 months. Patients provided subjective symptom reports at 6 and 12 months post intervention. No patients reported being worse off after the intervention, and nearly 60% had a favorable response at 12-month follow-up. Although BTX-A injection is expensive, the present findings also highlight that BTX-A treatments may result in fewer adverse effects than surgical treatment modalities.

Since PAES is a rare disease, patient selection and data collection is difficult, but all findings available so far suggest that more rigorous investigations are needed to confirm the effectiveness of BTX-A for treatment of functional PAES.

Use of BTX in Functional Vasospastic Disorders

Vasospastic disease is an inappropriate, reversible vascular constriction in the distal arteries caused by a variety of stimuli, most commonly cold or emotional stress. Vasospasm induces ischemia that results in pain, ulcerations, and disuse, often rendering the patient debilitated and depressed [30].

Raynaud's phenomenon is defined as reversible ischemia of digital arteries induced by cold exposure and stress. Raynaud's disease is an idiopathic cause of Raynaud's phenomenon, whereas Raynaud's syndrome is defined as a secondary sequel of associated diseases including lupus, scleroderma, rheumatoid arthritis, Sjogren syndrome, lymphoma, leukemia, lead exposure, diabetes mellitus, and drug-related causes including beta-blockers or oral contraceptives [31].

Either primary or secondary vasospastic disorders resulting in arterial insufficiency may cause episodic digital asphyxia. Therapeutic options include general preventive measures such as avoiding tobacco and caffeine consumption, preventing exposure to cold, and reducing or eliminating emotional stress. Medical therapy is usually necessary, but effectiveness varies. Calcium antagonists are used as first-line treatment as they reduce the number and severity of the episodes [32]. Other medical treatment options include aspirin or dipyridamole to inhibit platelet aggregation, topical nitrates, phosphodiesterase inhibitors, prostaglandin analogs, endothelin receptor antagonists, and short-term heparin anticoagulation for refractory cases [33–36]. In cases with intractable pain, surgical denervation with sympathectomy is the preferred therapeutic choice.

Based on the effectiveness of BTX-A in the management of focal dystonic and spastic syndromes as well as its recent in vitro differential effects on vasoconstriction and vasodilation, Sycha et al. proposed the use of BTX-A for the treatment of Raynaud's phenomenon. In 2004, they published the results of their pilot study on two patients [37]. They treated primary and secondary Raynaud's phenomenon patients with intradigital BTX-A injections; the clinical response and the superficial blood flow was assessed using laser Doppler interferometry. Their data confirmed beneficial effects on clinical symptoms and also objectively showed an increased blood flow on Doppler scans. Interestingly, there was also some suggestion of mild systemic effect on noninjected fingers. After this pilot study, the use of BTX-A in Raynaud's phenomenon increased, and more studies were published confirming the effectiveness of BTX in management of Raynaud's phenomenon.

After the incidental finding that a patient treated for palmar hyperhidrosis by BTX showed elimination of symptoms of Raynaud's syndrome for 3 months, van Beek et al. hypothesized that BTX-A induced digital artery neuromuscular blockade [38]. They reported the use of BTX-A in 11 patients with Raynaud's syndrome presenting with intractable pain at rest, impending infarction, infarction, and ischemic ulcerations that were refractory to conventional oral and parenteral therapy. Their protocol was to inject all the fingers and palm of the symptomatic hand with an equal distribution of Botox into each injection site. Only if the thumb were symptomatic would it be injected at its base. Each hand was injected with 200 U of BTX. Targeted anatomic sites included the superficial palmar arch, common digital arteries, and proper digital arteries. Through multiple injection sites, 8–12 U of BTX solution was injected into each of the 8–10 areas previously marked. A total of 11 patients were followed with an average follow-up of 9.6 months, the longest being 30 months. All patients had relief of digital pain at rest from 9–10/10 to a level of 0–2/10. They all reported decreased episodes of vasospasm and cyanosis. All small digital ulcerations healed spontaneously. Skin temperature was recorded and all patients demonstrated 1.0–4.0 °C improvement in their skin surface temperature. None of the patients suffered any systemic complications related to the BTX. In this study, BTX was thought to have dual action: inhibition of vasospasm by blocking cold-induced vasoconstriction and prevention of α_2 receptor recruitment to vascular smooth muscle in cold conditions. Because of the complexity of surgical digital artery sympathectomy along with its associated high risk of persistent symptoms, the authors concluded that the therapeutic use of BTX-A injections represents an attractive alternative therapy.

Fregene et al. tried to identify patient subgroups that would most benefit from injection therapy and to define a uniform pattern for injection technique [39]. A total of 26 patients were treated with a range of 10–100 U of BTX-A, with a significant decrease in pain scores in all groups along with significant improvement in transcutaneous oxygen saturations and ulcer healing. However, they were unable to find a specific injection site statistically superior to others.

Neumeister et al. published a retrospective analysis of 19 patients with Raynaud's phenomenon [30]. All patients suffered from ischemic pain at rest. Sixteen patients (84%) noticed an immediate increase in perfusion of the fingers and a significant reduction in pain. A laser Doppler examination evaluated and verified the increase in digital blood flow. BTX did not benefit the three patients with advanced connective tissue disease. They reported that a fascinating aspect of BTX injection was the almost immediate and dramatic reduction in pain. One would not expect such a decrease in pain to be a result only of restoring blood flow, because many patients had ulcerations that should have remained tender until healed. Digit sensibility was not affected. They concluded that BTX might act through modulation of the innervations of the vessels or by blockade of the chronic neuropathic pain pathways.

In a 3-year follow-up study by Medina et al., a total of 15 patients with severe Raynaud's phenomenon who required infiltration with BTX-A were recruited [40]. The infiltration protocol comprised reconstitution of a vial containing 100 units of BTX-A in 5 mL of saline serum (diluted to 20 IU/mL) and injection of BTX-A (4–8 IU of BTX, depending on the severity) at the base of the lateral aspects of all the fingers, except the first finger, since this is least frequently affected (Fig. 7.2). Thirty minutes after injection of BTX, six patients already showed a response, and four of these were noted as "very good." This immediate response had been observed by other authors, with particular significance when it came to a reduction in pain. The reduction in the number of weekly vasospasm episodes was significant 1 month after the treatment, decreasing from an average of 30 to an average of 14. The average decrease in pain intensity – which was the earliest and most striking response – was also statistically significant. In addition, five patients continued to improve

Fig. 7.2 Injection sites of BTX in Raynaud's disease at the base of the lateral aspects of all the fingers, except the first. (Figure is derived from the article Medina et al. [40], with permission of the publisher)

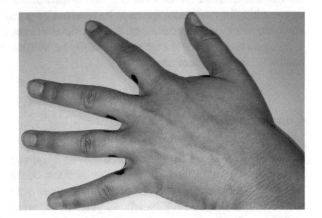

beyond the first month, reaching the maximum response at 6 months. For the others, after 6 months, both the number of episodes and the severity of pain remained stable with respect to the data recorded 1 month after the treatment. They concluded that BTX was a safe, accessible, and effective therapeutic alternative for the treatment of severe Raynaud's phenomenon, allowing the nonresponders to conventional treatments to maintain a good quality of life, through annual injections before the winter period.

Different from the other studies, Weum et al. performed precise administration of BTX around the radial artery using a single ultrasound-guided injection for vasospastic disorders [41]. Ten patients with the diagnosis of either primary or secondary Raynaud were included in their pilot study. Under ultrasound guidance, 20 IU BTX-A was administered around the radial artery and its adherent veins 3–5 cm proximal to the wrist. One patient reported temporary reduced grip strength, most likely due to leakage of BTX to the flexor pollicis longus muscle. All patients reported reduced number of vasospastic episodes, warmer hands, and reduced pain. This novel approach could be a promising treatment approach for vasospastic disorders of the hands in patients with primary and secondary Raynaud.

Use of BTX in Other Vascular Pathologies

In a case report published by Danielson et al., chemodenervation with BTX-A injection into the anterior scalene muscle effectively improved subclavian artery blood flow in a patient with thoracic outlet syndrome. This report suggested expansion of the role of BTX beyond a therapeutic option to include its use as a diagnostic test and predictor for surgical intervention [42].

With the proven effects of BTX on vasospastic disorders highlighted, theoretically BTX has potential applications for other vasospastic conditions of the hand, including frostbite, regional pain syndrome, reflex sympathetic dystrophy, vasopressor-induced digital ischemia, and extravasation injuries [38]. Any pathology resulting in vasospasm seems to be resolved by perivascular injection of BTX; however, since documentation of the beneficial effects is mandatory in order to propose its use as a novel treatment modality in additional conditions, randomized controlled trials are necessary.

Conclusion

Although BTX is approved for treatment of blepharospasm, cervical dystonia, hyperhidrosis, moderate-to-severe glabellar lines, ocular strabismus, and torticollis by the US Food and Drug Administration, there are also off-label uses, as discussed in this chapter [30]. Nearly 40 years of experience is available for the use of BTX in plastic surgery and ophthalmology, but its use in cardiovascular disorders is relatively new and in its infancy/crawling period. Recently published articles and ongoing studies show a promising role for use of BTX in a variety for cardiovascular disorders; its application will probably be extended as the mechanism of action, and effects of BTXs become better known and established in properly designed studies.

Acknowledgment We thank Ipek Duman, MD, for her collaboration in our previous studies performed by botulinum toxin and Niyazi Gormus, MD, Prof. Dr., chief of our clinic, for his endless support in our clinical and scientific studies.

References

1. Lamanna C, el-Hage AN, Vick JA. Cardiac effects of botulinal toxin. Arch Int Pharmacodyn Ther. 1998;293:69–83.
2. Carlson MD, Geha AS, Hsu J, Martin PJ, Levy MN, Jacobs G, et al. Selective stimulation of parasympathetic nerve fibers to the human sinoatrial node. Circulation. 1992;85:1311–7.
3. Furukawa Y, Wallick DW, Carlson MD, Martin PJ. Cardiac electrical responses to vagal stimulation of fibers to discrete cardiac regions. Am J Physiol. 1990;258:1112–8.
4. Tsuibo M, Furukawa Y, Kurogouchi F, Nakajima K, Hirose M, Chiba S. Botulinum neurotoxin A blocks cholinergic ganglionic neurotransmission in the dog heart. Jpn J Pharmacol. 2002;89:249–54.
5. Nisanoglu V, Erdil N, Aldemir M, Ozgur B, BeratCihan H, Yologlu S, et al. Atrial fibrillation after coronary artery bypass grafting in elderly patients: incidence and risk factor analysis. Thorac Cardiovasc Surg. 2007;55:32–8.
6. Ahlsson A, Bodin L, Fengsrud E, Englund A. Patients with postoperative atrial fibrillation have a doubled cardiovascular mortality. Scand Cardiovasc J. 2009;43:330–6.
7. Eckardt L, Hausler KG, Ravens U, Borggrefe M, Kirchof P. ESC guidelines on atrial fibrillation: summary of the most relevant recommendations and modifications. Herz. 2016;41:677–83.
8. Andrade JG, Macle L, Nattel S, Verma A, Caims J. Contemporary atrial fibrillation management: a comparison of the current AHA/ACC/HRS, CCS, and ESC guidelines. Can J Cardiol. 2017;33:965–76.
9. Amar D, Zhang H, Miodownik S, Kadish AH. Competing autonomic mechanisms precede the onset of postoperative atrial fibrillation. J Am Coll Cardiol. 2003;42:1262–8.
10. Pokushalov E, Kozlov B, Romanov A, Strelniov A, Bayramova S, Sergeevichev D, et al. Long-term suppression of atrial fibrillation by botulinum toxin injection into epicardial fat pads in patients undergoing cardiac surgery: one-year follow up of a randomized pilot study. Circ Arrhythm Electrophysiol. 2015;8:1334–41.
11. Romanov A, Pokushalov E, Ponomarev D, Bayramova S, Shabanov V, Losik D, et al. Long-term suppression of atrial fibrillation by botulinum toxin injection into epicardial fat pads in patients undergoing cardiac surgery: three-year follow up of a randomized study. Heart Rhythm. 2019;16:172–7.
12. Waldron NH, Cooter M, Haney JC, Schroder JN, Gaca JG, Lin SS, et al. Temporary autonomic modulation with botulinum toxin type A to reduce atrial fibrillation after cardiac surgery. Heart Rhythm. 2019;16:178–84.
13. Fatahian A. Botulinum toxin injection into epicardial fat pads: a promising potential modality for prevention of postoperative atrial fibrillation after cardiac surgery. Braz J Cardiovasc Surg. 2019;34:643.
14. Rosenfeldt FL, He GW, Buxton BF, Angus JA. Pharmacology of coronary artery bypass. Ann Thorac Surg. 1999;67:878–88.

15. Murakami E, Iwata H, Imaizumi M, Takemura H. Prevention of arterial graft spasm by botulinum toxin: an in-vitro experiment. Interact Cardiovasc Thorac Surg. 2009;9:395–8.
16. Hayashi M, Shimizu Y, Sato M, Yokoyama T, Yosimoto S. Changes in the blood flow of the femoral artery by botulinum toxin in rats. Ann Plast Surg. 2014;73:98–101.
17. Tanyeli O, Duman I, Dereli Y, Gormus N, Toy H, SAhin AS. Relaxation matters: comparison of in-vitro vasodilatory role of botulinum toxin-A and papaverine in human radial artery grafts. J Cardiothorac Surg. 2019;14:15.
18. Duman I, Tanyeli O, Dereli Y, Oltulu P, Toy H, Sahin AS. Effects of botulinum toxin A and papaverine in preventing spasm of human saphenous vein and internal mammary artery grafts: an in vitro study. 67th International Congress of the European Society of Cardiovascular and Endovascular Surgery, Strasbourg, France. J Cardiovasc Surg. 2018;59(Suppl 2):21–2.
19. Nahabedian MY, Momen B, Manson PN. Factors associated with anastomotic failure after microvascular reconstruction of the breast. Plast Reconstr Surg. 2004;114:74–82.
20. Clemens MW, Higgins JP, Shaw Wilgis EF. Prevention of anastomotic thrombosis by botulinum toxin A in an animal model. Plast Reconstr Surg. 2009;123:64–70.
21. Janz BA, Thomas PR, Fanua SP, Dunn RE, Wilgis EF, Means KR Jr. Prevention of anastomotic thrombosis by botulinum toxin B after acute injury in a rat model. J Hand Surg Am. 2011;36:1585–91.
22. Di Marzo L, Cavallaro A. Popliteal vascular entrapment. World J Surg. 2005;29:43–5.
23. Turnipseed WD. Popliteal entrapment in runners. Clin Sport Med. 2012;31:321–8.
24. Pillai J. A current interpretation of popliteal vascular entrapment. J Vasc Surg. 2008;48:61–5.
25. Shahi N, Arosemena M, Kwon J, Abai B, Salvatore D, diMuzio P. Functional popliteal artery entrapment syndrome: a review of diagnosis and management. Ann Vasc Surg. 2019;59:259–67.
26. Turnipseed WD. Functional popliteal artery entrapment syndrome: a poorly understood and often missed diagnosis that is frequently mistreated. J Vasc Surg. 2009;49:1189–95.
27. Hislop M, Kennedy D, Cramp B, Dhupelia S. Functional popliteal artery entrapment syndrome: poorly understood and frequently missed? A review of clinical features, appropriate investigations, and treatment options. J Sports Med. 2014;2014:105953.
28. Gandor F, Tisch S, Grabs AJ, Delaney AJ, Bester L, Darveniza P. Botulinum toxin A in functional popliteal entrapment syndrome: a new approach to a difficult diagnosis. J Neural Transm. 2014;121:1297–301.
29. Hislop M, Brideaux A, Dhupelia S. Functional popliteal artery entrapment syndrome: use of ultrasound guided Botox injection as a non-surgical treatment option. Skelet Radiol. 2017;46:1241–8.
30. Neumeister MW, Chambers CB, Herron MS, Webb K, Wietfeldt J, Gillespie JN, et al. Botox therapy for ischemic digits. Plast Reconstr Surg. 2009;124:191–200.
31. Herrick AL. Pathogenesis of Raynaud's phenomenon. Rheumatology. 2005;44:587–96.
32. Thompson AE, Pope JE. Calcium channel blockers for primary Raynaud's phenomenon: a meta-analysis. Rheumatology. 2005;44:145–50.
33. Matucci-Cerinic M, Denton CP, Frust DE, Mayes MD, Hsu VM, Carpentier P, et al. Bosentan treatment of digital ulcers related to systemic sclerosis. Results from RAPIDS-2 randomised, double-blind placebo-controlled trial. Ann Rheum Dis. 2011;70:32–8.
34. Wigley FM, Wise RA, Seibold JR, McCloskey DA, Kujala G, Medsger TA Jr, et al. Intravenous iloprost infusion in patients with Raynaud phenomenon secondary to systemic sclerosis. A multicentric placebo-controlled, double-blind study. Ann Intern Med. 1994;120:199–206.
35. Nguyen VA, Eisendle K, Gruber I, Hughe B, Reider D, Reider N. Effect of the dual endothelin receptor antagonist bosentan on Raynaud's phenomenon secondary to systemic sclerosis: a double-blind prospective, randomized, placebo-controlled pilot study. Rheumatology. 2010;49:583–7.

36. Uroskie J, Schmidt C, Baratz MF. Vascular disorders of the hand and upper extremity. In: Beredjiklian P, Bozentka DJ, editors. Review of hand surgery. Philadelphia: Saunders; 2004. p. 63–78.
37. Sycha T, Graninger M, Auff E, Schnider P. Botulinum toxin in the treatment of Raynaud's phenomenon: a pilot study. Eur J Clin Investig. 2004;34:312–3.
38. Van Beek AL, Lim PK, Gear AJL, Marc RP. Management of vasospastic disorders with botulinum toxin A. Plast Reconstr Surg. 2007;119:217–26.
39. Fregene A, Ditmars D, Siddiqui A. Botulinum toxin type A: a treatment option for digital ischemia in patients with Raynaud's phenomenon. J Hand Surg. 2009;34:446–52.
40. Medina S, Zubiaur AG, Casillas NV, Rodriguez IP, Ruiz L, Izquierdo C, et al. Botulinum toxin type A in the treatment of Raynaud's phenomenon: a three-year follow-up study. Eur J Rheumatol. 2018;5:224–9.
41. Weum S, Weerd L. Ultrasound -guided sympathetic block of the radial artery with botulinum toxin to treat vasospasm. Plast Reconstr Surg Glob Open. 2018;6:e1836.
42. Danielson K, Odderson IR. Botulinum toxin type A improves blood flow in vascular thoracic outlet syndrome. Am J Phys Med Rehabil. 2008;87(11):956–9.

Chapter 8
Botulinum Toxin A in Abdominal Wall Reconstruction

Allaeys Mathias and Berrevoet Frederik

Abstract Reconstruction of large abdominal wall defects is often a challenge for both surgeons and patients. Preoperative conditioning prior to surgery can be crucial for success. Administration of botulinum toxin A (BTA) in the lateral abdominal wall for stretching the musculature seems to provide myofascial advancement and enlargement of the torso diameter. Although the use of BTA has increased since its introduction in 2009, the current evidence on both its safety and efficacy, as well as on its exact role in the treatment algorithm of these types of hernias, remains undetermined. In this chapter, we aim to give a complete overview on the current evidence on the use of BTA in abdominal wall reconstruction.

Keywords Abdominal wall repair · Incisional hernia · Botulinum toxin A · Giant hernia · Loss of domain

Introduction

Abdominal wall surgery encompasses the treatment of fascial defects. These lead to an abnormal bulge of the peritoneum (i.e., the hernia sac), which contains visceral structures. Primary hernias are mostly categorized by location, varying from the frequent inguinal, umbilical, and epigastric hernias to the somewhat less common Spigelian (at the semilunar line) and lumbar defects (Petit and Grynfeltt). These hernias always present in distinct anatomical regions with known structural weakness.

An incisional hernia, however, will always present as a result of a previous surgical intervention, in which the aponeurotic layers of the incision heal incompletely. This leads to a fascial defect that will gradually enlarge over time due to physiological intra-abdominal pressure changes and fibrosis of the lateral abdominal wall

A. Mathias · B. Frederik (✉)
Department of General and HPB Surgery and Liver Transplantation, University Hospital of Ghent, Ghent, Belgium
e-mail: Frederik.Berrevoet@Ugent.be

© Springer Nature Switzerland AG 2020
B. Jabbari (ed.), *Botulinum Toxin Treatment in Surgery, Dentistry, and Veterinary Medicine*, https://doi.org/10.1007/978-3-030-50691-9_8

muscles. So one can understand that virtually any location in the abdominal wall can present with an incisional hernia. Due to a median laparotomy, being the most commonly used access in open abdominal surgery, midline incisional hernias comprise the bulk of these defects.

When the linea alba is cut during midline laparotomy and afterward fails to heal completely, the insertion of the lateral oblique muscles is lost. This results in passive unloading of the lateral abdominal wall, because the normal force across the myofascial structure is lost. The work by Dubay et al. showed that the disruption of this equilibrium of loading forces induces pathologic fibrosis, disuse atrophy, and changes in muscle fiber-type composition in the internal oblique muscles [1]. This will then subsequently lead to lateral retraction of the abdominal wall and hernia width progression with therapeutic consequences as well, as the forces to bring the midline back together become much stronger, leading to a higher tension repair and thus increasing the risk of recurrence after hernia repair.

As one of the most frequent complications after abdominal surgery, incisional hernias have a reported incidence of up to 20%, with this number going as high as 35% in high-risk patients [2]. These hernias cause significant morbidity, impair quality of life, and form a substantial economic burden [3]. Predisposing factors for hernia formation are diabetes mellitus, obesity, cachexia, increasing patient age, male sex, chronic obstructive pulmonary disease (COPD), history of or surgery for abdominal aortic aneurysm, anemia, smoking, corticosteroids, upper midline incision, previous median laparotomy, previous incisional hernia, emergency surgery, and prior local wound infection [4, 5].

When ventral hernias become very large, with a laterolateral diameter of around and over 15 cm, surgery becomes more and more challenging (Fig. 8.1). Repair is then associated with a higher rate of impaired wound healing, a longer hospital stay, a higher rate of reoperations and readmissions, and increased recurrence rates.

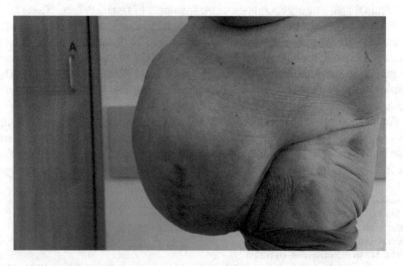

Fig. 8.1 Clinical example of a giant ventral hernia with loss of domain

For research purposes and unification, the European Hernia Society proposed a classification system in 2009. Here, hernias are subdivided according to localization (five midline regions and three lateral regions), width of the defect, and whether or not the defect has been repaired before [6]. This, however, does not suffice as an adequate guide for clinical and surgical strategy decision-making. In 2014, a definition was proposed of what entailed a complex abdominal wall hernia [7]. Again, size and location were factored in, but also contamination and soft tissue condition, patient's history as well as risk factors, and the clinical scenario. This somewhat illustrates that hernia repair comprises more than simply closing a fascial defect. Patients who present with large and complex abdominal wall defects are frequently patients with an extensive medical and surgical history and concomitant comorbidities, placing them at risk for a higher rate of surgical and nonsurgical complications.

Surgical Technique

As stated above, the abdominal flank muscles exert a continuous lateral force, which impedes bringing the fascial edges together (i.e., the primary goal in incisional hernia surgery). In a standard retromuscular repair, the medial edges of the posterior rectus sheath are cut, and the retromuscular plane is developed onto the semilunar line. This creates a retromuscular pocket where a mesh is then placed. Cutting the fascial envelope of the rectus sheath also flattens and widens the rectus muscle, which leads to a medial gain of around 5 cm (Fig. 8.2) [8]. Generally speaking, in a hernia defect width larger than 10 cm, a standard retromuscular dissection will not suffice. The wider the defect becomes, the lower the rate of primary fascial closure and the higher the rate of recurrence. Surgery for these larger defects also predisposes to a higher risk for local wound complications and places the patient at risk for respiratory complications. Furthermore, a large ventral hernia can lead to significant loss of domain, where a large portion of the visceral contents (>25%) sits outside of the abdominal cavity [9]. When tackling these hernias and reducing the contents into the abdomen, these patients have an elevated risk of developing intra-abdominal hypertension and subsequent abdominal compartment syndrome.

Bridging, in contrast, is a technique in which the anterior aponeurotic layers can not be fully approximated, and in which cases a mesh is placed on top of the anterior fascia and fixed with a large overlap, thus "bridging" the defect. Although not always possible, this is best avoided, since it leads to more bulging (pseudohernia) and possibly higher recurrence rates. It also does not reconstitute the functional core anatomy of the abdominal wall.

Various extra surgical strategies exist to overcome the problem of bridging the defect. In component separation techniques, one of the lateral abdominal muscles and its aponeurosis is cut to provide added medialization of the anterior fascia. This can either be the external oblique muscle (anterior component separation (Fig. 8.3); Ramirez et al. [10]) or the transversus abdominis muscle (transverse abdominis release or TAR (Fig. 8.4); Novitsky et al. [11]). Both of these techniques flatten and

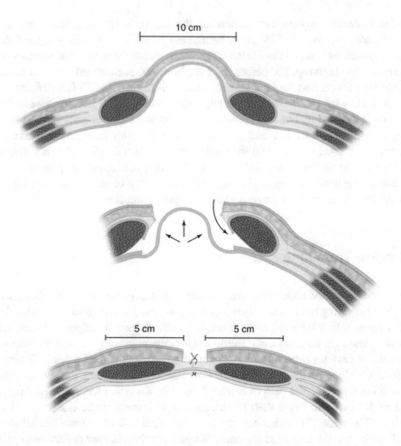

Fig. 8.2 A standard retromuscular hernia repair, as described by Jean Rives and René Stoppa. (From book: Hernia Surgery Current Principles. ©Springer International Publishing Switzerland 2016. Online ISBN 978-3-319-27470-6 – Reproduced with permission from Springer publishing)

stretch the remaining two lateral wall muscles, making it easier to bring the midline together.

In progressive pneumoperitoneum (PPP), the abdomen is gradually distended by daily insufflation of room air through a surgically placed catheter. This is usually achieved over a period of 7–14 days, after which the hernia repair is carried out subsequently. PPP primes the abdominal cavity for the added volume of visceral contents when reducing the hernia, thus reducing the rate of postoperative intra-abdominal hypertension and increasing the rate of anterior fascial closure.

Botulinum Toxin A in Hernia Repair

Botulinum toxin A (BTA) is known to induce flaccid paralysis in directly targeted muscle groups. This effect gradually begins after 2–3 days of administration, with a maximum effect after 2–4 weeks. After 3 months, the paralytic effect will then

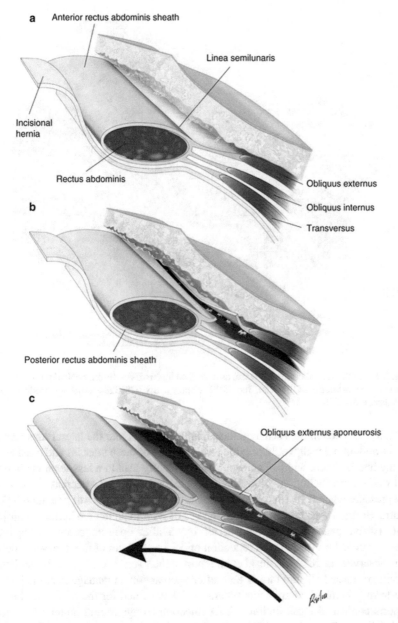

Fig. 8.3 Anterior component separation, as described by Ramirez. (From book: Minimally Invasive Component Separation for the Repair of Large Abdominal Wall Defects. ©Springer International Publishing AG 2017. Online ISBN 978-3-319-55868-4. Reproduced with permission from Springer Publishing)

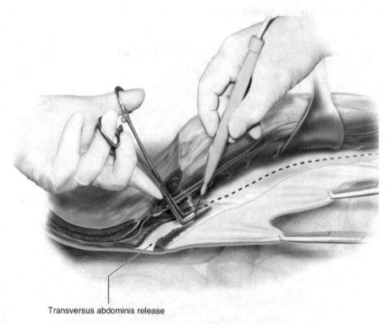

Transversus abdominis release

Renard Y, Lardière-Deguelte S, de Mestier L, et al. Management of large incisional hernias with loss of domain:
A prospective series of patients prepared by progressive preoperative pneumoperitoneum.
Surgery. 2016;160(2):426-435. doi:10.1016/j.surg.2016.03.033

Fig. 8.4 Transversus abdominis release, as described by Novitsky. (From book: Atlas of abdominal wall reconstruction. ©Elsevier, Inc. 2017. eBook ISBN 9780323428019 – reproduced with permission from Elsevier)

steadily start declining. As a hypothesis, injecting BTA into the lateral musculature of the abdominal wall would provide an elongation of these muscles and a reduction of the hernia defect width. This would subsequently lead to a less-tension abdominal wall reconstruction. In 2006, Kakmak et al. demonstrated a decrease in abdominal pressure when BTA was injected into the abdominal muscles of a rat model [12]. Ibarra-Hurtado was the first to report the use of BTA in an in vivo hernia repair [13, 14]. Twelve patients undergoing hernia repair after open abdomen management were treated. An overall mean reduction of 5.25 ± 2.32 cm of the transverse defect was observed. In 2012, Zielinski et al. reported their series of 18 patients, achieving a primary fascial closure rate of 83% after open abdomen management [15]. Here, the term "chemical components separation" was coined for the first time. Further reports confirmed these findings: BTA injection elongates and flattens the lateral abdominal wall muscles and decreases the hernia defect measures, in both open and laparoscopic-assisted hernia repairs [16–19].

There are only a few observational studies, mostly retrospective, evaluating the effects of BTA administration in hernia surgery and no prospectively randomized trials or even comparative studies. The number of reported patient series is low and very heterogeneous in terms of dosage, injection technique, hernia characteristics, final operative technique, and type of mesh used. These issues were highlighted by

Motz et al. [20] The reviewed studies used either 500 U total of BTA administered via five injections per laterality of the abdomen [13, 16, 21], or 300 U total administered via three injections per side [17, 22], or a total of 200 or 300 U administered via three injections per side [23]. The BTA was diluted to different concentrations with 0.9% saline depending on the individual protocols of each study, ranging from 2 U/mL [17, 22, 23] to 10 U/mL [21] to 100 U/mL [16]. Injection location was confirmed with either ultrasound guidance [16, 17, 22, 23] or electromyography [13, 21]. Four studies describe injecting equal amounts of BTA in the muscle bellies of the external oblique, internal oblique, and transversus abdominis [17, 21–23]. One study described injecting between the external and internal oblique [16], and one study did not specify the level of injection [13]. Two studies administered injections of BTA between 1 and 4 weeks before hernia repair [17, 23], whereas three administered BTA 4 weeks before surgery [13, 16, 21]. One study did not control for time from administration to surgery, with the majority of patients receiving BTA on the day of surgery [22].

In spite of this limited data, it becomes clear that BTA administration provides several useful effects. Hernia defect size reduction was reported in three studies [13, 16, 21], and two studies showed significant lengthening of the lateral abdominal wall musculature [17, 23], with all of these findings having been objectively confirmed through CT scans (Fig. 8.5). Primary fascial closure rates, as reported in 4 studies range from 95.7% up to 100% [13, 15, 20, 22]. Zendejas et al. published a fascial closure rate of only 40.9%, but this r is probably due to the short period of time between BTA administration and final surgery [22].

In 2018, Bueno-Lledó et al. demonstrated that the combination of BTA injection and progressive pneumoperitoneum is highly effective in the repair of complex incisional hernia repair [21]. A retrospective series of 70 patients with prospectively collected data was presented. Only patients with a "volume of incisional hernia" (VIH)-to-"volume of abdominal cavity" (VAC) ratio greater than 20% were included. All patients underwent BTA injection 4 weeks prior to surgery, as well as 500–1000 cc of PPP daily for 1–2 weeks. Despite the fact that the average VIH

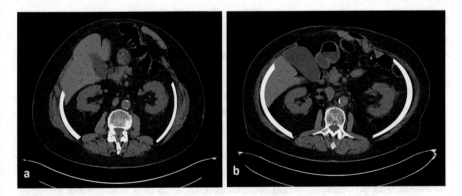

Fig. 8.5 Abdominal CT scan (**a**) before BTA application and (**b**) after BTA application, showing flattening and lengthening of the lateral abdominal wall muscles

increased, the VIH/VAC ratio decreased dramatically, with an average reduction of 16.6%. Although the width of the transverse fascial defect was not diminished significantly, primary fascial closure was achieved in nearly all patients (95.7%). And at an average follow-up of 34.5 months, only four patients presented with a recurrence (5.7%).

All of together these findings have led to the fact that BTA is now widely accepted as a beneficial adjunct in abdominal wall reconstruction, being particularly useful in patients with large ventral hernias with or without loss of domain, and in contaminated settings that prohibit the use of synthetic mesh. Comparative studies could establish this further (e.g., comparing patients injected with BTA to a control group and even comparing these to classical surgical component separation and patients treated with PPP). However, in reality this study setup is difficult to manage, as patients with complex ventral hernia require a detailed surgical treatment plan, with the use of all possible adjuncts to maximize the change of success. A complex ventral hernia repair, in most cases, is a one shot surgery, and study designs in which patients would be refused beneficial treatment strategies might be difficult to justify.

Botulinum Toxin A and Postoperative Pain

A somewhat less known effect of BTA is that it provides analgesia, since it not only blocks the release of acetylcholine but also prevents the release of calcitonin gene-related peptide and substance P, which are pain-modulating molecules. After a case report by Smoot [24] that paved the way, Zendejas et al. established these analgesic properties in a series of 22 patients undergoing incisional hernia repair. These patients were retrospectively matched to 66 control subjects. The patients receiving BTA injections used significantly less opioid analgesia (expressed in morphine equivalents) and also reported significantly less pain (visual analog scale – VAS) when compared to the controls. However, no significant difference in hospital stay was noted [21].

Botulinum Toxin A in Hernia Prevention

The lateral muscle complex (external oblique, internal oblique, and transverse abdominis) yields a continuous lateral retraction force, which is opposed by the linea alba. When performing a median laparotomy, the linea alba is incised and at the end of the procedure reapproximated. This linea alba incision needs time to remodel and scar together. The hypothesis could be made that if the lateral complex could be paralyzed during the early remodeling phase of the linea alba, the rate of incisional hernia formation would decline. In 2015, Lien et al. showed that injecting botulinum toxin A (BTA) into the abdominal muscles of a rat model, the rate and size of incisional hernia formation after midline laparotomy was significantly lower when compared to rats that were injected with saline [25]. As for the role of BTA in hernia prevention in humans, no data exists. Up to this point, Zielinski et al. were the only ones to publish their use of BTA as an adjunct to achieve primary fascial closure in open abdomen management rather than hernia repair [15]. Unfortunately, no data was published on the rate of hernia formation afterward.

When used as an adjunct in complex ventral hernia repair, BTA administration and its prolonged postoperative effect is thought to protect against subsequent incisional breakdown of the repair and to minimize the risk of dehiscence during the early healing phase [19, 26]. In cases in which the risk of recurrence is considered to be high, an additional administration of BTA in the postoperative phase may provide additional protection.

Administration Technique and Safety

Administration of BTA is generally well tolerated, with only rarely reported side effects. Intravascular injection is to be avoided at all cost, since this can lead to a generalized botulism-like syndrome [27]. Up to now, no serious adverse events have been reported in the literature following BTA administration for hernia repair. Lesser side effects such as bloating, and weaker cough and sneeze, generally run a benign course and do not cause significant clinical issues. Most of these symptoms can be managed with the use of an abdominal binder.

In a report by Nielsen et al. [28], including 37 patients who underwent BTA administration prior to hernia repair, patients were retrospectively evaluated for short-term outcome and complications related to the use of BTA. They found BTA to be a safe adjunct to large ventral hernia repair, demonstrating that the overall complication rate after abdominal wall reconstruction was comparable to studies who reported on complex ventral hernia repair without the use of BTA. One patient reported pain immediately after the injection, which resolved spontaneously. Theoretically, since the abdominal wall muscles play a role as accessory respiratory muscles, a higher rate of respiratory complications could be expected. But even in patients with known COPD, administration of BTA did not cause any exacerbations, although caution is still advised in this population of patients.

Although never reported in hernia repair, primary non-response has been documented in up to 10% in the general population [27]. Secondary non-response, due to BTA antibody formation, is a factor to be taken into account when administering BTA for hernia repair in patients chronically receiving the product with short intervals for other indications [29]. Of course, failure to properly handle the product (e.g., storage temperature requirements and dilution technique) can also prohibit the desired clinical effect.

As to which guidance technique should be used to confirm injection into the three specific muscle layers, no consensus exists. Most papers describe the use of ultrasound to identify the correct muscle bellies and guide the injection needle. EMG guidance has also been described [13, 21], but the most suitable technique has not been established. Ultrasound guidance seems to have the upper hand, probably due to its accessibility, low cost, and ease of use.

The same uncertainty is true for the ideal dose of BTA. Dosages ranging from 100 to 500 units have been reported. Most studies achieved satisfactory relaxation with 300–500 units. In two studies, 100 units were administered, but with conflicting results [30]. In their series, Rodriguez-Acevedo et al. showed no statistically significant difference in muscle elongation between patients who had been injected with 200 versus 300 units of BTA [23].

Our Rationale and Method

For us, BTA administration is not a single means to treat an incisional hernia, but rather a tool in a wider armamentarium. It is an adjunct to increase the effectiveness of already established techniques. In our algorithm, patients presenting with a hernia wider than 18 cm are eligible for BTA administration. Below this range, standard surgical component separation usually suffices. When a substantial loss of domain is present (VIH/VAC ratio >20%), PPP is added to the equation [31].

For the moment, no consensus exists on the method or timing of administration, the guidance technique, the number of BTA units to be used, the solution agent, the timing of surgery, etc. Below, we describe our preferred method, which was adapted from Zielinski et al. [15]

Administration of botulinum toxin A (BTA) is done in an ambulatory setting, approximately 28–42 days before surgery. In collaboration with a dedicated radiologist, the injection is done by ultrasound guidance. The patient is placed in the lateral decubitus position, and three injection sites are identified around the midaxillary line, between the subcostal margin and the iliac crest (Fig. 8.6). The procedure is then repeated on the other side of the abdomen.

Three hundred units of BTA in total (Botox, Allergan, Dublin, Ireland) are diluted in 150 ml of 0.9% saline. Using ultrasound guidance, the three lateral muscle bellies (transversus abdominis, internal oblique, and external oblique) are distinguished, and approximately 8.3 ml is injected into each muscle (Fig. 8.7). This process is then mimicked for all six injection sites.

Patients are educated about the progressive feeling of abdominal distension and a weaker cough and sneeze. These symptoms are always self-limiting.

14 to 28 days before the planned surgery, a clinical examination and repeat CT scan are performed, to evaluate the elongation of the lateral muscle complex and whether or not secondary measures (progressive pneumoperitoneum) are to be taken to improve the estimated chance of anterior fascial closure.

The surgery is started with dissection of the hernia sac, keeping as much of this tissue as possible. A standard retromuscular dissection is performed, and the medial gain is evaluated (i.e., can the midline be approximated). If not sufficient, and depending on hernia width and localization, either an anterior or posterior component separation is carried out.

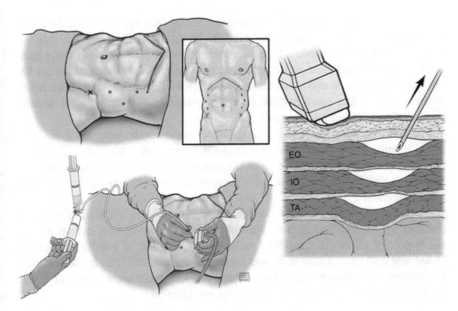

Fig. 8.6 BTA application by ultrasound guidance in ambulatory setting. (From article: Zendejas et al. [22]. ©Société Internationale de Chirurgie 2013 – Reproduced with permission from World Journal of Surgery)

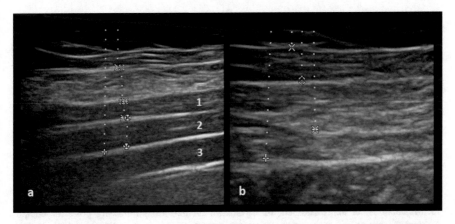

Fig. 8.7 Ultrasound with identification of lateral muscles [1], external oblique [2], internal oblique [3], transversus abdominis, in (**a**) an ideal image (**b**) fibrotic changes in the abdominal wall making identification of the different muscle bellies unreliable

Conclusion

In the last decade, there has been an increased interest for BTA in the field of hernia repair. Although the amount of scientific data is low, reports that have been published show promising results. BTA injection into the lateral abdominal muscle complex flattens and elongates these muscles. In this way, transverse hernia defect width decreases and the abdominal capacity increases. With no serious adverse events reported, it is a minimally invasive procedure with a potentially large gain. Many questions still need to be answered however. No consensus exists on the method of application and whether ultrasound guidance or EMG-controlled injection is superior. The exact needed dosage is unknown, just as the ideal waiting period before proceeding to surgery.

We feel that when considering progressive pneumoperitoneum for giant incisional hernias, BTA administration should always be added to the mix. However, the combination of these interventions is not mandatory but rather complementary. The single identifiable role of these components in complex hernia surgery remains to be established.

Nevertheless, BTA administration shows great promise in our field of work. As challenging surgeries become feasible with the adjunct of temporary muscle paralysis, hopefully future data registries will solidify the role of botulinum toxin in abdominal wall reconstruction or even hernia prevention. And with the added effect of significantly reduced postoperative pain, this long-term comorbidity of hernia repair could possibly be prevented or maybe even treated.

References

1. DuBay DA, et al. Incisional herniation induces decreased abdominal wall compliance via oblique muscle atrophy and fibrosis. Ann Surg. 2007;245:140–6.
2. Deerenberg EB, et al. A systematic review of the surgical treatment of large incisional hernia. Hernia. 2015;19:89–101.
3. Gillion J-F, et al. The economic burden of incisional ventral hernia repair: a multicentric cost analysis. Hernia. 2016;20:819–30.
4. Bosanquet DC, et al. Systematic review and meta-regression of factors affecting midline incisional hernia rates: analysis of 14 618 patients. PLoS One. 2015;10(9):e0138745.
5. Walming S, et al. Retrospective review of risk factors for surgical wound dehiscence and incisional hernia. BMC Surg. 2017;17(1):19.
6. Muysoms F, et al. Classification of primary and incisional abdominal wall hernias. Hernia. 2009;13(4):407–14.
7. Slater NJ, et al. Criteria for definition of a complex abdominal wall hernia. Hernia. 2014;18(1):7–17.
8. Mujander A, et al. Assessment of myofascial medialization following posterior component separation via transversus abdominis muscle release in a cadaveric model. Hernia. 2018;22:637–44.
9. Tanaka E, et al. A computerized tomography scan method for calculating the hernia sac and abdominal cavity volume in complex large incisional hernia with loss of domain. Hernia. 2010;14:63–9.
10. Ramirez OM, et al. "Components separation" method for closure of abdominal-wall defects: an anatomic and clinical study. Plast Reconstr Surg. 1990;86:519–26.
11. Novitsky YW, et al. Transversus abdominis muscle release: a novel approach to posterior component separation during complex abdominal wall reconstruction. Am J Surg. 2012;204:709–16.

12. Kakmak M, et al. Effect of paralysis of the abdominal wall muscles by botulinum A toxin to intraabdominal pressure: an experimental study. J Pediatr Surg. 2006;41:821–5.
13. Ibarra-Hurtado T, et al. Use of botulinum toxin type A before abdominal wall hernia reconstruction. World J Surg. 2009;33:2553–6.
14. Renard Y, Lardière-Deguelte S, de Mestier L, et al. Management of large incisional hernias with loss of domain: a prospective series of patients prepared by progressive preoperative pneumoperitoneum. Surgery. 2016;160(2):426–35. https://doi.org/10.1016/j.surg.2016.03.033.
15. Zielinski M, et al. Chemical components separation with botulinum toxin A: a novel technique to improve primary fascial closure rates of the open abdomen. Hernia. 2013;17:101–7.
16. Ibarra-Hurtado T, et al. Effect of botulinum toxin type A in lateral abdominal wall muscles thickness and length of patients with midline incisional hernia secondary to open abdomen management. Hernia. 2014;18:647–52.
17. Farooque F, et al. Preoperative abdominal muscle elongation with botulinum toxin A for complex incisional ventral hernia repair. ANZ J Surg. 2015;86:79–83.
18. Elstner K, et al. Laparoscopic repair of complex ventral hernia facilitated by pre-operative chemical component relaxation using Botulinum Toxin A. Hernia. 2016;20:209–19.
19. Elstner K, et al. Preoperative chemical component relaxation using Botulinum toxin A: enabling laparoscopic repair of complex ventral hernia. Surg Endosc. 2017;31:761–8.
20. Motz BM, et al. Chemical components separation: concepts, evidence, and outcomes. Plast Reconstr Surg. 2018;142(3 Suppl):58S–63S.
21. Bueno-Lledó J, et al. Preoperative combination of progressive pneumoperitoneum and botulinum toxin type A in patients with loss of domain hernia. Surg Endosc. 2018;32(8):3599-3608. doi:10.1007/s00464-018-6089-0
22. Zendejas B, et al. Outcomes of chemical component paralysis using Botulinum Toxin for incisional hernia repairs. World J Surg. 2013;37:2830–7.
23. Rodriguez-Acevedo O, et al. Preoperative botulinum toxin A enabling defect closure and laparoscopic repair of complex ventral hernia. Surg Endosc. 2018;32:831–9.
24. Smoot D, et al. Botox A injection for pain after laparoscopic ventral hernia: a case report. Pain Med. 2011;12:1121–3.
25. Lien SC, et al. Contraction of abdominal wall muscles influences incisional hernia occurrence and size. Surgery. 2015;158(1):278–88.
26. Tomazini Martins R, et al. Limitations of electromyography in the assessment of abdominal wall muscle contractility following botulinum toxin A injection. Front Surg. 2019;9(6):16.
27. López-Cano M, Armengol-Carrasco M. Chemical component separation using botulinum toxin. In: Hernia surgery: current principles. Cham: Springer; 2016. p. 421–36.
28. Nielsen MO, et al. Short-term safety of preoperative administration of botulinum toxin A for the treatment of large ventral hernia with loss of domain. Hernia. 2020;24(2):295–9.
29. Dressler D, Saberi FA. Safety of botulinum toxin short interval therapy using incobotulinumtoxin A. J Neural Transm. 2017;124:437–40.
30. Soltanizadeh S, et al. Botulinum toxin A as an adjunct to abdominal wall reconstruction for incisional hernia. Plast Reconstr Surg Glob Open. 2017;5(6):e1358.
31. Yurtkap Y, van Rooijen MMJ, Roels S, et al. Implementing preoperative Botulinum toxin A and progressive pneumoperitoneum through the use of an algorithm in giant ventral hernia repair [published online ahead of print, 2020 Jun 3]. Hernia. 2020. https://doi.org/10.1007/s10029-020-02226-2.

Chapter 9
Use of Botulinum Toxin A in Postmastectomy Breast Reconstruction

Allen Gabriel and G. Patrick Maxwell

Abstract Botulinum toxin A has been successfully used in a variety of areas to temporarily obliterate muscle mobility for either functional or aesthetic gain. Tissue expander-based breast reconstruction has been plagued with pain and discomfort. This chapter describes the use of botulinum toxin A in managing pain and discomfort in the breast reconstruction patients.

Keywords Breast reconstruction · Botox · Neurotoxin · Botulinum toxin A · Pain · Tissue expanders · Breast implants · Breast cancer

Introduction

Implant-based breast reconstruction is the most frequently performed reconstructive technique following breast ablative surgery. Breast reconstruction with tissue expanders (two-stage) and direct to implant (DTI) offers patients satisfying aesthetic results with minimal donor site morbidity. Each year, the number of breast cancer survivors who choose postmastectomy breast reconstruction keeps rising, and a majority will choose expander/implant reconstruction [1]. Evolved over the past few decades into a highly successful and rewarding method of reconstruction, implant-based breast reconstruction is a precise and demanding method.

Postmastectomy reconstruction with a tissue expander and implant can involve a staged approach. The first stage consists of the placement of a tissue expander deep

A. Gabriel (✉)
Department of Plastic Surgery, Loma Linda University Medical Center, Loma Linda, CA, USA

Peacehealth Plastic Surgery, Vancouver, WA, USA

G. P. Maxwell
Department of Plastic Surgery, Loma Linda University Medical Center, Loma Linda, CA, USA

© Springer Nature Switzerland AG 2020

B. Jabbari (ed.), *Botulinum Toxin Treatment in Surgery, Dentistry, and Veterinary Medicine*, https://doi.org/10.1007/978-3-030-50691-9_9

to the pectoralis major muscle or into the prepectoral space. This may be done immediately following the mastectomy or as a delayed procedure. The purpose of the expander is to create a soft and precise pocket to contain the permanent implant. The expander during immediate reconstruction is not for expansion purposes but rather a pocket-creating device (PCD). This is followed by a period of weekly tissue expansions that can sometimes last months depending on the patient. In the second stage, the tissue expander is removed in a surgical procedure and replaced with a permanent breast implant. Despite the well-recognized advantages of this success-ful breast reconstruction technique, the subpectoral placement of a tissue expander is associated with significant pain and discomfort in the immediate postoperative period and during the phase of tissue expansion. Pectoralis major muscle spasm is a frequently reported problem during tissue expansion and in certain instances has led to premature removal of expanders [2]. Legeby et al. showed that women who underwent prosthetic breast reconstruction had higher pain scores and took more analgesics than those who did not choose postmastectomy reconstruction [3]. Therefore, numerous methods and technical variations have been attempted to decrease pain associated with subpectoral placement of tissue expanders and implants, all with questionable success [4–9].

Botulinum toxin A is a neurotoxin approved for the treatment of several condi-tions including wrinkles, strabismus, headaches, and cervical dystonia. In the past decade, the use of botulinum toxin A for pain relief in a wide array of clinical condi-tions has been reported. Botulinum toxin A is a neurotoxin produced by *Clostridium botulinum* bacteria and modulates the release of neuropeptides such as substance P and calcitonin gene-related protein and inhibits neurogenic inflammation, which likely underlies its independent antinociceptive effect [10]. In particular, the sensory function of substance P is thought to be related to the transmission of pain informa-tion into the central nervous system. The analgesic action of botulinum toxin A was initially thought to be related to its effects on muscular contraction but has since been supplanted by in vitro studies of the inhibition of substance P by botulinum toxin A in embryonic rat dorsal neurons [11]. The presence of analgesic properties of botulinum toxin A is increasingly supported by several clinical observations: pain relief with botulinum toxin A injections has been reported for migraine headaches [12], chronic pelvic pain [13], chronic tennis elbow [14], and postoperative pain control for painful joint arthroplasty [15], among others. Furthermore, botulinum toxin A has been used to treat various painful muscle spasms, such as paravertebral muscle spasm [16], fibromyalgia-myofascial pain [17], and temporomandibular joint pain [18]. The profound number of biological and clinical applications of botu-linum toxin A is exhibited in the literature today.

The antinociceptive action of botulinum toxin A in breast cancer survivors who elect to pursue breast reconstruction with tissue expanders and implants is not fully utilized. Layeequee et al. reported muscular infiltration of botulinum toxin by direct visualization for mastectomy, and tissue expander placement significantly reduced postoperative pain and discomfort without complications; interestingly, the neuro-toxin group in this study used significantly less narcotic medication within 24 hours of administration [19]. Figus et al. reported the effects of botulinum toxin A injections on muscle spasms in women undergoing breast reconstruction with latissimus dorsi flaps and subpectoral implants [20]. Others have also demonstrated objectively some pain relief with the use of botulinum toxin into the pectoralis major muscle [21, 22]. All of these studies have used a dose range of 75–100 units per pectoralis major or latissimus dorsi muscle groups. In our study, we evaluated 30 patients following mastectomies with immediate expander/ADM reconstruction and divided them into two groups [23]. The neurotoxin group ($n = 15$) received 40 units of neurotoxin (botulinum toxin A, Allergan, Inc., Irvine, CA) into each pectoralis major muscle through four serial injections, and the placebo group ($n = 15$) received four serial injections of 0.9% NaCl. We found no significant difference between the two groups in terms of age, laterality, expander size, and complications ($p = 0.46–0.66$). However, there was a significant difference between the two groups in the VAS (Visual Analog Scale) score demonstrating decreased pain in the neurotoxin group ($p < 0.05$). In addition, there was a significant increase in the volume of expansion per visit in the neurotoxin group as compared to the placebo group ($p < 0.05$). There was no significant difference in narcotic use in the first 3 days after surgery; however, there was a significant decrease in use of narcotics from 7 to 45 days in the neurotoxin group ($p < 0.05$). There were no complications associated with the use of neurotoxin [23].

The early significant pain control with the neurotoxin, as documented by Layeeque et al., can be explained by the antinociceptive effect of the drug. Botulinum toxin A injections have an independent antinociceptive effect [24], in addition to the well-known anticholinergic effect (responsible for muscle-paralyzing action), which has been utilized to treat several syndromes associated with painful muscle spasms. This dual action was noted in cervical dystonia [25] and headache studies [26]. The antinociceptive effect is likely due to inhibition of neurogenic inflammation [10], which is mediated by CGRP and substance P and blockade of local glutamate release that leads to local edema [27]. A recent systematic review summarized evidence from randomized clinical control trials that supports the antinociceptive effect of botulinum toxin A in osteoarticular pain including patients with tennis elbow, low back pain, temporomandibular joint pain, carpal tunnel syndrome, and plantar fasciitis [28].

Discussion

Noninvasive aesthetic procedures are continuously on the rise, and every year there is an increase in uptake of botulinum toxin as one of the most popular procedures performed in the United States and perhaps the world. In addition to the well-known anticholinergic effect (responsible for muscle-relaxation action), there is also increasing evidence of the antinociceptive effect, likely due to inhibition of neurogenic inflammation [10], which is mediated by CGRP and substance P and blockade of local glutamate release that leads to local edema [27]. It is difficult to quantify the utilization of botulinum toxin for its therapeutic uses as currently there is no

tracking method of this modality and one may be surprised that the therapeutic utilization may be as high as the aesthetic market growth.

In breast reconstruction, our study provides the evidence related to the efficacy
of botulinum toxin A in the pectoralis major muscle for the improvement of pain
and enhanced tissue expansion in patients undergoing immediate breast reconstruction [23]. This observation aligns well with previously observed efficacy of botulinum toxin A in reduction of pain in several disease processes. Several patients had
a sustained pain relief and improved experience with tissue expansion after botulinum toxin A treatment. Pain relief was especially noticeable in the postoperative
period after 3 days and up to day 45, with a significant difference in the amount of
narcotics and muscle relaxants/anxiolytics necessary to provide adequate pain control. No data was collected beyond 45 days for pain control as all patients had
already completed expansion and were no longer on narcotics. It is very intriguing
that Layeequee et al. showed significantly reduced postoperative pain within the
24 hours of administration [19]. Even though not discussed, this clinical finding
may be explained by the in vitro finding of the effect of substance P inhibition by
botulinum toxin A in embryonic rat dorsal neurons [11].

It is also important to understand the anatomy of the muscle and ensure that the
tail of the pectoralis major is injected followed by at least three other locations, for
maximum effect [29] (Fig. 9.1).

By relaxing the muscle, and decreasing the pain associated with stretch of muscle, more efficient expansions can be performed. With the advent of tabbed expanders in early 2011, the need for injection of serratus anterior muscle was introduced

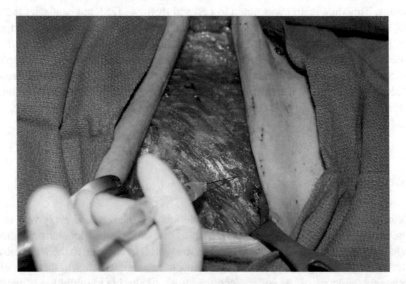

Fig. 9.1 Intraoperative portrayal of proper injection into the pectoralis major muscle in a 55-year-
old female with left breast cancer undergoing skin-sparing mastectomy. Botulinum toxin A is first
injected into the tail of the pectoralis major muscle to maximally paralyze the muscle, where the
nerve enters the muscle

to minimize the long-term discomfort when sutures are placed in the serratus anterior fascia or muscle [23]. Of course, pain tolerance per patient varies, and as tissue expanders can be firm and uncomfortable when fully expanded, we believe that by relaxing the muscle, the discomfort of this area is minimized. Furthermore, a shorter span of time necessary to complete the expansion phase of breast reconstruction can shorten the entire reconstructive timeline, all the while providing maximal comfort for the patient.

For the past 20 years, implant-based breast reconstruction has been performed primarily with subpectoral implant placement via the dual-plane approach. The coverage and support provided by the pectoralis major muscle has not only minimized implant-related complications but has mitigated the risk of capsular contracture and produced a more natural-looking breast. However, a concern with this approach is the risk of functional impairment of the pectoralis muscle and animation deformities, both of which are a direct consequence of muscle elevation [30]. The muscle discomfort can be at times controlled with neurotoxin injection into the tail of the pectoralis major muscle, but this is not a sustainable solution long term. Therefore, in the last 6 years, the trend has been to change the implant site to a prepectoral placement to help resolve some of these concerns [30].

Even though the pectoralis major muscle is not included in prepectoral reconstruction, neurotoxin injection into serratus anterior and pectoralis major muscles should still be considered. This can be beneficial, since numerous tacking sutures are placed in these muscles. These tacking sutures can lead to severe muscle spasms in the postoperative period and sometimes until the expander is replaced with an implant. In addition, in the site where the axilla is violated, the injection of neurotoxin into the pectoralis major can help with postoperative discomfort.

Botulinum toxin A has not been approved by the US Food and Drug Administration for paralysis of pectoralis major muscle in breast reconstruction. Therefore, this constitutes an "off-label" use and should be considered only after a full understanding of risks/benefits by the patients and care providers. In the systematic review of the literature, limited studies researching the effect of botulinum toxin A on pain during expander-based reconstruction have been published [19, 21]. Altieri et al. showed improved pain control starting at day 7 in the neurotoxin cohort, which is consistent with our findings, but the amount of botulinum toxin A was not specified [31]. Layeeque et al. also showed improved pain control in the neurotoxin group, but this was observed immediately at postoperative 1 with decreased narcotic use [19]. The same group described the safety of nipple-sparing mastectomy in 2011 and revealed that all 293 patients received neurotoxin into the pectoralis major muscle to reduce postoperative pain, decrease hospital stay, and facilitate expansion [32]. Our data does not support a decrease in hospital stay but rather supports decreased pain and ease of expansion. These investigators, much like our group, have incorporated neurotoxin injection into the reconstructive algorithm in all patients undergoing expander-based reconstruction.

The role of botulinum toxin is expanding every year in aesthetic and therapeutic markets. There are many benefits of its use that have been well described [11–18, 23–26, 28].

We believe that as more surgeons are innovative and understand the potential benefits of botulinum toxin, the more clinical applications will be identified. Even though many of these therapeutic treatments are "off label," the use and advantages cannot be overlooked. Unfortunately, industry will not be able to obtain an "on-label" use of an existing FDA-approved product for every clinical scenario, given the stringent government study requirements for an on-label approval. It will be up to every physician to describe the potential benefit of its use and have the patient consent to the procedure. One example is the rapidly expanding use of botulinum toxin in management of large hernias [33].

Despite its simplicity, implant-based breast reconstruction requires integration of severable variables, the most important being careful postoperative management to minimize complications and maximize patient satisfaction and end result. Intramuscular injection of botulinum toxin A is a potential clinical tool for plastic surgeons to navigate successful postoperative management. The use of this neurotoxin can be utilized in both aesthetic and reconstructive procedures involving the pectoralis major muscle and can be further expanded in other areas of the body that require relaxation of muscle for pain control.

References

1. American society of plastic surgeons 2013 plastic surgery statistics report 2013. Accessed 22 Dec 2014, at http://www.plasticsurgery.org/Documents/news-resources/statistics/2013-statistics/plastic-surgery-statistics-full-report-2013.pdf.
2. Disa JJ, Ad-El DD, Cohen SM, Cordeiro PG, Hidalgo DA. The premature removal of tissue expanders in breast reconstruction. Plast Reconstr Surg. 1999;104:1662–5.
3. Legeby M, Segerdahl M, Sandelin K, Wickman M, Ostman K, Olofsson C. Immediate reconstruction in breast cancer surgery requires intensive post-operative pain treatment but the effects of axillary dissection may be more predictive of chronic pain. Breast. 2002;11:156–62.
4. May JW Jr, Bucky LP, Sohoni S, Ehrlich HP. Smooth versus textured expander implants: a double-blind study of capsule quality and discomfort in simultaneous bilateral breast reconstruction patients. Ann Plast Surg. 1994;32:225–32; discussion 32–3
5. McCarthy CM, Cordeiro PG, Disa JJ, Mehrara BJ, Pusic AL. The impact of breast reconstruction on the oncologic efficacy of radiation therapy. Ann Plast Surg. 2008;61:585.
6. Pusic AL, Cordeiro PG. An accelerated approach to tissue expansion for breast reconstruction: experience with intraoperative and rapid postoperative expansion in 370 reconstructions. Plast Reconstr Surg. 2003;111:1871–5.
7. Raposio E, Santi PL. Topical application of DMSO as an adjunct to tissue expansion for breast reconstruction. Br J Plast Surg. 1999;52:194–7.
8. Sinow JD, Cunningham BL. Intraluminal lidocaine for analgesia after tissue expansion: a double-blind prospective trial in breast reconstruction. Ann Plast Surg. 1992;28:320–5.
9. Turan Z, Sandelin K. Local infiltration of anaesthesia with subpectoral indwelling catheters after immediate breast reconstruction with implants: a pilot study. Scand J Plast Reconstr Surg Hand Surg. 2006;40:136–9.
10. Meng J, Wang J, Lawrence G, Dolly JO. Synaptobrevin I mediates exocytosis of CGRP from sensory neurons and inhibition by botulinum toxins reflects their anti-nociceptive potential. J Cell Sci. 2007;120:2864–74.

11. Mustafa G, Anderson EM, Bokrand-Donatelli Y, Neubert JK, Caudle RM. Anti-nociceptive effect of a conjugate of substance P and light chain of botulinum neurotoxin type A. Pain. 2013;154:2547–53.
12. Dodick DW, Turkel CC, DeGryse RE, et al. OnabotulinumtoxinA for treatment of chronic migraine: pooled results from the double-blind, randomized, placebo-controlled phases of the PREEMPT clinical program. Headache. 2010;50:921–36.
13. Abbott JA, Jarvis SK, Lyons SD, Thomson A, Vancaille TG. Botulinum toxin type A for chronic pain and pelvic floor spasm in women: a randomized controlled trial. Obstet Gynecol. 2006;108:915–23.
14. Placzek R, Drescher W, Deuretzbacher G, Hempfing A, Meiss AL. Treatment of chronic radial epicondylitis with botulinum toxin A. A double-blind, placebo-controlled, randomized multi-center study. J Bone Joint Surg Am. 2007;89:255–60.
15. Singh JA, Mahowald ML, Noorbaloochi S. Intraarticular botulinum toxin A for refractory painful total knee arthroplasty: a randomized controlled trial. J Rheumatol. 2010;37:2377–86.
16. Foster L, Clapp L, Erickson M, Jabbari B. Botulinum toxin A and chronic low back pain: a randomized, double-blind study. Neurology. 2001;56:1290–3.
17. Lang AM. Botulinum toxin therapy for myofascial pain disorders. Curr Pain Headache Rep. 2002;6:355–60.
18. Tan EK, Jankovic J. Treating severe bruxism with botulinum toxin. J Am Dent Assoc. 2000;131:211–6.
19. Layeeque R, Hochberg J, Siegel E, et al. Botulinum toxin infiltration for pain control after mastectomy and expander reconstruction. Ann Surg. 2004;240:608–13; discussion 13–4.
20. Figus A, Mazzocchi M, Dessy LA, Curinga G, Scuderi N. Treatment of muscular contraction deformities with botulinum toxin type A after latissimus dorsi flap and sub-pectoral implant breast reconstruction. J Plast Reconstr Aesthet Surg. 2009;62:869–75.
21. Zhibo X, Miaobo Z. Botulinum toxin type A infiltration for pain control after breast augmentation. Plast Reconstr Surg. 2009;124:263e–4e.
22. Ferraro G, Altieri A, Grella E, D'Andrea F. Botulinum toxin: 28 patients affected by Frey's syndrome treated with intradermal injections. Plast Reconstr Surg. 2005;115:344–5.
23. Gabriel A, Champaneria MC, Maxwell GP. The efficacy of botulinum toxin A in post-mastectomy breast reconstruction: a pilot study. Aesthet Surg J. 2015;35:402–9.
24. Jabbari B. Botulinum neurotoxins in the treatment of refractory pain. Nat Clin Pract Neurol. 2008;4:676–85.
25. Jankovic J, Schwartz K. Botulinum toxin injections for cervical dystonia. Neurology. 1990;40:277–80.
26. Gobel H, Heinze A, Heinze-Kuhn K, Jost WH. Evidence-based medicine: botulinum toxin A in migraine and tension-type headache. J Neurol. 2001;248(Suppl 1):34–8.
27. Cui M, Li Z, You S, Khanijou S, Aoki K. Mechanisms of the antinociceptive effect of subcutaneous Botox: inhibition of peripheral and central nociceptive processing. Arch Pharmacol. 2002;365:R17.
28. Singh JA. Botulinum toxin therapy for osteoarticular pain: an evidence-based review. Ther Adv Musculoskelet Dis. 2010;2:105–18.
29. Jost W. Pictorial atlas of botulinum toxin injection: dosage, localization, application. Germany: Quintessence Pub Co; 2012.
30. Sigalove S, Maxwell GP, Sigalove NM, et al. Prepectoral implant-based breast reconstruction and postmastectomy radiotherapy: short-term outcomes. Plast Reconstr Surg Glob Open. 2017;5:e1631.
31. Altieri A, Brongo S, Mele CM, Amoroso A, D'Andrea F. The botulinum toxin in breast reconstruction. Rivista Italiana di Chirurgia Plastica. 2006;38:127–30.
32. Boneti C, Yuen J, Santiago C, et al. Oncologic safety of nipple skin-sparing or total skin-sparing mastectomies with immediate reconstruction. J Am Coll Surg. 2011;212:686–93; discussion 93–5.
33. Smoot D, Zielinski M, Jenkins D, Schiller H. Botox A injection for pain after laparoscopic ventral hernia: a case report. Pain Med. 2011;12:1121–3.

Chapter 10
Botulinum Toxins for Treatment of Pain in Orthopedic Disorders

Christian Wong, Shahroo Etemad-Moghadam, and Bahman Jabbari

Abstract A considerable number of orthopedic disorders are accompanied by pain which can be a clinical challenge for clinicians and a major problem for patients. Botulinum neurotoxins (BoNTs) have been recently shown to possess analgesic effects leading to their extensive use in various situations, including pain control for orthopedic issues. This chapter presents information on BoNT treatment of five orthopedic disorders with available placebo-controlled studies. The recommendations of the Assessment Subcommittee of the American Academy of Neurology are applied to establish an evidence-based level of efficacy for these disorders that include chronic lateral epicondylitis, refractory pain following total knee arthroplasty, painful local arthritis, anterior knee pain related to vastus lateralis imbalance, and orthopedic contracture and/or pain release (French and Gronseth, Neurology 71:1634–8, 2008; Gronseth and French, Neurology 71:1639–43, 2008).

According to the studies discussed in the following sections, an "A" level of evidence has been provided for chronic lateral epicondylitis, defining BoNT-A as being "effective" for this disorder. In painful local arthritis and issues related to orthopedic contracture and/or pain release including distraction osteogenesis and correction of scoliosis, the level of evidence is "B" demonstrating BoNT-A therapy to be "probably ineffective." For refractory pain after total knee arthroplasty, anterior knee pain related to vastus lateralis imbalance, and other problems related to orthopedic contracture and/or pain release, the level of evidence is determined as "C" or "possibly effective." Some of the studies providing these levels of evidence are of class III and IV types, and the number of class I studies in a few of these disorders is limited. Further class I/II studies are required to support a definitive analgesic role of BoNTs in orthopedic disorders.

C. Wong
Department of Orthopaedics, University Hospital of Hvidover, Copenhagen, Denmark

S. Etemad-Moghadam
Dental Research Center, Dentistry Research Institute, Tehran University of Medical Sciences, Tehran, Iran

B. Jabbari (✉)
Department of Neurology, Yale University School of Medicine, New Haven, CT, USA
e-mail: bahman.jabbari@yale.edu

© Springer Nature Switzerland AG 2020
B. Jabbari (ed.), *Botulinum Toxin Treatment in Surgery, Dentistry, and Veterinary Medicine*, https://doi.org/10.1007/978-3-030-50691-9_10

Keywords Lateral epicondylitis · Tennis elbow · Anterior knee pain ·
Patellofemoral syndrome · Osteoarthritis · Arthritis · Botulinum toxin · Botulinum
neurotoxin · OnabotulinumtoxinA · AbobotulinumtoxinA · IncobotulinumtoxinA ·
RimabotulinumtoxinB

Introduction

Refractory pain associated with orthopedic disorders is a major problem for many
individuals and has therefore led to the development of multiple studies attempting
to provide accessible and simple management options for this issue. The efficacy of
botulinum neurotoxin (BoNT) injection in relieving this type of pain has been a
topic of interest in the past two decades. In this chapter, five such disorders with
available blinded, placebo-controlled studies and case series will be discussed.
These include chronic lateral epicondylitis, refractory pain following total knee
arthroplasty, painful local arthritis, anterior knee pain related to vastus lateralis
imbalance, and orthopedic contracture and/or pain release.

Chronic Lateral Epicondylitis (CLE)

Lateral epicondylitis (LE), also known as tennis elbow in athletes, is described as
elbow pain resulting from overuse of the joint [1]. It is seen more often among
heavy workers, and a prevalence of 4–7/1000 patients per year has been reported for
this relatively common disorder [17, 43]. Degeneration of the extensor tendons is
presently regarded as a responsible factor for the clinical symptoms of LE [30];
however, despite limited pathological evidence, the role of inflammation is still an
ongoing discussion. The idea of tendinopathy and tendon degeneration is confirmed
by studies using ultrasound for examination of the affected joints [11]. According to
Smidt et al. [40], 83% of acute LE patients return to normal within 12 months.
Nevertheless, a minor percentage of individuals develop the chronic form (CLE)
and unfortunately do not respond to drugs. Management of these chronic types
involves abstaining from applying heavy load to the damaged elbow, bracing, physical therapy, pharmacotherapy, and surgery. Cyclooxygenase inhibitors, nonsteroidal
anti-inflammatory drugs, GABAergic analgesics (gabapentin and pregabalin), and,
in more severe cases, opioids are commonly used medications in the management
of CLE. Steroid and nonsteroid pharmaceutical substances are introduced into painful areas via injection.

A total of 141 randomized controlled trials (RCTs) were systematically reviewed
by Krogh et al. [21] to compare the efficacy/safety of injection therapies in CLE
patients. Seventeen RCTs using eight different treatments including corticosteroids,
BoNTs, autologous blood, platelet-rich plasma (PRP), hyaluronic acid, prolother-

apy, polidocanol, and glycosaminoglycan polysulfate were selected. Despite the reported efficacy of injection therapy, most of the evaluated studies demonstrated issues related to blinding of the patient and/or health-care provider, allocation concealment, selective or attrition reporting, and company interest. These posed difficulties in accurate and definitive interpretation of the data.

The results of a more recent meta-analysis [24] comparing BoNT therapy with nonsurgical methods reported data on 321 LE patients participating in six randomized trials. The results indicated significant pain reduction in subjects treated with BoNT-A in comparison to those receiving placebo. This toxin was less effective in the short term (2–4 weeks) when compared to corticosteroids but showed identical effects after 8 weeks. Grip strength decreased in the first 2–4 weeks after BoNT-A injections, which lasted for 8–12 weeks and was more conspicuous compared to that produced by corticosteroid administration.

Botulinum Neurotoxin Studies in CLE

Of the eight reported RCTs in CLE, four were blinded, placebo-controlled trials, three were blinded comparator studies, and one was an experimental investigation on a series of patients.

Placebo-Controlled Studies

In a double-blind, placebo-controlled study on the efficacy of BoNT-A therapy in CLE, Wong et al. [46] showed significant analgesic effects of abobotulinumtoxinA (aboA) in 49 women and 11 men with this condition. The primary outcome of injection was reported as "pain reduction." A total of 60 U aboA diluted in 1 ml normal saline was used in this RCT. For both placebo (saline) and aboA, the injection point was directed toward the painful area, 1 cm from the lateral epicondyle, and the needle was inserted "deeply into the subcutaneous tissue and muscle." Measurements were based on 0–100 mm visual analog scale (VAS) scores and demonstrated pain reduction on the 4th and 12th weeks of the study period. The 40.2 mm VAS score reduction in the toxin group compared to the 15.7 mm decrease in the placebo group was statistically significant. These findings were also replicated at 12 weeks where significant differences in mean VAS scores were found between the aboA (23.5 mm) and saline subjects (43.5 mm), in favor of BoNT. Grip strength was measured as a secondary outcome, and despite a slight decrease in both groups, it was not significantly different between the test and control patients at any timepoint. The most common adverse effect was paralysis of finger extension, which occurred in four patients on week 4 of the study.

Hayton et al. [19], in another blinded and controlled trial, compared pain, quality of life, and hand grip, between aboA and placebo (saline), in 40 CLE patients unresponsive to steroids. These outcomes were measured with VAS scale, short-form SF12, and Jamar dynamometer, respectively. Assessments were made at baseline and 3 months after injection of 50 U aboA or saline. All injections were intramuscularly administered, 5 cm distal to the maximum point of tenderness at the lateral epicondyle, in line with the middle of the wrist. No differences in neither of the outcomes were reported between aboA and saline at 3 months.

Placzek et al. [33] conducted a double-blinded, placebo-controlled RCT in 16 centers to evaluate the effectiveness of BoNT treatment in chronic tennis elbow. A total of 130 CLE subjects were injected with either 60 units aboA diluted in 0.9% saline or the same volume placebo (saline). Half the solution was administered intramuscularly, 3–4 cm distal from the tender epicondyle, and the other half was injected after partially pulling the needle out and applying a horizontal rotation. This method provided different depths of infiltration. VAS was used to determine the level of pain before injections (baseline) and at 2, 6, 12, and 18 weeks. Satisfaction of both patients and blinded clinicians was measured at the same timepoints using a global assessment score of 0–4, which indicated "substantially worse" to "substantially better" outcomes, respectively. Furthermore, finger extension strength of all patients was assessed through a vigorimeter. The results demonstrated that aboA administration caused significant reduction of pain at all studied timepoints after injection (Table 10.1).

A randomized placebo-controlled study by Espandar et al. [14] aimed to assess BoNT efficacy in CLE patients using injection sites that were calculated by anatomical measurements. A total of 48 patients with chronic refractory LE received either 60 units of aboA or the same volume normal saline. Based on a cadaver study [25], 33% of the arm length inferior to the lateral epicondyle was selected for injection. This area forms the point where the posterior interosseous nerve innervates the extensor carpi ulnaris and extensor digitorum. Pain intensity at rest was considered as the primary outcome (0–100 mm, VAS score), which was measured postinjection at 4, 8, and 16 weeks. Secondary outcomes consisted of pain intensity during maximum pinch and maximum handgrip in addition to grip strength (kg). The primary outcome decreased significantly in the aboA group in comparison to

Table 10.1 Comparison of clinical pain scores between groups

Visit	Score[a]		p value[b]
	Botulinum	Placebo	
Injection	8.43 ± 0.24 (68)	8.55 ± 0.21 (62)	0.920
Week 2	5.24 ± 0.38 (68)	6.85 ± 0.35 (61)	0.003
Week 6	4.53 ± 0.37 (68)	5.69 ± 0.37 (61)	0.020
Week 12	3.76 ± 0.36 (68)	5.02 ± 0.41 (61)	0.023
Week 18	2.88 ± 0.35 (68)	4.29 ± 0.41 (57)	0.009

From Placzek et al. [33]. Printed with permission from the *Journal of Bone and Joint Surgery*
[a]The values are given as the mean clinical pain score and the standard error of the mean with the number of patients in parentheses
[b]The level of significance of the difference between the botulinum and placebo groups as assessed with the Mann–Whitney U test

the control group at 4, 8, and 16 weeks with VAS scores of 14.1 mm, 11.5 mm, and 12.6 mm, respectively ($p = 0.01$). Similarly, pain intensity during maximum pinch was significantly lower in patients injected with BoNT-A than those receiving saline ($p = 0.004$). Grip strength during follow-up diminished in the aboA group compared to the controls, but the difference was not significant in between-group comparisons. Weakness of finger extension interfering with functioning at work was reported in aboA patients at week 4 which resolved by the 8th week in one patient and the 16th week in the rest of the participants in the test group.

Ruiz et al. [36] studied the pain reduction and functional performance of 12 CLE patients after receiving injections of 10–30 U/muscle incobotulinumtoxinA (incoA). The toxin was diluted with 1 ml normal saline and administered into the extensor carpi ulnaris (20 U), extensor digiti minimi (10 U), extensor digitorum longus (30 U), and extensor carpi radialis brevis (20 U) muscles of all subjects. If more than one muscle was involved, injections were administered into each of the muscles, but none of the patients received the maximum allowed dose of 80 U. In order to locate the muscles for injection, the participant was asked to perform specific movements while the epicondyle was palpated. Ultrasound was used to confirm the correct selection of the insertion point. Pain intensity based on VAS scores (0, best, to 10, worst) was significantly diminished from 6.9 ± 1.8 at baseline to 4.3 ± 2.6, 4.0 ± 2.9, and 4.3 ± 3.9 after injections at the 1-, 3-, and 6-month timepoints, respectively. Likewise, hand functionality evaluated by the QuickDASH scale (0, best, to 100, worst) showed significant improvement from baseline (60.1 ± 20.9) to 1 month (47.6 ± 22.2), 3 months (44.5 ± 24.2), and 6 months (36.3 ± 32.3). Following injections, 87.5% of the patients were affected with third finger weakness, which disappeared after 45–90 days, but no adverse effects were reported at follow-up visits. Three patients required an additional dose of BoNT-A, and five subjects were required to undergo surgery due to insufficient recovery of normal functionality after toxin injection.

Comparator Studies

In a small double-blind study by Lin et al. [23], pain (VAS), handgrip (dynamometry), and quality of life (World Health Organization's brief questionnaire) were compared between patients receiving 50 units onabotulinumtoxinA (onaA) and those injected with 40 mg triamcinolone acetonide. The extensor carpi radialis brevis near the common origin of the wrist and finger extensors of the affected elbow was selected as the site of injection for both substances, and assessments were made at baseline and weeks 4, 8, and 12. In a total of 19 affected elbows in 16 subjects, pain reduction was observed at week 4 in both groups, but the reduction was significantly greater in patients injected with steroid ($p = 0.02$). The other two timepoints were also associated with pain improvement, but the difference between Botox and triamcinolone acetonide was not significant either at 8 or 12 weeks. Interestingly, the analgesic effect of BoNT-A increased with time, but the level of pain reduction decreased in the steroid group ($p > 0.05$). Grip strength showed mild decrease and increase in the Botox and steroid groups, respectively, and demonstrated significant differences between the two groups at 4 and 8 weeks. There was no significant difference in quality of life between the groups, and no debilitating adverse effects were found in the participants.

Guo et al. [18] in a double-blind, randomized, active drug-controlled trial compared the effect of low-dose onabotulinumtoxinA (20 units, 1 ml) and the commonly used steroid injection of triamcinolone acetonide (40 mg, 1 ml) in 26 patients with CLE. Additionally, the antinociceptive impact of BoNT-A was compared between two different injection sites which included the most tender point of the common extensor muscles (Botox-Tend group) and 1 cm distal to the painful lateral epicondyle (Botox-Epic and Steroid groups). The primary outcome was intensity of pain measured by VAS before intervention and at 4, 8, 12, and 16 weeks after treatment. The only significant difference in pain improvement among the three groups was found at week 4, in favor of steroid administration. All interventions were similar in VAS score reduction after 8, 12, and 16 weeks of injection. Secondary outcomes including grip strength analyzed by dynamometry and functionality determined through the Patient-Rated Tennis Elbow Evaluation Questionnaire were significantly better for the steroid group at 4 weeks. However, no significant differences were observed at the other timepoints. Primary and secondary outcomes were worse when BoNT-A was administered to the tender points of the muscles (Botox-Tend group), compared to steroid injections at week 4 but not the other timepoints. These outcomes were not significantly different between Botox-Epic and steroid groups (4, 8, 12, and 16 weeks). No severe adverse events were reported, except that two patients in the Botox-Tend group had either extension lag or diminished strength of the middle finger, which were temporary. The authors concluded that low-dose BoNT-A and steroids injected into the lateral epicondyle both successfully decreased pain and improved upper limb function for at least 16 weeks.

In a double-blind randomized trial, Lee et al. [22] compared the analgesic impact of small and large doses of BoNT-A in CLE. Sixty patients with this condition were randomly assigned to receive a single dose of either a 10I U or 50I U BoNT-A (Meditox), diluted in 0.7 ml dextrose solution (30%) and 0.3 ml mepivacaine (2%). Injections were administered under ultrasound guidance in the common wrist extensor tendon, using the peppering technique (Fig. 10.1). Outcome measures were assessed at baseline and every month for 6 months and included pain intensity (numeric rating scale from 0 to 10), grip strength (kg, dynamometer), and questions about weakness in the wrist or fingers. The results indicated significant pain reduction in both groups at all timepoints, which was significantly higher in patients receiving the high-dose treatment at all timepoints except months 5 and 6. However, "successful pain treatment" did not differ between the groups. This parameter was defined as more than, or equal to, 50% decrease in pain intensity scores at 6 months [change in numeric rating scale (%) = (pretreatment score – six-month post-treatment score/pretreatment score × 100)]. Similar results were obtained for grip strength, except that between-group differences were absent only at month 5. Motor weakness was significantly more pronounced in the high-dose group but did not cause debilitation. In general, it was concluded that BoNT-A administered at high doses yields better results, compared to lower doses of this toxin.

BoNT studies in CLE are summarized in Table 10.2.

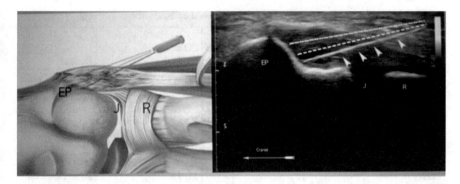

Fig. 10.1 Schematic (left) and ultrasound image (right) demonstrating injection of botulinum toxin A into the common wrist extensor tendon. Arrowheads, needle; EP, epicondyle; J, joint; R, radius. (From [22], with permission from Oxford University Press)

Comment

Table 10.2 categorizes BoNT studies in CLE, based on the level of evidence criteria described by the Assessment Subcommittee of the American Academy of Neurology [15, 16]. Accordingly, three class I and three class II studies using botulinumtoxinA and one class IV study utilizing incobotulinumtoxinA have all reported effectiveness of BoNT-A. However, there was one class III study with onaA [19] who contradicted these results and found BoNT to be ineffective against pain in CLE patients. Predicated on this information, it is safe to say that treatment of CLE with botulinumtoxinA meets level A evidence or in other words could be considered "effective" for treating CLE. The problem with the abovementioned class III study was the limited number of subjects selected for evaluation, and more importantly it only used one efficacy assessment at only one timepoint (3 months). Previous experience with the application of BoNT indicates that its effect is temporary and often disappears within 3 months. In the comparator study by Lin et al. [23], results were based on only 16 patients which is too small and may lead to type II statistical error. On the other hand, Gou et al. [18] evaluated the efficacy of BoNT with a larger number of subjects, reducing this type of error and leading to the conclusion that triamcinolone is as effective as botulinumtoxinA but without its side effects on finger function.

At present, favorable findings on BoNT injections used for the treatment of CLE exist in the literature, which are based on blinded studies. However, an important problem is that the favorable effects are accompanied by weakness in finger extension that develops after BoNT injection. To deal with this issue, larger blinded studies using different neurotoxins and methods are required so that patients can benefit from the positive outcomes of this toxin without enduring its negative effects.

Table 10.2 Blinded studies of BoNT-A in chronic lateral epicondylitis

Study	Class	# of pts	Type	Toxin	Dose (u)	PO at week(s)	SO	Results
Wong et al. [46]	II	60	DBPC	AboA	60	VAS: 12	Handgrip	$p < 0.001$ (VAS)
Hayton et al. [19]	III	40	DBPC	AboA	50	VAS	SF12, handgrip	NS
Placzek et al. [33]	I	130	DBPC	AboA	60	VAS: 2, 6, 12, 16	PPS	$p < 0.05$ (VAS) all weeks, PPS $p < 0.05$
Espandar et al. [14]	II	48	DBPC	AboA	60	VAS: 4, 8, 16 MP, MG		$p = 0.01$ (VAS) $p = 0.04$ (MP)
Lin et al. [23]	II	16	Comp	OnaA and triamcinolone	50	VAS: 4, 8, 12		$p = 0.02$ (VAS) week 4 triamcinolone >onaA
Gou et al. (2017)	I	36	Comp	OnaA (two sites) and triamcinolone	20	VAS: 4, 8, 12, 16	handgrip, PTEE	$p = 0.01$ (VAS) and all SO at week 4 in favor of triamcinolone
Lee et al. [22]	I	60	Comp	Meditox small and large doses	10 and 50	NRS, grip strength, weakness in wrist/ finger: 1, 2, 3, 4, 5, and 6 months		$p < 0.05$ (NRS) 1, 2, 3, 4 months; $p < 0.05$ grip strength (kg) all times except month 5 all in favor of 50 U; $p = 0.044$ motor weakness more prevalent in 50 U

Study class according to definition of the Assessment Subcommittee of AAN [15, 16]
DBPC double blind, placebo controlled, *AboA* abobotulinumtoxinA, *onaA* onabotulinumtoxinA, *PO* primary outcome, *SP* secondary outcome, *PPS* patient and physician satisfaction scale (0–4), *MP* maximum pinch, *MG* maximum grip, *ns* not significant, *PTEE* Patient-Rated Tennis Elbow Questionnaire, *NRS* numeric rating scale

Refractory Pain Following Total Knee Arthroplasty (TKA)

A significant source of chronic pain in adults is chronic, advanced osteoarthritis of the knee which responds poorly to medication. A successful modality for improving pain and quality of life in patients with this problem is total knee arthroplasty [29], which is very commonly performed in the USA, estimated as 500,000 cases annually. This number is proposed to have a sixfold increase by 2030, reaching 3.48 million/year [39].

Unfortunately, the procedure is not always satisfactory for the patients, and almost a quarter of them complain of various issues after treatment [2]. Furthermore, an additional 7–44% continue to have persistent pain following the procedure [4, 47]. The mechanism of TKA-related pain depends on the active contribution of known pain transmitters. In contrast to normal joints, elevated levels of substance P have been demonstrated in the joint fluid of patients with chronic osteoarthritis who have been subjected to TKA [35]. Considering that the chronic pain which develops after this treatment is resistant to drug therapy, novel treatment strategies are clearly welcome in this area of pain medicine.

Singh et al. [39] conducted a randomized, double-blind, placebo-controlled study to evaluate the efficiency of intra-articular (IA) injection of onaA, in relieving TKA-induced pain. The 54 patients enrolled in this study were mostly male (84%) with a mean age of 67 years and had undergone complete arthroplasty of the knee. Their mean TKA-related pain duration was 4.5 years, which exceeded 6 months and was moderate or severe (>6 on 0–10 VAS). For the BoNT injections, 100 units of onaA was reconstituted in 5 ml of 0.9% saline without preservative and injected IA. The primary outcome was the proportion of patients who experienced a reduction of two or more points of the numerical VAS scale (0–10), which was compared between the BoNT and placebo groups at 2 months. VAS and Western Ontario and McMaster Universities (WOMAC) Osteoarthritis Index physical function were assessed at baseline and at 2, 3, and 4 months. The patient and physician's global impression of change were also determined at the same timepoints.

The proportion of patients who reported VAS-based pain reduction was significantly larger in the group who received onaA (71%) compared to the saline group (35%), at the 2-month timepoint ($p = 0.028$). A significant difference in duration of meaningful pain relief was found between the onaA and placebo groups recorded as 39.6 ± 50.4 days and 15.7 ± 22.6 days, respectively ($p = 0.045$). Similar significant differences in favor of onaA was reported in physician global assessment of change ($p = 0.003$), Short-Form 36 pain subscale score ($p = 0.049$), the physical function subscale ($p = 0.026$), stiffness subscale ($p = 0.004$), and total scores ($p = 0.024$) of WOMAC Osteoarthritis Index at all timepoints. There were no serious treatment-associated adverse events in the onaA group. Local pain due to injection and mild temporary weakness around the joint was observed in some of the participants, but they were not significantly different between the two groups.

One of the major challenges in the discipline of pain medicine is postsurgical pain. Due to its numerous attributes, BoNT therapy has emerged as a successful option for a heterogeneous group of conditions related to postsurgical pain such as that arising from mastectomy, hemorrhoidectomy, cholecystectomy, hernia repair, and post-adductor release surgery in children with cerebral palsy. Its mechanism of action is multifaceted, and elements like local accumulation of pain transmitters, damage to terminal nerve endings, local inflammation, etc., may be responsible for or play a role in its clinical effects.

Comment

The RCT by Singh et al. [39] can be categorized as a class II study with level C evidence, indicating that BoNT treatment for TKA-induced pain could be "possibly effective," based on the criteria and guidelines of the American Academy of Neurology's Subcommittee on Assessment of the efficacy of randomized clinical trials [15, 16]. Further high-quality (classes I and II) studies are suggested to confirm these encouraging results and help provide a better understanding of the role of BoNT treatment in the refractory pain associated with TKA.

Painful Local Arthritis

Arthritis is regarded as one of the most common debilitating health conditions worldwide. It can involve a variety of joints including the knee, which afflicts 46 million people in the USA.

In a recent review, Cheng et al. [10] reported data gathered from systematic reviews and clinical trials pertaining to the efficacy of IA administration of different agents for the treatment of arthritic knee pain. Accordingly, steroids and hyaluronate both effectively reduced pain, but the pain relief obtained from hyaluronate lasted longer. Among steroids, triamcinolone hexacetonide demonstrated superior results compared to triamcinolone acetonide and was suggested as a good option for IA use. Other effective substances included tropisetron, a 5-HT3 receptor antagonist, and tanezumab, a monoclonal antibody against nerve growth factor, which were given a 2B+ efficacy level, similar to BoNT-A. A variety of IA radioisotopes have also been reported to be partially effective, but there is uncertainty regarding their long-term safety and efficiency.

Mahowald et al. [26] presented their 1-year clinical experience on onaA injection for the treatment of arthritis and arthritic pain in nine shoulders, three knees, and three ankles in 11 patients. All participants had a history of failed treatments involving intra-articular administration of steroids and/or viscosupplement agents. Shoulder and limb joints were injected with 50–100 units and 25–50 units of onaA, respectively. Comparing pain at baseline and time of maximum relief, a significant ($p = 0.02$) mean maximum reduction of 55% was found in limb joints. The decrease was even greater in shoulder joints reaching 72% ($p < 0.001$). Similarly, significant improvements in lower extremity function (36%) and shoulders (67% in flexion, 42% in abduction) were reported at follow-up ($p = 0.044$, $p = 0.001$, and $p = 0.01$, respectively). Limb improvements occurred between 4 and 10 weeks postinjection. No significant adverse events were observed.

Castiglione et al. [8] conducted a prospective, open-label study of five patients with post-hemiplegic shoulder pain. OnaA (100 units), aboA (500 units), and incoA (100 units) were used to inject the glenohumeral painful joints in two, one, and two patients, respectively. At 2 and 8 weeks, VAS was used to determine the level of pain at rest and pain during passive arm abduction. All subjects at both timepoints reported significant improvement of shoulder pain at rest ($p = 0.001$) and at arm abduction ($p < 0.001$). No difference in the level of pain relief was observed at 2 and 8 weeks.

McAlindon et al. [28] conducted a phase 2, multicenter, double-blind, randomized, placebo-controlled parallel-group study on 158 patients with knee osteoarthritis. Those with nociceptive pain, assessed through a painDETECT questionnaire ($\leq$12), were enrolled. All subjects received IA injections under ultrasound guidance after aspiration of synovial fluid effusion (if present). The injections included onaA with doses of 400 U or 200 U or normal saline which were administered in a total volume of 2 ml to patients allocated in a 1:1:2 ratio. The duration of follow-up was 24 weeks. On week 8, the "daily average numeric rating scale pain score," measured over a 7-day period, was recorded for the study knee. The results showed a two-point decrease for all treatments which was maintained during the entire follow-up. However, there were no significant between-group differences for any of the injected substances. These findings were repeated for all secondary outcome measures including WOMAC physical function scores and the patient global impression of change (PGIC).

In a double-blind, randomized, placebo-controlled, 12-week study by Arendt-Nielsen et al. [3], efficacy of BoNT therapy was evaluated in painful osteoarthritis of the knee. A total of 121 patients with this condition were randomly injected with botulinumtoxinA (200 U, 2 ml) or placebo (2 ml, 0.9% saline) and followed for 12 weeks. Injections were performed under ultrasound guidance. The test and control groups consisted of 61 and 60 subjects, respectively, and were further divided into nociceptive ($n = 68$) and non-nociceptive ($n = 53$) subgroups based on the painDETECT questionnaire. Outcomes were measured using quantitative sensory testing, WOMAC, average daily pain, and PGIC. No significant between-group differences were demonstrated for mechanistic pain biomarkers. However, the nociceptive subgroup demonstrated significant improvements in the above parameters.

Comparator Studies

In a study by Boon et al. [7], 60 knee osteoarthritis patients, unresponsive to conventional treatments and physical therapy, were recruited to compare different doses of onaA with steroids. All participants had a minimum VAS score of 6/10 and functional impairment of the knee. Injections of onaA were administered with either low (100 units) or high (200 units) doses, and its efficacy was compared with 40 units of methylprednisolone acetate. Evaluations were made at 8 and 26 weeks, and of the 60 participants, all competed the 8 weeks, while only 32 patients went through the entire study period. VAS-based pain reduction was considered as the primary outcome, which despite showing effectiveness for all three substances at week 8 reached significant levels only in the low-dose onaA group ($p = 0.01$). Secondary outcomes included quality of life determined via Short-Form 36,

WOMAC Arthritis Index, patient global assessment using a three-question format, and a 40-meter timed walk. Statistically significant decreases in pain and stiffness subsets of the WOMAC Arthritis Index scores were found in all groups. Side effects consist of local swelling and pain at the site of injection, dry mouth, and balance problems which were mild and did not differ among the groups. However, local swelling and pain at the site of injection along with balance problems were more common in the high-dose onaA group ($p > 0.05$).

In a single (assessor) blind, prospective study, Sun et al. [42] recruited 75 patients with symptomatic ankle osteoarthritis to compare the safety/effectiveness of IA "onaA" and "hyaluronate plus rehabilitation exercise." Single doses of BoNT-A (100 units) were administered to 38 subjects, while the rest received IA injections of hyaluronate along with physiotherapy for 30 min per session, three times a week for 1 month. The total score of the Ankle Osteoarthritis Scale (AOS) was regarded as the primary outcome of the study, and its endpoint assessment was 6 months. This patient-rated measure is based on two nine-item pain and disability subscales resulting in a final score of 0–10, denoting "none" to "worst" pain or disability. Several secondary outcomes were considered, and those related purely to pain included VAS and global patient satisfaction, which were determined before injection (baseline) and at 2 weeks and 1, 3, and 6 months. A minimum decrease of 30% in pain score was defined as significant. For ankle joint injections, the needle was inserted 1 cm anterior to the distal medial malleolus and advanced posteriorly and slightly upward toward the middle of the ankle joint above the talus to deliver 100 units of onaA or 2 ml sodium hyaluronate. In cases accompanied by effusion, aspirations were performed before injections. According to the measured pain subset of AOS and VAS scores, all patients reported a significant reduction of $\geq 50\%$. In onaA subjects, VAS scores decreased from 4 at baseline to 1.8 on week 2, which continued to decline to 1.7 on the third month of the study. Pain alleviation was similar between the two groups with no significant differences. Similarly considerable improvement in the disability scores was observed in both groups, which even lasted for 6 months in a number of participants. None of the patients experienced any serious side effects.

Bao et al. [5] in a single-center, placebo-controlled, single-blinded study randomized 60 patients with knee osteoarthritis into three injection groups including saline (placebo), onaA, and hyaluronate. The articular cavity of the knee was located using color Doppler ultrasound, which positioned the injection point at the level of the suprapatellar bursa. A dose of 100 U onaA in 2.5 ml saline and the same volume placebo were used, while the hyaluronate group received injections once a week for 5 weeks. Exercise therapy was administered in all groups, and outcomes were recorded at baseline and 4 and 8 weeks. WOMAC Index questionnaire score, VAS, and Medical Outcomes Study 36-Item Health Survey (SF-36) constituted the outcome measures. In the group receiving onaA, WOMAC, VAS, and both physical and mental components of SF-36 improved significantly compared to both placebo and hyaluronate groups at 4 and 8 weeks.

Comment

Two blinded class I studies [3, 28], one small blinded class II trial [26], three blinded comparator studies, and a small open-label study showed conflicting results regarding the efficacy of intra-articular injection of BonT-A in the treatment of arthritic joint pain. Two class I studies did not confirm the positive impact of BoNT, whereas one contradicted this finding and reported positive effects for this toxin [5]. Among the three comparator studies, one [7] had a considerable number of dropouts (30%) and reported a superior response to low dose compared to high doses of onaA, without adequate justification. On account of the high amount of subject dropout, this study can best be defined as class III. Of the two other comparator studies, both were single-blinded. One showed similar effects between BoNT-A and the other intervention [42], while the other study [5] reported favorable effects of BoNT therapy.

Therefore, the level of evidence for BoNT efficacy in the treatment of painful arthritis (AAN guidelines [15, 16]) is B (probably ineffective) based on the availability of two class I studies. Further controlled studies are required to substantiate these negative claims – especially considering one positive class I study.

Anterior Knee Pain Related to Vastus Lateralis Imbalance

A common complaint among the general population is anterior knee pain with a suggested incidence of 22/1000 individuals/year [6]. One of its major causes is patellofemoral syndrome, which is known as anterior knee pain that occurs mostly in young women, without any significant relevant pathology [32]. A probable source of anterior knee pain and the patellofemoral syndrome can be an imbalance of the vastus lateralis muscles [34].

Based on this probable source, a double-blind, placebo-controlled trial on 24 patients with anterior knee pain was conducted by Singer et al. [38] to study the effectiveness of BoNT in pain relief. The vastus lateralis muscles randomly received 4 ml aboA (500 units) or placebo (saline) in eight sites (0.5 ml/site) under electromyographic guidance (Fig. 10.2). The primary outcomes were measured at 3 months using Anterior Knee Pain Scale and VAS to assess improvements in "knee pain-related disability" and "activity-induced knee pain," respectively. Significant improvement of the former was only found in patients injected with aboA. Similarly, "activity-induced knee pain" in the BoNT group showed clinically significant decreases in mean VAS for kneeling, stair walking, squatting, and level walking. In the placebo subjects, there was only a decline in stair walking, which was not statistically significant. The authors concluded that aboA had a significant favorable impact on chronic anterior knee pain due to vastus lateralis imbalance.

Chen et al. [9] conducted an unblind, prospective, case-control study on the efficacy of BoNT-A for the treatment of knee pain due to patellofemoral pain syn-

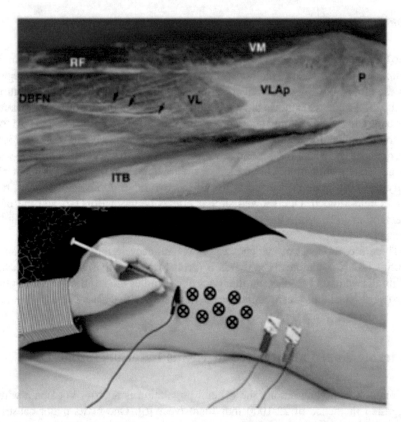

Fig. 10.2 Dissection showing the distal branch of the femoral nerve to vastus lateralis (small arrows), with the iliotibial band (ITB) reflected posteriorly (upper panel). As illustrated in the lower panel, multiple injection sites, using EMG guidance, were employed to ensure spread of injectate within the distal VL muscle. VLA p, vastus lateralis aponeurosis of the knee joint capsule; RF, rectus femoris muscle; VM, vastus medialis; p, patella. (Original figure is reprinted from Singer et al. [48], which has been made available under Creative Commons Attribution License)

drome. Case selection consisted of patients affected with this syndrome in both knees, so that the contralateral knee could be used as control. OnaA (10 U/0.1 ml diluted in saline) was injected into the vastus lateralis muscle of the knee in 12 subjects. The knee with the worse pain received BoNT-A under electromyographic guidance, and the control knee was left untreated. The dose was administered at one injection site, where the needle was inserted about 3–5 cm above the patella, on an oblique angle just lateral to the midline. Assessment involved changes in WOMAC score, which was evaluated at baseline and after 4, 8, and 12 weeks of onaA administrations to record pain, stiffness, and functional status of the knees. Additionally, muscle force was determined by an isokinetic dynamometer at the same timepoints. According to the WOMAC results obtained at 12 weeks, the BoNT-A-injected knees demonstrated a clinically significant reduction in mean pain (-1.8, $p = 0.014$) and function scores (-6.6, $p = 0.029$). Despite the decrease in stiffness scores, the difference on week 12 was not significant. The isokinetic test demonstrated a significant reduction in flexion moment (12.1 Nm, $p = 0.041$) but not in extension moment, after BoNT-A treatment. The control knee did not achieve significant changes in WOMAC scores but demonstrated an increased flexion moment as in the treated knee. The authors concluded that injection of onaA could improve anterior knee pain, function, and isokinetic torque caused by vastus lateralis imbalance.

Comment

The abovementioned class II and III studies define a C level of evidence (possibly effective) for anterior knee pain with vastus lateralis imbalance (AAN assessment of evidence, [15, 16]).

Orthopedic Contracture and/or Pain Release

Intramuscular injections of botulinum toxins are well-known options for the treatment of spasticity. Spasticity is a complex issue and a common symptom observed in a variety of neurologic conditions like stroke, multiple sclerosis, brain/spinal cord injury, and cerebral palsy. Despite the fact that spasticity responds well to drug therapy, it can cause unwanted adverse events and has a short response period. One of the FDA-approved applications of BoNT is its intramuscular injections to treat spasticity. However, the efficacy of BoNT therapy in pain related to this issue is less determined, and evidence level is more unclear [20]. The practice of intramuscular injection using BoNT has led to the development of new areas and additional options for treatment of other orthopedic-related issues. Scientific studies are beginning to evaluate the role of BoNT in treating these problems which include orthopedic contracture and/or pain release.

Smith et al. [41] investigated the efficacy of a single injection of onabotulinumtoxinA for improving flexion contracture after total knee arthroplasty in a prospective, randomized, double-blinded, placebo-controlled trial. Patients with flexion contracture after total knee arthroplasty were randomized to receive either 100 units of onabotulinumtoxinA diluted in 2 ml saline (nine knees) or the same volume of 0.9% saline (six knees). Injections were administered into the hamstrings, and all subjects were assessed at 1, 6, and 12 months. Extension significantly improved at all timepoints in both BoNT and control groups. Significant difference in extension between the two groups was noted 1 month postinjection in favor of BoNT-A. After a mixed model regression analysis, onaA also showed significant improvement compared to placebo on month 12 of the study period. Due to the fact that improvements were encountered in both groups, the authors concluded that the significant difference between the BoNT and placebo groups was of limited clinical significance.

Eibach et al. [12] presented a case report of a 47-year-old male with tetraplegia due to cerebral palsy. The patient required a total hip joint arthroplasty because of hip arthrosis. OnaA guided by CT fluoroscopy was injected preoperatively into hip flexor and adductor muscles (200 U in iliopsoas and 50 U bilateral in adductor magnus). This was performed in order to minimize the risk of postoperative luxation. Seven days after treatment, the patient had a reduction in spasticity, I think preoperatively is correct flexion and adduction contracture and was pain-free. Santamato et al. [37] reported the application of BoNT-A in a 34-year-old woman with persistent painful contracture in the adductor magnus muscle after total hip arthroplasty. OnaA (150 UM) was injected preoperatively into adductor magnus muscles of the hip under electromyographic guide. Seven days after treatment, the patient had a reduction in pain evaluated by VAS, and on day 20 Harris hip score and external rotation of the hip showed considerable improvement. The clinical effects were maintained at the 2-month follow-up. Both the abovementioned case studies reported no adverse events.

Eleopra et al. [13] conducted a prospective, randomized double-blind multicenter study to evaluate the effectiveness of intramuscular botulinumtoxinA injections in 46 patients with hip osteoarthritis. The rationale was to relieve pressure in the arthritic hip joint to improve pain and range of motion. AboA or saline was injected randomly into the adductor muscles of the affected arthritic hip joint. The total dose of abobotulinumtoxinA was 400 U in 2 ml of saline, with 250 U being injected in the adductor longus muscle and 150 U in the adductor magnus muscle under electromyographic guidance. The control group received the same volume of saline without the aboA. Evaluation was performed before injection and after 2, 4, and 12 weeks. After the fourth week, the BoNT-A group showed significant differences in pain level (VAS) and Harris hip scores compared to the controls and also in all timepoints compared to baseline (Fig. 10.3). Otherwise, there were no significant differences during follow-up neither in primary nor secondary outcome parameters such as Medical Research Council scale for muscle strength and Short Form scale (SF-36) scores. No adverse events were detected in either treatment groups. A pilot study by Marchini et al. [27] was conducted prior to the RCT by the same group [13], which included a series of 39 patients with the same treatment regime and scientific design, except for the fact that it was a longitudinal prospective series without a control group. Their results demonstrated a significant improvement in pain level evaluated by VAS and in Harris hip score after 2, 4, and 12 weeks and also in SF-36 scores after 4 and 12 weeks.

In a prospective randomized triple-blind, single-center study, Wong et al. [45] used intramuscular botulinumtoxinA injections for correction of neuromuscular scoliosis in 10 severely handicapped, tetraplegic children with cerebral palsy (gross motor function classification system 3–5). The randomization was based on a crossover design with two consecutive 6-month study periods. Radiologic examinations were performed before and 6 weeks after BoNT-A injections. OnaA (10 U/0, 1 ml) was administered in the iliopsoas, quadratus lumborum, and erector spinae muscles under ultrasound guidance using 100 U, 50 U, and 30 U, respectively. In the "control period," the participants received the same volume of saline without the onaA

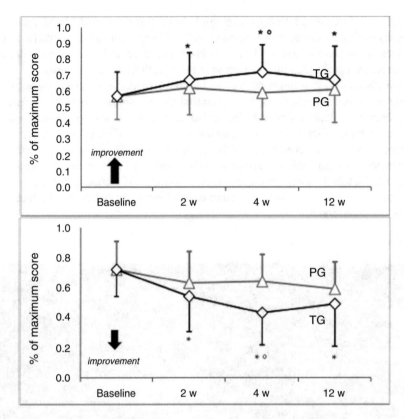

Fig. 10.3 Harris hip score (upper) and visual analog scale (lower) before injection and 2, 4, and 12 weeks after. Values are given as mean ± standard deviation and represent percentage of maximum score (100). PG, placebo group (*n* = 15); TG, treated group (*n* = 31); (*), significant difference with baseline; (0), significant difference with placebo group. (Original figure is reprinted from Eleopra et al. [13], which has been made available under Creative Commons Attribution License)

in the target muscles. Primary outcome parameter consisted of change in the radiological parameter for scoliotic curve severity of Cobb's angle, and no significant improvement was detected. Similarly, no clinical improvements were reported. The study was terminated at an interim analysis after the death of one patient. This occurred after two hand surgical procedures and several months after BoNT-A injection therapy termination. No other severe adverse events were detected. A follow-up study was conducted by Wong et al. [44] on a consecutive series of nine adolescent patients with idiopathic scoliosis to investigate the possible role of spinal muscular forces/pulls in the induction of spinal deformity. A single ultrasound-guided injection of onaA (10 U/0, 1 ml) with a maximum dose of 100 U was administered to the psoas part of the iliopsoas muscle on the concave side of the lumbar spine. Radiological examination (Fig. 10.4) evaluating curve severity and rotation as a primary outcome parameter was carried out before and 6 weeks after injections.

Significant, but not clinically meaningful, improvement was detected for curve severity of Cobb's angle. However, no significant improvement was found for radiological derotation evaluated ad modem Nash and Moe. Adverse events were not detected, except for temporary soreness at the injection site in two cases.

Park et al. [31] in a single-center, double-blind, randomized, placebo-controlled study examined the effects of botulinumtoxinA on clinical outcomes of femoral lengthening. Bilateral femoral distraction osteogenesis was performed on 44 patients with familial short stature. OnabotulinumtoxinA (200 U) was administered intraoperatively into seven points of the quadriceps muscle, and an equal volume of sterile normal saline was injected in the other thigh. The patients were evaluated at 4, 8, 12, 24, and 48 weeks. No improvement in range of motion of the hip or knee and also no difference in maximal thigh circumference or distraction-induced pain levels were observed.

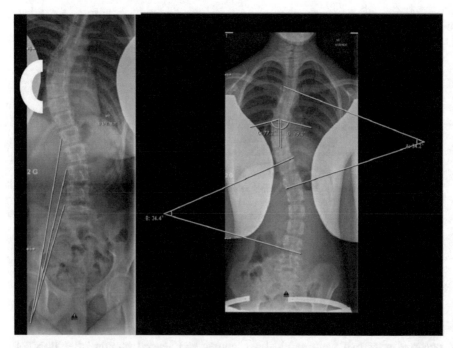

Fig. 10.4 Radiographic image of scoliosis depicting the psoas major on the concave side of a thoracic scoliosis; the stronger thoracic muscles are marked with C and are located in the convex side of the scoliosis (left). Measurements of thoracic and lumbar Cobb's angle and concave and convex rib vertebra angle (right). (Original figure is reprinted from Wong et al. [44], which has been made available under Creative Commons Attribution http://creativecommons.org/licenses/by/4.0/, http://creativecommons.org/publicdomain/zero/1.0/)

Comment

Intramuscular injection therapy using BoNT for orthopedic contracture and/or pain release in relation to arthroplasty and joint arthritis has been evaluated in one class I [13] and four class IV studies. This defines a C level of evidence (possibly effective) for this indication (AAN assessment of evidence, [15, 16]). One class I study for femoral distraction osteogenesis and one class I and one class III study for scoliosis correction define a level B evidence considered as probably ineffective.

Conclusion

The favorable findings of RCTs using BoNT therapy for orthopedic disorders discussed in the preceding chapter have set the stage for conducting additional controlled studies in this essential area of orthopedic surgery. Most likely, with the advent of improved methods and administration of optimum dosage, BoNT injection has the potential to become a valuable option for treatment of refractory pain in orthopedic disorders.

References

1. Ahmad Z, Siddiqui N, Malik SS, Abdus-Samee M, Tytherleigh-Strong G, Rushton N. Lateral epicondylitis: a review of pathology and management. Bone Joint J. 2013;95-B:1158–64.
2. Anderson JG, Wixson RL, Tsai D, Stulberg SD, Chang RW. Functional outcome and patient satis- faction in total knee patients over the age of 75. J Arthroplast. 1996;11:831–40.
3. Arendt-Nielsen L, Jiang G-L, Degryse R, Turkel CC. Intra-articular onabotulinumtoxinA in osteoarthritis knee pain: effect on human mechanistic pain biomarkers and clinical pain. Scand J Rheumatol. 2017;46(4):303–16.
4. Baker PN, van der Meulen JH, et al. The role of pain and function in determining patient satisfac- tion after total knee replacement: data from the National Joint Registry for England and Wales. J Bone Joint Surg Br. 2007;89:893–900.
5. Bao X, Tan JW, Flyzik M, Ma XC, Liu H, Liu HY. Effect of therapeutic exercise on knee osteoarthritis after intra-articular injection of botulinum toxin type A, hyaluronate or saline: a randomized controlled trial. Rehabil Med. 2018;50(6):534–41.
6. Boling M, Padua D, Marshall S, Guskiewicz K, Pyne S, Beutler A. Gender differences in the inci- dence and prevalence of patellofemoral pain syndrome. Scand J Med Sci Sports. 2010;20:725–30.
7. Boon AJ, Smith J, Dahm DL, Sorenson EJ, Larson DR, Fitz-Gibbon PD, Dykstra DD, Singh JA. Efficacy of intra-articular botulinum toxin type A in painful knee osteoarthritis: a pilot study. PM R. 2010;2:268–76.
8. Castiglione A, Bagnato S, Boccagni C, Romano MC, Galardi G. Efficacy of intra-articular injec- tion of botulinum toxin type A in refractory hemiplegic shoulder pain. Arch Phys Med Rehabil. 2011;92:1034–7.
9. Chen JT, Tang AC, Lin SC, Tang SF. Anterior knee pain caused by patellofemoral pain syndrome can be relieved by Botulinum toxin type A injection. Clin Neurol Neurosurg. 2015;129(Suppl 1):S27–9.

10. Cheng OT, Souzdalnitski D, Vrooman B, Cheng J. Evidence-based knee injections for the manage- ment of arthritis. Pain Med. 2012;13:740–53.
11. Connell D, Burke F, Coombes P, McNealy S, Freeman D, Pryde D, Hoy G. Sonographic examina- tion of lateral epicondylitis. AJR Am J Roentgenol. 2001;176:777–82.
12. Eibach S, Krug H, Lobsien E, Hoffmann KT, Kupsch A. Preoperative treatment with Botulinum Toxin A before total hip arthroplasty in a patient with tetraspasticity: case report and review of literature. NeuroRehabilitation. 2011;28(2):81–3.
13. Eleopra R, Rinaldo S, Lettieri C, Santamato A, Bortolotti P, Lentino C, Tamborino C, Causero A, Devigili G. AbobotulinumtoxinA: a new therapy for hip osteoarthritis. A prospective randomized double-blind multicenter study. Toxins (Basel). 2018;10(11):448.
14. Espandar R, Heidari P, Rasouli MR, Saadat S, Farzan M. Use of anatomic measurement to guide injection of botulinum toxin for the management of chronic lateral epicondylitis. CMAJ. 2010;182:768–73.
15. French J, Gronseth G. Lost in a jungle of evidence: we need a compass. Neurology. 2008;71:1634–8.
16. Gronseth G, French J. Practice parameters and technology assessments: what they are, what they are not, and why you should care. Neurology. 2008;71:1639–43.
17. Hamilton PG. The prevalence of humeral epicondylitis: a survey in general practice. J R Coll Gen Pract. 1986;36:464–5.
18. Guo YH, Kuan TS, Chen KL, Lien WC, Hsieh PC, Hsieh IC, Chiu SH, Lin YC. Comparison between steroid and 2 different sites of botulinum toxin injection in the treatment of lateral epicondylalgia: a randomized, double-blind, active drug-controlled pilot study. Arch Phys Med Rehabil. 2017;98(1):36–42.
19. Hayton MJ, Santini AJ, Hughes PJ, Frostick SP, Trail IA, Stanley JK. Botulinum toxin injection in the treatment of tennis elbow. A double-blind, randomized, controlled, pilot study. J Bone Joint Surg Am. 2005;87:503–7.
20. Jabbari B. Botulinum toxin treatment of pain disorders Springer New York Heidelberg Dordrecht London©. New York: Springer Science+Business Media; 2015.
21. Krogh TP, Bartels EM, Ellingsen T, Stengaard-Pedersen K, Buchbinder R, Fredberg U, Bliddal H, Christensen R. Comparative effectiveness of injection therapies in lateral epicondylitis: a sys- tematic review and network meta-analysis of randomized controlled trials. Am J Sports Med. 2013;41:1435–46.
22. Lee SH, Choi HH, Chang MC. The effect of botulinum toxin injection into the common extensor tendon in patients with chronic lateral epicondylitis: a randomized trial. Pain Med. 2019; https://doi.org/10.1093/pm/pnz323.
23. Lin YC, Tu YK, Chen SS, Lin IL, Chen SC, Guo HR. Comparison between botulinum toxin and corticosteroid injection in the treatment of acute and subacute tennis elbow a prospective, ran- domized, double-blind, active drug-controlled pilot study. Am J Phys Med Rehabil. 2010;89:653–9.
24. Lin YC, Wu WT, Hsu YC, Han DS, Chang KV. Comparative effectiveness of botulinum toxin versus nonsurgical treatments for treating lateral epicondylitis: a systematic review and meta-analysis. Clin Rehabil. 2018;32(2):131–45.
25. Liu J, Pho RWH, Pereira BP, Lau HK, Kumar VP. Distribution of primary motor nerve branches and terminal nerve entry points to the forearm muscles. Anat Rec. 1997;248:456–63.
26. Mahowald ML, Singh JA, Dykstra D. Long term effects of intra-articular botulinum toxin A for refractory joint pain. Neurotox Res. 2006;9(2–3):179–88.
27. Marchini C, Acler M, Bolognari MA, Causero A, Volpe D, Regis D, Rizzo A, Rosa R, Eleopra R, Manganotti P. Efficacy of botulinum toxin type A treatment of functional impairment of degenerative hip joint: preliminary results. J Rehabil Med. 2010;42(7):691–3.
28. McAlindon TE, Schmidt U, Bugarin D, Abrams S, Geib T, DeGryse RE, Kim K, Schnitzer TJ. Efficacy and safety of single-dose onabotulinumtoxinA in the treatment of symptoms of osteoarthritis of the knee: results of a placebo-controlled, double-blind study. Osteoarthr Cartil. 2018;26(10):1291–9.

29. Nashi N, Hong CC, Krishna L. Residual knee pain and functional outcome following total knee arthroplasty in osteoarthritic patients. Knee Surg Sports Traumatol Arthrosc. 2014;23(6):1841–7.
30. Nirschl RP, Ashman ES. Elbow tendinopathy: tennis elbow. Clin Sports Med. 2003;22:813–36.
31. Park H, Shin S, Shin HS, Kim HW, Kim DW, Lee DH. Is botulinum toxin type A a valuable adjunct during femoral lengthening? A randomized trial. Clin Orthop Relat Res. 2016;474(12):2705–11.
32. Petersen W, Ellermann A, Gösele-Koppenburg A, Best R, Rembitzki IV, Brüggemann GP, Liebau C. Patellofemoral pain syndrome. Knee Surg Sports Traumatol Arthrosc. 2014;22:2264–74.
33. Placzek R, Drescher W, Deuretzbacher G, Hempfing A, Meiss AL. Treatment of chronic radial epicondylitis with botulinum toxin A: a double-blind, placebo-controlled, randomized multicenter study. J Bone Joint Surg Am. 2007;89:255–60.
34. Powers CM. Patellar kinematics, part I: the influence of vastus muscle activity in subjects with and without patellofemoral pain. Phys Ther. 2000;80:956–64.
35. Pritchett JW. Substance P, level in synovial fluid may predict pain relief after knee replacement. J Bone Joint Surg Br. 1997;79:114–6.
36. Ruiz AG, Díaz GV, Fernández BR, Ruiz De Vargas CE. Effects of ultrasound-guided Administration of Botulinum Toxin (IncobotulinumtoxinA) in patients with lateral epicondylitis. Toxins (Basel). 2019;11(1):46.
37. Santamato A, Ranieri M, Panza F, Solfrizzi V, Frisardi V, Lapenna LM, Moretti B, Fiore P. Botulinum toxin type A in the treatment of painful adductor muscle contracture after total hip arthroplasty. Orthopedics. 2009;32(10):774–6. https://doi.org/10.3928/01477447-20090818-29.
38. Singer BJ, Silbert PL, Song S, Dunne JW, Singer KP. Treatment of refractory anterior knee pain using botulinum toxin type A (Dysport) injection to the distal vastus lateralis muscle: a ran- domized placebo controlled crossover trial. Br J Sports Med. 2010;65:640–5.
39. Singh JA, Mahowald ML, Noorbaloochi S. Intraarticular botulinum toxin A for refractory painful total knee arthroplasty: a randomized controlled trial. J Rheumatol. 2010;37:2377–86.
40. Smidt N, Van der Windt DA, Assendelft WJ, Deville WL, Korthals-de Bos IB, Bouter LM. Corticosteroid injections, physiotherapy, or a wait-and-see policy for lateral epicondylitis: a randomised controlled trial. Lancet. 2002;359:657–62.
41. Smith EB, Shafi KA, Greis AC, Maltenfort MG, Chen AF. Decreased flexion contracture after total knee arthroplasty using Botulinum toxin A: a randomized controlled trial. Knee Surg Sports Traumatol Arthrosc. 2016;24(10):3229–34.
42. Sun SF, Hsu CW, Lin HS, Chou YJ, Chen JY, Wang JL. Efficacy of intraarticular botulinum toxin A and intraarticular hyaluronate plus rehabilitation exercise in patients with unilateral ankle osteoarthritis: a randomized controlled trial. J Foot Ankle Res. 2014;7(1):9. https://doi.org/10.1186/1757-1146-7-9.
43. Verhaar JA. Tennis elbow. Anatomical, epidemiological and therapeutic aspects. Int Orthop. 1994;18:263–7.
44. Wong C, Gosvig K, Sonne-Holm S. The role of the paravertebral muscles in adolescent idiopathic scoliosis evaluated by temporary paralysis. Scoliosis Spinal Disord. 2017;12:33.
45. Wong C, Pedersen SA, Kristensen BB, Gosvig K, Sonne-Holm S. The effect of botulinum toxin A injections in the spine muscles for cerebral palsy scoliosis, examined in a prospective, randomized triple-blinded study. Spine (Phila Pa 1976). 2015;40(23):E1205–11.
46. Wong SM, Hui AC, Tong PY, Poon DW, Yu E, Wong LK. Treatment of lateral epicondylitis with botulinum toxin: a randomized, double-blind, placebo-controlled trial. Ann Intern Med. 2005;143:793–7.
47. Wylde V, Hewlett S, Learmonth ID, Dieppe P. Persistent pain after joint replacement: prevalence, sensory qualities, and postoperative determinants. Pain. 2011;152:566–72.
48. Singer BJ, Silbert BI, Silbert PL, Singer KP. The role of botulinum toxin type A in the clinical management of refractory anterior knee pain. Toxins (Basel). 2015;7(9):3388–404.

Chapter 11
Botulinum Toxin for Pediatric Patients, Who? For What? When?

Sanaz Attaripour Isfahani and Katharine Alter

Abstract It is unanimously accepted in medicine that children are not simply miniature adults and require specialized medical care. In children with chronic diseases, treatment strategies are often limited by this population's vulnerability, capacity for understanding the disease/consequences of treatment, research procedures, and alternative options. Still, this vulnerability should not deprive them of a strong and specifically targeted research which may enhance outcomes and quality of life.

In this chapter, we review the existing knowledge on the treatment strategies involving botulinum toxin in the pediatric population. A major movement in medicine in the past two decades has been the transition to less invasive therapeutics. Following this movement, in this chapter, our focus is on the indications of botulinum toxin that may supplement noninvasive and surgical procedures to improve outcomes. While the indications for the use of botulinum toxin in children are numerous, approvals from regulatory agencies remain fewer than in the adult population. Ongoing research into the indications for botulinum toxin in children is likely to level this playing field.

Keywords Pediatrics · Botulinum toxin · Chemo-denervation · Growth and development · Cerebral palsy · Surgery · Rehabilitation

In 1981, Dr. Alan B. Scott used botulinum neurotoxin (hereafter BoNT) clinically in the human population for the first time. He concluded that BoNT is a safe and efficacious alternative for the surgical correction of the misaligned eyes in patients

S. Attaripour Isfahani (✉)
Department of Neurology, University of California, Irvine, Irvine, CA, USA
e-mail: sattarip@hs.uci.edu

K. Alter
Rehabilitation Medicine, Functional and Applied Biomechanics Section Clinical Center,
National Institutes of Health, Bethesda, MD, USA
e-mail: kalter@cc.nih.gov

© Springer Nature Switzerland AG 2020   217
B. Jabbari (ed.), *Botulinum Toxin Treatment in Surgery, Dentistry,
and Veterinary Medicine*, https://doi.org/10.1007/978-3-030-50691-9_11

with strabismus [1]. None of the 18 patients in the first cohort studied by him were in their childhood, but in 1989, he and his colleagues reported a case series consisting of 356 pediatric patients with strabismus and reported that both the drug and the injection procedure were safe and effective in this age population [2].

Around 30 years have passed since the first FDA approval of a serotype A BoNT [3], onabotulinumtoxinA (brand name Botox®). The first FDA approval for the use of botulinum toxin was in 2016 when abobotulinumtoxinA (brand name Dysport®) was approved in pediatric patients 2–17 years of age for the treatment of lower limb spasticity. Its use is also approved in the treatment of cervical dystonia in patients older than 16 and strabismus and blepharospasm in patients 12 years of age and older [4]. In 2019, three additional FDA approvals for the treatment of pediatric spasticity (ages 2–17 years) were added including onabotulinumtoxinA and abobotulinumtoxinA for upper limb spasticity and onabotulinumtoxinA for lower limb spasticity [5, 6].

Although there are no FDA-approved uses of BoNT in very young children, the safety of use in children younger than 2 years has been studied [7]. In a cohort of patients with clubfoot in British Columbia Children's Hospital, Canada, a total of 239 patients and 361 feet were enrolled in the study and 523 injections of onabotulinumtoxinA were performed. A case of transverse myelitis was the only adverse event reported and toxin was not deemed to be a causal factor.

The risks of BoNT injections for children are not specifically different from the adult population. However, the Blackbox warning from the FDA contains an extra phrase about a higher risk of the spread of the toxin beyond treatment areas in children treated for spasticity. This risk exists with therapeutic doses and even subtherapeutic doses of the toxin. The list of the potential risks provided by the FDA may at first glance appear overwhelmingly long, but there is substantial evidence supporting a reasonable safety profile for use of botulinum toxin in the pediatric population in different clinical scenarios [8–10], which justifies its use in the suitable clinical context.

During childhood, development and growth are actively ongoing, and abnormal tone can adversely affect these processes. Therefore, the impact of toxin in early life is considered to be of paramount importance [11].

Koman et al. treated spasticity in cerebral palsy using BoNT injections, while the surgical orthopedic intervention was delayed until the children attained a more stable gait pattern (age 6–10) [12]. This delay allows for continued maturation and acquisition of milestones providing the patient's treating team with additional opportunities to revise the treatment plan as the patient grows. The decreased tone with BoNT gives rise to greater muscle lengthening and improves the position and – as a result – the function until the surgery becomes a safer option.

Cerebral palsy is the most common cause of motor disorders in children with a prevalence of 2–3 per 1000 live births. It is the most frequently studied pediatric application of BoNT.

In 2009, Heinen et al. [13] updated the 2006 European consensus on the use of botulinum toxin for children with CP. The consensus recommends the use of BoNT in combination with all other possible treatment modalities, including physical therapy, constraint-induced movement therapy (CIMT), orthoses, casting, splinting, intrathecal baclofen, or other pharmacological and surgical interventions.

In 2013, Novak et al. published a systematic review on the best available intervention evidence for children with cerebral palsy (CP). Of the outcomes assessed, 16% (21 out of 131) were graded "do it" (green go), 58% (76 out of 131) "probably do it" (yellow measure), 20% (26 out of 131) "probably do not do it" (yellow measure), and 6% (8 out of 131) "do not do it" (red stop). Botulinum toxin injection was among the 15 green light interventions. BoNTs received a "green light recommendation," meaning it should be considered when appropriate [14].

BoNT in the realm of cerebral palsy has been studied from a variety of aspects: botulinum toxin's potential as an intervention in addition to or as an alternative to serial casting, various surgical interventions, different rehabilitation techniques, selection of patients before surgery, and impact on pain management following surgery. Its effects on function and various spasticity measures have been studied as well.

Botulinum Toxin in Cerebral Palsy

CP and Lower Limb Spasticity

Lower limb spasticity can limit ambulation, a crucial body function and one of the determinants of the degree of independence in patients with cerebral palsy. Abnormal gait patterns vary in severity and often change over time.

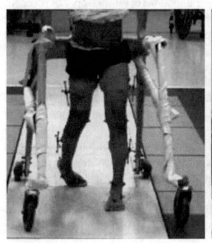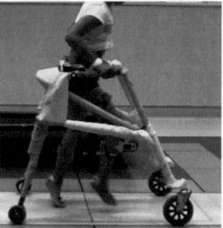

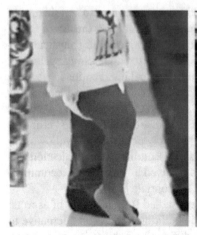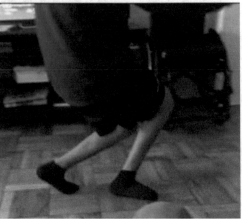

In non-ambulatory patients, lower limb spasticity significantly interferes with positioning and caring for patients with cerebral palsy.

In 26 children with cerebral palsy and a dynamic contracture of lower limb muscles interfering with positioning or walking, botulinum toxin A was injected into each affected muscle group. The range of dosages varied from 5 to 28 units per kilogram of body weight with the total dosages per patient ranging from 100 to 440 units of toxin. The outcome was measured by repeated clinical examination and gait analysis. Ambulatory status significantly improved. In some cases, the benefits even persisted after the tone-reducing effects of the toxin had worn off. The authors did not detect any systemic side effects attributable to the administration of the toxin [15].

In a larger randomized placebo-controlled trial, 114 pediatric patients with cerebral palsy and equinus deformity secondary to increased gastrocnemius/soleus muscle tone were assigned to two groups to receive injections of either BoNT or placebo. Patients in the BoNT group demonstrated improved gait function on observational gait analysis and range of motion of the ankle. No serious adverse events were reported [16].

In a head-to-head study of BoNT versus serial casting, the efficacy of botulinum toxin A injections was similar to serial fixed plaster casting in improving dynamic calf tightness in ambulant or partially ambulant children with cerebral palsy. Parents consistently favored botulinum toxin A and highlighted the inconvenience of serial casting [17].

In a 33-month longitudinal follow-up of a homogeneous group of patients with CP treated with BoNT, all patients exhibited progressive improvement in their gait pattern and none of them developed fixed contractures. No surgical correction was necessary, and no significant side effects were seen. All these patients had an equinus gait resulting from calf muscle spasticity without other muscle group involvement and all were treated with the same total dose (4 units/kg) at the same time interval (every 3 months) [18].

In a study on patients with cerebral palsy and gait abnormality who were candidates for muscle lengthening surgery, BoNT injection was performed preoperatively to evaluate for any deleterious effects of surgery on joint stability. BoNT temporarily weakens the muscle and muscle weakening is a known side effect of muscle tendon lengthening. In this study, preoperative BoNT-A test injections in all muscles considered for lengthening caused deleterious effects in 21% of patients. As a result, their lengthening surgery was canceled. In none of the rest of the patients after the surgery, gait function deteriorated. The percentage who showed deterioration of gait with BoNT injection was comparable with 18% who experienced negative outcome from the muscle lengthening surgery in a previous study which was used as a historical control. These data suggest that preoperative BoNT-A test injection can work reliably as a tool for predicting negative outcome after muscle lengthening surgery in patients with CP and can be helpful to avoid this negative outcome [19].

Contrary to the progressive improvement of gait reported in the latter study, there are reports of secondary nonresponsiveness to BoNT injections after initial success.

In a report on 12 patients (mean age 6.8 years, range 3–14 years) who received toxin injections for adductor spasm or spastic pes equinus, the formation of neutralizing antibodies became a limitation for long-term use of BoNT-A. Five patients were treated with Botox® and seven with Dysport®. Initially, all patients were documented to have a minimum of two beneficial treatments, but later on, they failed to show any clinical response to two consecutive sets of injections. Neutralizing antibodies were detected using a bioassay. Mean antibody titers were 8.7 mu/ml (range 1.8–10). Secondary nonresponses occurred after an average of 6 treatment visits (range 4–11 visits) and a treatment duration of 19 months (range 10–33 months) [20].

There are conflicting conclusions on whether BoNT delays or reduces the number of orthopedic surgeries in children with CP.

In a retrospective review of 424 children with cerebral palsy, the prevalence of orthopedic surgical procedures at different ages (3–9 years) and the time to the first surgical procedure were measured. Patients were divided into groups of patients who were managed according to best-practice guidelines in orthopedics and patients who had received botulinum toxin type A injections. The progression to orthopedic surgery was significantly lower in the group who received BoNT injections [21]. These conclusions are contradicted by a smaller study from 2009. In this study, BoNT injections consistently improved the spasticity of the lower limbs and functional outcome in CP patients, but the prevention of deformity did not seem to be part of the beneficial profile of the toxin [22].

In addition to clinical measurements, some other objective quantitative tools have been applied to assess the outcome of BoNT injections for the treatment of spasticity of lower limbs in cerebral palsy.

Energy expenditure measurement is proposed to be a tool for objective clinical evaluation of the functional outcome of some therapeutic interventions. BoNT-A injection into the gastrocnemius muscle was performed in 16 children with CP. In addition to reduced spasticity, improvement of ankle range of motion, and walking pattern, energy consumption was also reduced, which was assumed to act as a surrogate for functional improvement [23].

Real-time sonoelastography (RTS) was used in the medial gastrocnemius muscle after rehabilitation therapy with botulinum toxin type A injection in spastic CP, and it showed that intrinsic stiffness of the injected muscle decreases and this score was correlated with clinical evaluation of spasticity by the Modified Ashworth Scale [24]. In another study on changes in the deep tendon reflexes following BoNT injection, along with a reduction of Modified Ashworth Scale, the amplitude of compound motor action potential was decreased at 2 weeks, Hoffmann reflex amplitude was decreased at 4 weeks, and tendon reflex amplitude was decreased at 2 and 4 weeks. At 12 weeks, none of the neurophysiologic parameters differed from baseline [25].

In a study using ultrasonography (US) to investigate the architectural changes in gastrocnemius muscles after BoNT-A injection in children with cerebral palsy and equinus, architectural changes in both the medial and lateral heads of the gastrocnemius muscles of 20 legs were assessed using B-mode, real-time US. It was demonstrated that in addition to the significantly reduced spasticity at 1 and 3 months after injection, muscle architectural changes were induced by BoNT-A injection. The architectural changes were found to include reduced muscle thickness and fascicle angle of both heads of the muscle in neutral and resting ankle positions. The fascicle length of both the medial and lateral heads was significantly increased in a resting position but not in a neutral position [26].

Muscle histopathological changes following BoNT-A injection in treated medial gastrocnemius muscle of children with CP were studied and findings were compared with the vastus lateralis muscle biopsy taken during orthopedic surgery. Neurogenic atrophy was seen in the medial gastrocnemius between 4 months and 3 years post-BoNT-A injection. Type 1 fiber loss with type 2 fiber predominance was significantly related to the number of BoNT-A injections ($r = 0.89$, $P < 0.001$). The authors recommended considering rotating muscle selection or injection sites within the muscle or allowing a longer time between injections to minimize the long-term negative impacts of the toxin on the muscle structure [27].

CP and Hip Flexion Contracture and/or Deformity

In patients with cerebral palsy, hip flexion deformity secondary to iliopsoas spasticity may interfere with gait, impair sitting balance, or contribute to hip subluxation or dislocation. Twenty-eight patients (53 hips) with cerebral palsy were treated with BoNT-A injections to ameliorate iliopsoas spasticity. Selective neuromuscular blockade of the iliacus or psoas muscles or both was performed under ultrasound guidance for needle placement and active electromyographic stimulation was used to verify the needle position adjacent to active myoneural interfaces. The use of this technique resulted in improved hip range of motion with a non-surgical, minimally invasive method. No adverse events or complications were observed [28]. In a similar study, injecting BoNT to the iliopsoas muscles in 37 patients from 3 to 15 years of age with spastic iliopsoas cerebral palsy resulted in clinical benefits in gait and motor development [29].

Progressive hip subluxation leading to hip dislocation is a common and serious problem in children with CP (with natural risk for hip dislocation in a total population of children with CP being 15–30%). Retrospective chart review carried out on 194 patients with cerebral palsy concerning radiographic findings showed comparable effects of BoNT-A (Botox®) injection to soft-tissue surgery in this study. This finding suggests that toxin injection, if timely reinjected, may be an alternative to or replace soft-tissue surgery as a prophylactic procedure against progressive hip subluxation or dislocation in children. Age at intervention, functional level, and initial MP (Reimers hip migration percentage) before therapeutic intervention are factors affecting the outcomes [30]. Targeted BoNT-A injections reduced pain in children with significant spasticity and pain at the hip level. It might have impacted the quality of life of non-ambulant children with CP and a hip problem as well [31].

To assess whether preoperative botulinum neurotoxin A (BoNT-A) affects pain after major hip surgery in children with bilateral CP, a randomized, placebo-controlled trial was carried out. The patients were 2–15 years old and were diagnosed with hypertonic CP and were awaiting bony hip surgery. They were randomized into either BoNT-A or placebo injections into the muscles of the hip on a single occasion immediately before surgery. The pediatric pain profile (PPP) was assessed at baseline and weekly for 6 weeks. Use of BoNT-A immediately before bony hip surgery to reduce postoperative pain in children with CP did not reduce postoperative pain, nor affected the postoperative quality of life [32].

CP and Upper Limb Spasticity

Upper limb spasticity and dystonia often contribute to functional limitations in reaching, grasping, and related functional tasks.

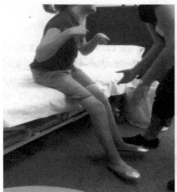
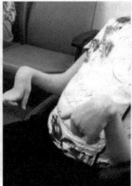
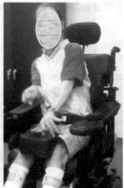

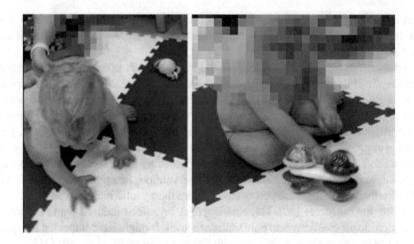

Thirty children with spastic hemiplegia were randomly assigned to receive either a BTA injection plus occupational therapy or occupational therapy alone. In children with at least moderate spasticity, BoNT injections improved the function of the upper extremity [33].

In another report of 32 children (1–18 years of age, average 6.9 years) with hemiplegic or quadriplegic cerebral palsy and spasticity, spasticity in the upper limb was measured using the Modified Ashworth Scale. Spasticity as measured by Ashworth scores for elbow and wrist extension decreased ($P < 0.02$) by 1 month after toxin injection, and the benefit continued for 3–4 months. Caregivers reported improvement in subjectively rated management, appearance, and function. Age had no significant relationship to benefits detected [34]. Improved manual function in children and adolescents with cerebral palsy has been demonstrated in several other studies with BoNT-A (Botox® and Dysport®) [35, 36] and botulinum toxin type B (Myobloc) [37].

CP and Cervical Dystonia

Two patients with dystonic cerebral palsy were scheduled for cervical spine fixation for progressive cervical myelopathy and received high-dose BoNT-A for muscle relaxation before the surgery. They both had severe cervical dystonia and surgery was to halt the gradual progression of myelopathy-related weakness. Because of marked dystonic posturing of the neck, the treating physicians had concerns about the placement of halo fixation during the surgery and tolerance and efficacy of this device and integrity of the spinal fusion postoperatively during recovery. Chemo denervation with high-dose botulinum toxin A was deemed to be safe and efficacious in tolerating halo fixation and facilitated postoperative spinal fusion [38].

CP and Scoliosis

A group of patients (10 patients, aged 2–18 years) with scoliosis and cerebral palsy were injected with either NaCl or BTX in selected spine muscles under ultrasound guidance in 6-month intervals. The study design was a prospective, randomized triple-blinded crossover. Radiological parameters and clinical results were evaluated. Due to a possible serious adverse event (pneumonia resulting in death in one patient), the study was terminated. No positive radiological or clinical effects were demonstrated by this treatment compared with Nalco injections, except for the parent's initial subjective but positive appraisal of the effect [39].

CP and Sialorrhea

In 22 patients with cerebral palsy and significant sialorrhea, who were injected in either only the submandibular gland or the submandibular and parotid glands under ultrasound localization, BTX-A (Botox®) was found to be a potentially safe and promising, minimally invasive treatment [40].

In a controlled clinical trial, single-dose BoNT injections into the submandibular salivary glands were compared with scopolamine treatment. Forty-five school-aged children were included. Salivary flow rates from all major glands were obtained at baseline and compared with measurements during the interventions. Intraglandular BoNT injections were concluded to significantly reduce salivary flow rate in the majority of drooling CP children, demonstrating high response rates up to 24 weeks. Compared with baseline, the mean decrease in the submandibular flow of saliva was 25% during scopolamine and 42% following BoNT injections [41].

Eight patients with cerebral palsy and severe drooling participated in a study where BoNT-A (Botox®) was injected into both submandibular and parotid glands. In addition to the severity of drooling, the morphologic change and the size of salivary glands were measured before injection and 3 weeks after injection using computed tomography of the neck. Statistically significant improvements were shown in the severity of drooling. Also, the size of the salivary glands was significantly decreased at 3 weeks after onabotulinum type A toxin injection. The decreased size of salivary glands may partially explain the mechanism underlying decreased drooling [42].

In another study, BoNT-A (Botox®) injection of the salivary glands is frequently shown to be effective and safe for the treatment of drooling in patients with either spastic or dyskinetic CP, based on the objective measurement of saliva production and subjectively reported symptoms. No significant advantage of injecting both submandibular and parotid glands over injecting parotid glands alone is demonstrated [43].

In regards to BoNT-B, 3000 MU injection of Myobloc into the salivary glands of children with cerebral palsy significantly improved the frequency and severity of sialorrhea. Each parotid and submandibular gland received 375, 750, and 1250 mouse units of the BoNT-B dose, respectively. Patients were randomized into three groups of low dose, medium dose, and high dose. The low-dose group received 62.6 MU/kg. The medium-dose group received 130.5 MU/kg and the high-dose group received 231.1 MU/kg of BoNT-B. The lower dose did not provide adequate benefit, and the higher dose did not show greater benefit and caused more side effects [44]. The dose for Myobloc (BoNT-B) is recommended to be 250–1000 U into the submandibular and 400–1000 U into the parotid glands [45].

Repeated doses of BoNT-A may cause muscle atrophy and loss of contractile tissue in target muscles and also in nontarget muscles that are far from the injection site [46].

Salivary gland atrophy could potentially be useful by decreasing the amount of secretions over time, while the same effects of botulinum toxin represent a significant problem in muscle [47].

In 2019, BoNT injections are frequently recommended than surgical procedures for the treatment of sialorrhea because of being less invasive and with fewer adverse effects compared with oral or topical anticholinergic medication. Still, adverse events have been reported. A case is reported by Yuan et al. where a patient with cerebral palsy developed serious acute sialadenitis and submandibular sialolithiasis after intraglandular botulinum neurotoxin injection for sialorrhea [48].

CP and Pain

Pain happens in more than half of children with CP and is the main cause of reduced quality of life. Postoperative pain in children with spastic cerebral palsy (CP) is often attributed to muscle spasm.

In addition to its effect in reducing muscle contraction, BoNTs are reported to reduce pain associated with CP. BoNT has been shown to reduce pain, length of stay, and analgesic use when BoNT was injected before adductor lengthening orthopedic surgery in patients with spastic CP. The authors proposed that these findings may have implications for the management of pain secondary to muscle spasm in other clinical settings [49].

Due to valid concerns about whether this patient population is adequately capable of communicating their level of pain, the authors proposed a new method of pain measurement. The method is based on the physiologic response to pain (r-FLACC) and increased muscle tone during passive joint movement [50].

Guidance Techniques

For anatomically correct application to the salivary glands, sonography is considered the standard procedure by most clinicians [51]. However, a Phase III clinical trial of incobotulinumtoxinA for sialorrhea in adults suggests that both sonography and anatomic guidance led to effective reductions in saliva production [52]. The full prescribing information on Myobloc® states that manual and ultrasound guidance are equally effective [53].

In cases of spasticity, for some time, the palpation of anatomical landmarks was assumed to be sufficiently accurate for precise injection into spastic muscles. But in a study by Chin et al, the accuracy of manual needle placement technique was compared with electrical stimulation. Needle placement by palpation in children failed the targeted muscles in between 22% (gastrocnemius muscle) and 88% (tibialis posterior muscle) of injections [54].

Ultrasound techniques were recommended by Berweck et al. for visually controlled, anatomically precise injection of botulinum toxins in spasticity secondary to cerebral palsy in the pediatric population as it is easy, quick, painless, and relatively widely accessible [55].

Botulinum toxin injection guided by electrical stimulation vs palpation and 2 weeks of physiotherapy were compared in 65 children with spastic hemiplegic or diplegic cerebral palsy. Botulinum toxin injection guided by electrical stimulation plus physiotherapy was demonstrated to be the best in improving spasticity and functional performance in children with cerebral palsy [56].

In a systematic review of the available randomized controlled trials of BoNT for limb spasticity, trials from 1990 to 2016 were included. In the category of injection localization technique, they reported level 1 evidence for using ultrasound, electromyography, and electrostimulation being superior to manual needle placement [57].

Another systematic review of different injection guidance techniques explored the effectiveness of BoNT-A for the treatment of focal spasticity and dystonia. This review also demonstrated that instrumented guiding using ultrasonography, electrical stimulation, and electromyogram is more effective than manual needle placement for the treatment of spastic equinus in children with cerebral palsy. Three studies provided strong evidence (level 1) of similar effectiveness of US and ES for spastic equinus in children with cerebral palsy, but there was poor evidence or no available evidence for EMG or other instrumented techniques [58].

Why Toxin Injection Was Stopped?

A review of medical records focusing on the clinical characteristics of 70 children with CP who had received at least one "BoNT-A" injection in an outpatient clinic for movement disorders, but who had stopped treatment at the time of evaluation, determined their reasons for discontinuation: 11% did not need any further treatment because of lasting functional benefits, 18% underwent elective orthopedic surgery, 47% showed a secondary nonresponse (75% had developed neutralizing antibodies and 25% were antibody negative), and 8% reported side effects such as excessive local weakening or emotional stress due to repeated injections. Noncompliance was responsible for 10% of treatment discontinuation and nonmedical reasons, e.g., relocation was reported in 6% [59].

Adverse Effects of BoNT in CP

In an epidemiological study on the adverse drug reactions in children with CP, most events seemed to be linked to a systemic spread of BoNT-A. The most commonly reported adverse reactions were asthenia and fatigue, followed by dysphagia and aspiration. The study suggests a higher risk of adverse reactions in children who receive BoNT-A compared with adults [60]. Naidu et al. reported systemic adverse events following botulinum toxin A (BoNT-A) therapy in children with cerebral palsy. The authors report on the incidence of bladder and bowel incontinence and respiratory symptoms after BoNT-A injections (1980 episodes) in the lower limbs of 1147 children with various types of cerebral palsy. They found that the incidence of (serious) adverse events was low, with 16 episodes of incontinence of the bowel, representing about 1% of all injection episodes [61].

Three patients developed transient constipation after receiving therapeutic doses of BoNT-A to treat spasticity of the lower limbs (two patients) and the upper limbs (one patient). Constipation was observed within the first week after treatment [62].

In summary, the preponderance of the evidence indicates that BoNT injections in children with cerebral palsy is safe and effective in reducing spasticity and sialorrhea. Additional systematic studies are needed to determine:

- When BoNT therapy should begin
- The optimal treatment interval
- The optimal dose per condition/muscle
- Maximum recommended total dose
- Most effective guidance method(s)
- Efficacy of BoNT for other conditions
- If long-term use of BoNT in growing children has deleterious effects on muscle development [63]

Other Conditions with Spasticity

In addition to numerous applications of BoNT in spasticity secondary to cerebral palsy, it has been studied in spasticity secondary to other conditions like idiopathic toe walking, brachial plexus palsy due to obstetric complications, hereditary spastic paraplegia, and congenital muscular torticollis.

Idiopathic Toe Walking

Idiopathic toe walking (ITW) or habitual toe walking is a diagnosis of exclusion.

A variety of treatment strategies such as physiotherapy, serial casting, and open or percutaneous lengthening of the Achilles tendon and even nontreatment have been proposed. In patients treated with Achilles tendon lengthening, only about one-third of patients were reported to achieve a normal gait and one-fourth had an unchanged walking pattern [64].

BoNT has been studied in isolation or in addition to other modalities for the treatment of ITW. A study on BoNT treatment of ITW was completed in a group of children aged 5–13 years. They underwent 3D gait analysis before treatment and then 3 weeks and 3, 6, and 12 months after treatment. A classification of toe walking severity was made before treatment and after 12 months. The parents also rated the perceived amount of toe walking prior to treatment and 6 and 12 months after treatment. A total of 6 units/kg bodyweight of onabotulinum toxin A was injected in the calf muscles and an exercise program was also pursued. The gait analysis demonstrated improvement of gait with decreased plantarflexion angle at initial contact and during swing phase and increased dorsiflexion angle during midstance at all posttreatment testing instances. In parents' perception of toe walking, 3 out of 11 children had ceased toe walking completely, 4 decreased toe walking, and 4 continued toe walking. The authors concluded that a single injection of BTX in combination with an exercise program can improve the walking pattern in children with ITW seen at gait analysis, but the obvious goal of ceasing toe walking only reached in less than half of patients [65]. In a randomized controlled trial carried out at the same institution, on a larger group of patients, 47 children were randomized to undergo 4 weeks of treatment with casts either as the sole intervention or casting after receiving injections of botulinum toxin A into the calves. 3D gait analysis and parent-rated questionnaires showed no differences in any outcome parameter between the groups before treatment or at 3 or 12 months after cast removal. Adding onabotulinum toxin A injections before cast treatment for idiopathic toe walking was not shown to improve the outcome of cast-only treatment [66].

To compare a combination of repeated BoNT and conservative treatment versus conservative treatment alone, children 2–9 years of age were randomized into the conservative (14 patients) or BoNT group (16 patients). The conservative treatment included firm shoes, night splints, a home stretching program, and physiotherapy. The BoNT group had all the same conservative treatments in addition to calf muscle BoNT injections with repeated injections every 6 months if needed. Adding BoNT injections did not significantly enhance the goal to walk either flat foot or with heel strike at 24 months posttreatment in either evaluation by physiotherapist (blinded and unblinded) or parents. The most prominent improvement was noted during the first year of both therapies [67].

Birth-Related Brachial Plexus Birth Injury

In neonates with brachial plexus birth injury, early life bony deformities and abnormal active and passive range of motion will result in limitation of function. Several authors have reviewed the literature on the therapeutic role of botulinum toxin in the treatment of deformities and abnormalities of posture, tone, and function secondary to birth-related injuries of the brachial plexus [68, 69]. BoNT, specifically type A toxin, is shown to reduce contractures in internal rotation and adduction of the shoulder, flexion and extension of the elbow, and pronation of the forearm. This treatment should be started early on as the benefits are less prominent as patients age. The risks of treatment with toxin are deemed to be low.

A multicenter randomized controlled trial is designed to evaluate the effectiveness of BoNT in the shoulder internal rotator muscles of 12-month-old babies in limiting the progression of posterior subluxation of the glenohumeral joint. The study also included a sham procedure. Deformity of the glenoid, range of motion of glenohumeral joint, and functionality of the upper limb in addition to the tolerability of the treatment are defined as secondary objectives of this study. MRI of the joint will be obtained to measure the deformity and clinical evaluations and clinical scores (Mini-Assisting Hand Assessment) will be used to assess the outcome [70].

Hereditary Spastic Paraplegia

Muscle weakness in hereditary spastic paraplegia (HSP) remains relatively mild but spasticity of the lower limbs is progressive.

In adult patients who receive BoNT in different muscle groups, the outcome has been conflicting. In a group of adult patients with a diagnosis of HSP, BoNT-A (Dysport®, 500–750 MU) injections did not improve the motor function for HSP but fatigue improved [71]. Bilateral botulinum toxin A treatment and subsequent stretching of the hip adductors improved gait in a different group of adult patients with pure hereditary spastic paraplegia [72]. Data on the use of BoNT injections for children with hereditary spastic paraplegia is limited. In a report on 12 pediatric patients with HSP, botulinum toxin A injection to lower limbs was concluded to provide prolonged functional improvement despite the progressive nature of the disease. The mean age of participants was 4.8 ± 2.5 years and they underwent up to 6 sessions of BoNT-A injections to the hamstrings, adductors, and gastrocnemius muscles. Both muscle tone and motor function improved ($P < 0.001$). This effect was found to last for up to 10 months [73].

Congenital Muscular Torticollis

Congenital muscular torticollis (CMT) is the most common cause of torticollis in childhood. This condition is usually recognized and successfully treated in infancy, but it may present in late childhood or adulthood particularly if not treated. Treatment following early recognition seems to be crucial for the prevention of subsequent contractures and other complications [74]. Botulinum toxin type A is safe and effective in the treatment of children with congenital muscular torticollis (CMT) who fail to respond to physical therapy. In a retrospective case series of injection of BoNT-A for treatment of 27 children (6–18 months age) with congenital muscular torticollis who fail to improve with conservative management, BoNT-A was injected into their sternocleidomastoid or upper trapezius muscle, or both. Moreover, 74% had improved cervical rotation or head tilt after the injections. Only 7% experienced transient adverse events, mainly mild dysphagia and neck weakness [75]. In untreated or inadequately treated patients who are in their late childhood and adults, treatment can be tried as a clinical benefit might still be achievable [76].

In a recent retrospective analysis, 39 patients (average age of 14 months, ranging between 6.5 and 27.6 months) with CMT who failed to respond to conventional therapy who received BoNT treatment were identified. Almost half of them received multiple injections. Head tilt and range of motion of neck improved significantly ($P < 0.001$) and no patient required tendon lengthening surgery. No adverse effect was reported and caregivers reported satisfaction with the treatment [77].

Shortening of the sternocleidomastoid muscle (SCM) in congenital muscular torticollis is often secondary to muscle atrophy and interstitial fibrosis. Botulinum toxin type A with its antifibrotic effects regulates fibroblast and inhibits myofibroblast differentiation. This was studied in acquired muscular torticollis mimicking CMT in a rabbit model. Acquired muscular torticollis was induced by intra-SCM injection of anhydrous alcohol. Pre- and postinjection in vivo and in vitro studies showed that BoNT-A injection attenuated shortening and thickening of fibrotic SCM [78].

Urinary Dysfunction

Neurogenic and Non-Neurogenic Bladder

Until 2002, the treatment of children with neurogenic bladder was limited to the use of anticholinergic drugs and serial intermittent catheterization. Surgery used to be considered as the next step. In patients who do not respond to conventional therapy and those who cannot tolerate medication side effects or have compliance issues, this strategy can be considered [79]. Schulte-Baukloh et al. studied 17 children (average age of 10.8 years) with detrusor hyperreflexia urodynamically. Further, 85–300 U of BoNT-A (Botox®) was injected into 30–40 sites in the detrusor muscle. Follow-up urodynamic studies 2–4 weeks after injection demonstrated improvement in many of the measured indexes and increased maximal bladder capacity and detrusor compliance and decreased maximal detrusor pressure [80]. Not in line with the increased bladder compliance in this study, in another study on patients with meningomyelocele, bladder compliance remained poor. The authors conveyed if earlier treatment with BoNT may lead to an improvement in bladder compliance as well [81]. The mean age of patients in this study was 6.7 ± 5.3 years and mean bladder compliance was 7 ml/cmH$_2$O. While in the previous study, average detrusor compliance was 20.39 (range 4.5–40) which was increased to 45.18 mL/cmH$_2$O (range 5.3–100) ($P < 0.01$). Based on this comparison, it seems that the poorer baseline compliance is a prognostic factor for posttreatment bladder compliance rather than the age of the participants. In another study with follow-up over 4 years, 21.7% of children with severe low-compliance bladders did not respond to treatment with BoNT-A, while the clinical outcome in the rest of the cohort was more favorable [82]. In keeping with this report, preoperative bladder compliance was significantly lower in nonresponders in 37 cases of neurogenic detrusor overactivity who underwent BoNT-A intra-detrusor injection [83]. Another possibility for lack of improvement in patients with myelomeningocele is that patients with meningomyelocele often have mixed upper and lower motor neuron pathology affecting bladder function rather than solely the upper motor neuron effects seen in other populations (cerebral palsy, acquired brain injury) [84].

In a retrospective review of records on 7 children with neurogenic detrusor overactivity, patients were treated with 1–5 times intra-detrusor BoNT-A injections. The enrolled patients already failed to respond to timed bladder catheterizations and anticholinergic agents. With BoNT treatment, social continence was achieved from the first injection and no further recurrent lower UTIs occurred [85]. In another group of 7 children with neurogenic bladder secondary to spina bifida, BoNT-A injection improved urodynamics and clinical measures and effects lasted for about 9 months. Interestingly, urodynamic measurements and subjective outcome did not show a clear correlation [86]. Similar results were reproduced in a group of patients with myelomeningocele as the pure etiology of the overactive bladder [87]. BoNT injection resulted in postponed or prevented surgical intervention in a study where 20 pediatric patients with overactive bladder secondary to myelomeningocele were enrolled and injected with 5 IU/kg (maximum 300 IU) of BoNT-A (Botox®) at 10–30 sites [88]. Repeated intra-detrusor BoNT injection was found to be safe and effective in children with acquired neurogenic bladder [89].

Intravesical BoNT-A injection with a dosage of 12.5 IU/kg with a maximum dose of 200 IU did not cause any major systemic side effects. Six out of 21 patients had slight hematuria only for 2–3 days and the treatment was thought to be useful and safe in children with an idiopathic overactive drug-resistant bladder [90]. Injection of BoNT-A (Dysport®) showed promise in another cohort of patients with idiopathic detrusor overactivity. The recommended dose of Dysport® was 13–14 IU/kg and a higher dose did not correlate with better clinical outcomes [91]. This was again observed in another study on fifty-three patients with a mean age of 8.5 years. While the clinical outcome was overall favorable, the poor urodynamic outcome resulted in only a 30% global success rate. The authors tried to find out prognostic factors and realized that patients with closed spinal dysraphism were significantly more likely to improve than patients with myelomeningocele ($P = 0.002$). The clinical success rate showed a correlation with maximum urethral closure pressure [92].

Reinjection might become necessary in about 6 months [93]. If repetitive injections become necessary, patients will continue to benefit from this treatment [75]. Even in case of an increment of antitoxin antibody titer, it does not seem to be permanent. In a study on BoNT-A (Dysport®), no clinical resistance to treatment was detected despite the presence of anti-Dysport® antibody [76]. Repetitive injections into the detrusor in children who were treated with 10 IU/kg BoNT-A up to a maximum of 300 IU did not cause increased fibrosis in the detrusor. Biopsies were taken endoscopically from the posterolateral bladder wall above the ureteral orifice [94].

In a study on pediatric patients with meningomyelocele with concomitant detrusor overactivity and bowel dysfunction, injection of 10 IU/kg of BoNT-A under cystoscopic guidance into the detrusor muscle resulted in decreased vesicoureteral reflux grade in 11 patients and even bowel dysfunction improved in 10 out of the 15 patients [95].

Detrusor injections of BoNT on postsynaptic muscular receptors in children and adolescents with neurogenic detrusor overactivity were studied in a group of patients who underwent bladder augmentation surgery because of neurogenic detrusor overactivity. Seven patients who had previously received 1–8 (average 3.86) onabotulinumtoxinA detrusor injections, where their detrusor pressure could not be maintained at tolerable levels because of low-compliance bladder, were compared with three patients who never had received that therapy (controls). Receptor analysis of muscarinic M2 and M3 and purinergic P2X1, P2X2, and P2X3 was performed on the bladder dome and nerve fiber density was analyzed. A downregulation of all examined receptors after BoNT-A injections was demonstrated. This downregulation was thought to be the cause of decreased force in the urinary bladder which eventually leads to an increase in urinary residue [96].

The outcome of BoNT injection to either the detrusor or urethral sphincter is promising in non-neurogenic bladder overactivity as well [97–99].

Long-term follow-up data (average 45 months, range 20–71) on intra-sphincteric BoNT-A injection in 12 children with dysfunctional voiding (mean age 10.5 years, range 4–19) showed significant improvement in voiding parameters in 8 of the 12 children (67%). Three of four patients who failed to improve were reported to have neuropsychiatric problems. The authors concluded that neuropsychiatric factors appear to have a negative impact on the success rate [100].

Dysfunctional Voiding

In patients with refractory voiding dysfunction and frequent urinary tract infections, botulinum-A toxin at a dose of 50–100 U was injected transperineally into the pelvic floor or external sphincter or both in all patients. Out of 20 patients (12 girls and 8 boys), nine reestablished a normal voiding curve and 8 showed improvement. Over the 9- to 14-month course of follow-up, the single injection provided lasting benefit. The authors concluded that toxin injection can break the circle of detrusor-sphincter dyssynergia and the period when it is sustained can be used for retraining the patient for normal voiding [101].

Intravesical electromotive BoNT-A administration (BoNTA-EMDA) in patients with myelomeningocele and neurogenic detrusor overactivity is a novel method of delivering the medication without a need for anesthesia or cystoscopy procedure. Results of a study on 24 patients demonstrated that BoNTA-EMDA with Dysport® is a feasible, safe, reproducible, cost-effective, long-lasting, and pain-free method on an outpatient basis, and effects are long term [102, 103]. The evidence is still controversial for use of this newer method as the results of the former study were not replicable in a second study on BoNT-EMDA [104].

Constipation, Achalasia, and GI Dysmotility Syndromes

Achalasia

Injection of botulinum toxin into the lower esophageal sphincter (LES) has been studied as an alternative to the established treatment for achalasia (esophageal pneumatic dilatation or surgical myotomy) in children [105]. Out of 26 patients, 19 initially responded to botulinum toxin and the effect lasted for 4.2 months ± 4.0 (SD). At the end of the study, three patients responded to repeat injections, three underwent pneumatic dilatation, eight underwent surgery, three underwent pneumatic dilatation with subsequent surgery, and three awaited surgery. Botulinum toxin was effective initially and postponed the other more invasive interventions. As one-half of patients would need an additional procedure within 7 months of the first BoNT injection, BoNT was recommended as a reasonable alternative for pediatric achalasia patients who are poor candidates for either pneumatic dilatation or surgery [106]. In another group of patients, botulinum toxin produced a sustained response beyond 6 months in less than half of 7 patients. The authors found an inverse relationship between the pretreatment pressure in the lower esophageal sphincter and the duration of response. The average time of response was 4 months (ranging between 1 and 14 months).

Clinical benefit from an intra-sphincteric BoNT injection in children with internal anal sphincter (IAS) achalasia was shown to be safe and effective in a retrospective review of medical records of 20 patients (8 male, mean 5.8 ± 4.2 years) with severe chronic constipation and IAS achalasia. Intra-sphincteric injections of botulinum toxin at a dose of 15–25 IU per quadrant (each patient received injection in four quadrants) were given. Patients were reassessed 4 weeks to 18 months after injection. Response to botulinum injection was rated excellent by the parents in 60% and by the physician in 35% of children. The duration of response ranged from 1 week to 18 months [107].

Six pediatric patients with cricopharyngeal achalasia who underwent cricopharyngeal BoNT injection were retrospectively reviewed and a prospective parental telephone survey was also performed to assess improvement and satisfaction. The age range was 3 months to 10 years. The number of injections ranged from one to three per patient.

Symptoms in 4 children were treated with injections alone. Two children benefited from injections but eventually needed myotomy. All parents were satisfied with the procedure. Only one child developed a transient worsening of aspiration [108].

Constipation

Following surgery for Hirschsprung disease, in some cases, anal myectomy of internal anal sphincter becomes necessary. This is to treat persistent constipation and obstructive symptoms secondary to the hypertonicity with nonrelaxation in the anal sphincter. Anal myotomy is at times ineffective or causes long-term incontinence. Intra-sphincteric BoNT injection was studied as an alternative for anal myotomy for these patients in a study on 18 children of 1–13 years of age. A total dose of 15–60 IU was injected into 4 quadrants of the sphincter. Repeated injection happened in 10 patients (1–5 additional injections).

Patients who demonstrated to have clinical improvement had a decrease in sphincter pressure of 8, while in the nonresponders, the pressure decrease was only 3. No major adverse effects were reported and only mild transient new encopresis after injection happened in 4 patients [109].

A retrospective review on 24 pediatric patients with intractable constipation showed significant improvement in constipation. Before the procedure, the patients were found to have either elevated internal anal sphincter (IAS) resting pressure or an absent or diminished rectoanal inhibitory reflex. They underwent OnabotulinumtoxinA (Botox®) injection into the IAS.

Twelve patients demonstrated benefits lasting at least 6 months. Transient postoperative incontinence was reported in five patients [110].

A double-blind randomized trial was carried out to compare BoNT injection with myectomy of the IAS for the treatment of chronic idiopathic constipation and soiling in children. Forty-two patients who failed to respond to laxative treatment and anal dilatation for chronic idiopathic constipation (4–16 years old) underwent anorectal manometry and anal endosonography and then randomized into the botulinum group (21 patients) and the myectomy group (21 patients). A validated symptom severity scoring system was used as the outcome (scores ranging from 0 to 65). At the 3-month and 12-month follow-up, both groups showed lasting clinical improvement. There was no complication reported in either group. BoNT was deemed to be equally effective as myectomy of the IAS for chronic idiopathic constipation and fecal incontinence in children. But as it is less invasive, its use is preferred over surgery [111].

The long-term outcomes of receiving BoNT therapy in children with a nonrelaxing IAS after surgically repaired Hirschsprung disease (HD) and IAS achalasia are reported in a retrospective review of 73 children (30 HD, 43 IAS achalasia). The mean follow-up term was 32.1 ± 2.9 months. Three-fourths of the children received multiple injections. Initial clinical improvement was seen in 90% of children after the first injection. Over one-half of children had an excellent or good outcome which was maintained for an average of 17 months from the time of the last BoNT injection. Ten percent developed transient fecal incontinence, and one patient developed significant pain after the injection. Initial short-term improvement after the first BoNT injection and having IAS achalasia rather than HD was shown to be predicting a favorable long-term clinical outcome [112].

The outcome of intra-sphincteric BoNT injections after the pull-through procedure (removal of the entire aganglionic colon, with an end-to-end anastomosis of the normal colon to the low rectum) for Hirschsprung disease was studied using operative records in biopsy-proven HD patients at Karolinska Institute. Serial treatment with BoNT was shown to improve the obstructive symptoms. A majority of patients need repeat injections; otherwise, laxatives or enemas will be required to manage the recurrent symptoms [113].

Prolonged chronic functional obstructive symptoms are common following successful surgical treatment of Hirschsprung disease (HD) and occur in 50% of children. Using neurostimulation-guided anal intra-sphincteric BoNT injections on postoperative obstructive symptoms in HD patients helps take the variability of the patient's anatomy secondary to curative surgery into consideration [114].

Chronic anal fissures with painful defecation and bloodstained stools can be seen in children of all ages. Constipation is a preceding or concomitant symptom. Treatment with botulinum toxin in the external sphincter produces a quick and effective alleviation of pain with the healing of chronic anal fissures in children. The treatment is not considered to carry any risks but requires light anesthesia. Recurrences are common but additional injections will provide clinical benefit [115]. Khout and Kadi emphasized that long-term follow-up studies are necessary to ensure the safety of this treatment and a need for blinded large-scaled randomized controlled studies to establish appropriate injection sites and dosages. They brought up a concern regarding the cost-effectiveness of botulinum toxin considering the need for repeat injections [116].

Complications associated with BoNT injection into the anal sphincters in children with severe defecation disorders are described in a retrospective review of pediatric patients who received onabotulinumtoxinA (Botox®) into the anal sphincter. Complications were reported in 0.7% of 1332 injections. Complications included urinary incontinence ($n = 5$), pelvic muscle paresis ($n = 2$), perianal abscess ($n = 1$), pruritus ani ($n = 1$), and rectal prolapse ($n = 1$). Patient age, weight, and diagnosis were not associated with an increased rate of complication in our institutional experience. All complications were self-limited and did not require intervention. There were no episodes of systemic botulinum toxicity. Overall, Botox injection into the anal sphincters in children with Hirschsprung disease, severe functional constipation, and internal anal sphincter achalasia was thought to be safe based on this review. Recommendations on dosing could not be ascertained and further study was recommended [117]. Complications of BoNT use for GI conditions in children also include one death but there are other significant complications ranging from minor pain to rash, other allergic reactions, pneumothorax, bowel perforation, and significant paralysis of tissues surrounding the injection site [118].

A group of children with chronic idiopathic constipation who failed to respond to medical treatment was randomized into a control group who received no injection and was only treated with stool softeners and a case group who received stool softener in addition to BoNT-A (Botox®) injection. Painful defecation reduced from 88% of patients before BoNT injection to 15% after injection. While in the control group, it was reduced from 90% to 86% after medical treatment ($P = 0.0001$). Hard stool was reduced from 80% to 28% in the BoNT group and from 81% to 78% in the control group. Defecation intervals for more than 3 days and soiling were also significantly different between the two groups [119].

Gastroparesis

Long-term clinical outcomes and predictive factors for endoscopic intra-pyloric botulinum injections (IPBIs) in children with gastroparesis refractory to medical therapy (mean age 9.98 ± 6.5 years; 23 female patients) were investigated in an open-label and retrospective study. IPBI failed in one-third of patients and was successful in the rest. One-third of the patients received multiple IPBIs. Exacerbation of vomiting happened in one patient only, which was transient. Older patients and those presenting with vomiting responded to the first-time injection and male patients responded better to repeat IPBIs [120].

Hyperhidrosis

Primary palmar hyperhidrosis in children and adolescents may be severe enough to affect school, social, and physical activities, causing emotional problems, stress in the patient's life, and compromised quality of life. Nine patients with palmar hyperhidrosis underwent treatment with botulinum A. Before the session and in the 1-, 3-, 6-, 9-, and 12-month post-session follow-ups, the patients were administered the Minor test, gravimetry, the Scales of Frequency and Severity, and the Questionnaire of Quality of Life. The mean age was 11 years, with seven girls and two boys. Each patient was administered at least one treatment of botulinum toxin in the palm of the hands (75–150 U for palm), with the mean number of sessions 2.2 (range 1–4). All sessions in the patients resulted in drying of the hands, with a mean duration of effect of 7 months. Botulinum toxin A controls excessive sweat in the palms of children and adolescents who have primary palmar hyperhidrosis, with an improvement in the quality of life.

Use of BoNT injections in the treatment of primary palmar hyperhidrosis in children with a disease that is severe enough to impact their quality of life is safe and effective and it should be considered before surgical interventions. This is based on the study on 9 patients (7 girls and 2 boys, mean age of 11) who received BoNT-A (75–150 U, 1–4 sessions) and were evaluated before and every 3 months after the treatment up to 1 year [121].

A review of 193 children with hyperhidrosis and physical, psychosocial, and consequence-related symptoms secondary to hyperhidrosis who received repetitive BoNT-A or BoNT-B injections were included. There were 176 out of 193 children who reported that their sweating disappeared completely and no severe adverse events occurred. BoNT-A or BoNT-B treatment for focal and multifocal hyperhidrosis in children with reduced quality of life is thought to be successful and safe based on this review [122].

Conclusions

Botulinum toxins are recognized as an effective therapy and approved for a wide variety of conditions in the adult population. As the results of ongoing high-quality studies in pediatric patients become available, additional approvals will likely occur for currently available and newly approved BoNT products in the USA and worldwide.

References

1. Scott AB. Botulinum toxin injection into extraocular muscles as an alternative to strabismus surgery. Ophthalmology. 1980;87(10):1044–9.
2. Scott AB, Magoon EH, McNeer KW, Stager DR. Botulinum treatment of strabismus in children. Trans Am Ophthalmol Soc. 1989;87:174–80; discussion 80–4.
3. Charles D, Gill CE. Neurotoxin injection for movement disorders. Continuum (Minneap Minn). 2010;16(1 Movement Disorders):131–57.
4. Escuder AG, Hunter DG. The role of botulinum toxin in the treatment of strabismus. Semin Ophthalmol. 2019;34(4):198–204.
5. Dysport package insert/prescribing information. Basking Ridge, NJ: Ipsen Biopharmaceuticals, Inc.
6. BOTOX® Prescribing Information, https://media.allergan.com, Allergan.
7. Chhina H, Howren A, Simmonds A, Alvarez CM. Onabotulinumtoxin A injections: a safety review of children with clubfoot under 2 years of age at BC Children's Hospital. Eur J Paediatr Neurol. 2014;18(2):171–5.
8. Ali SS, Bragin I, Rende E, Mejico L, Werner KE. Further evidence that onabotulinum toxin is a viable treatment option for pediatric chronic migraine patients. Cureus. 2019;11(3):e4343.
9. Mulpuri K, Schaeffer EK, Sanders J, Zaltz I, Kocher MS. Evidence-based recommendations for pediatric orthopaedic practice. J Pediatr Orthop. 2018;38(9):e551–e5.
10. Carraro E, Trevisi E, Martinuzzi A. Safety profile of incobotulinum toxin A [Xeomin((R))] in gastrocnemius muscles injections in children with cerebral palsy: randomized double-blind clinical trial. Eur J Paediatr Neurol. 2016;20(4):532–7.
11. Gaebler-Spira D, Revivo G. The use of botulinum toxin in pediatric disorders. Phys Med Rehabil Clin N Am. 2003;14(4):703–25.
12. Koman LA, Mooney JF 3rd, Smith BP, Goodman A, Mulvaney T. Management of spasticity in cerebral palsy with botulinum-A toxin: report of a preliminary, randomized, double-blind trial. J Pediatr Orthop. 1994;14(3):299–303.
13. Heinen F, Desloovere K, Schroeder AS, Berweck S, Borggraefe I, van Campenhout A, et al. The updated European Consensus 2009 on the use of Botulinum toxin for children with cerebral palsy. Eur J Paediatr Neurol. 2010;14(1):45–66.
14. Novak I, McIntyre S, Morgan C, Campbell L, Dark L, Morton N, et al. A systematic review of interventions for children with cerebral palsy: state of the evidence. Dev Med Child Neurol. 2013;55(10):885–910.
15. Cosgrove AP, Corry IS, Graham HK. Botulinum toxin in the management of the lower limb in cerebral palsy. Dev Med Child Neurol. 1994;36(5):386–96.
16. Koman LA, Mooney JF 3rd, Smith BP, Walker F, Leon JM. Botulinum toxin type A neuromuscular blockade in the treatment of lower extremity spasticity in cerebral palsy: a randomized, double-blind, placebo-controlled trial. BOTOX Study Group. J Pediatr Orthop. 2000;20(1):108–15.
17. Flett PJ, Stern LM, Waddy H, Connell TM, Seeger JD, Gibson SK. Botulinum toxin A versus fixed cast stretching for dynamic calf tightness in cerebral palsy. J Paediatr Child Health. 1999;35(1):71–7.
18. Garcia Ruiz PJ, Pascual Pascual I, Sanchez Bernardos V. Progressive response to botulinum A toxin in cerebral palsy. Eur J Neurol. 2000;7(2):191–3.
19. Rutz E, Hofmann E, Brunner R. Preoperative botulinum toxin test injections before muscle lengthening in cerebral palsy. J Orthop Sci. 2010;15(5):647–53.
20. Herrmann J, Mall V, Bigalke H, Geth K, Korinthenberg R, Heinen F. Secondary non-response due to development of neutralising antibodies to botulinum toxin A during treatment of children with cerebral palsy. Neuropediatrics. 2000;31(6):333–4.

21. Molenaers G, Desloovere K, Fabry G, De Cock P. The effects of quantitative gait assessment and botulinum toxin a on musculoskeletal surgery in children with cerebral palsy. J Bone Joint Surg Am. 2006;88(1):161–70.

22. Gough M. Does botulinum toxin prevent or promote deformity in children with cerebral palsy? Dev Med Child Neurol. 2009;51(2):89–90.

23. Balaban B, Tok F, Tan AK, Matthews DJ. Botulinum toxin a treatment in children with cerebral palsy: its effects on walking and energy expenditure. Am J Phys Med Rehabil. 2012;91(1):53–64.

24. Park GY, Kwon DR. Sonoelastographic evaluation of medial gastrocnemius muscles intrinsic stiffness after rehabilitation therapy with botulinum toxin a injection in spastic cerebral palsy. Arch Phys Med Rehabil. 2012;93(11):2085–9.

25. Jang DH, Sung IY, Kang YJ. Usefulness of the tendon reflex for assessing spasticity after botulinum toxin-a injection in children with cerebral palsy. J Child Neurol. 2013;28(1):21–6.

26. Park ES, Sim E, Rha DW, Jung S. Architectural changes of the gastrocnemius muscle after botulinum toxin type A injection in children with cerebral palsy. Yonsei Med J. 2014;55(5):1406–12.

27. Valentine J, Stannage K, Fabian V, Ellis K, Reid S, Pitcher C, et al. Muscle histopathology in children with spastic cerebral palsy receiving botulinum toxin type A. Muscle Nerve. 2016;53(3):407–14.

28. Willenborg MJ, Shilt JS, Smith BP, Estrada RL, Castle JA, Koman LA. Technique for iliopsoas ultrasound-guided active electromyography-directed botulinum a toxin injection in cerebral palsy. J Pediatr Orthop. 2002;22(2):165–8.

29. Liu JJ, Ji SR, Wu WH, Zhang Y, Zeng FY, Li NL. The relief effect of botulinum toxin-A for spastic iliopsoas of cerebral palsy on children. Eur Rev Med Pharmacol Sci. 2014;18(21):3223–8.

30. Yang EJ, Rha DW, Kim HW, Park ES. Comparison of botulinum toxin type A injection and soft-tissue surgery to treat hip subluxation in children with cerebral palsy. Arch Phys Med Rehabil. 2008;89(11):2108–13.

31. Lundy CT, Doherty GM, Fairhurst CB. Botulinum toxin type A injections can be an effective treatment for pain in children with hip spasms and cerebral palsy. Dev Med Child Neurol. 2009;51(9):705–10.

32. Will E, Magill N, Arnold R, Davies M, Doherty G, Fairhurst C, et al. Preoperative botulinum neurotoxin A for children with bilateral cerebral palsy undergoing major hip surgery: a randomized double-blind placebo-controlled trial. Dev Med Child Neurol. 2019;61(9):1074–9.

33. Fehlings D, Rang M, Glazier J, Steele C. An evaluation of botulinum-A toxin injections to improve upper extremity function in children with hemiplegic cerebral palsy. J Pediatr. 2000;137(3):331–7.

34. Friedman A, Diamond M, Johnston MV, Daffner C. Effects of botulinum toxin A on upper limb spasticity in children with cerebral palsy. Am J Phys Med Rehabil. 2000;79(1):53–9; quiz 75–6.

35. Rosblad B, Andersson G, Pettersson K. Effects of botulinum toxin type A and a programme of functional activity to improve manual ability in children and adolescents with cerebral palsy. Scand J Plast Reconstr Surg Hand Surg. 2007;41(5):250–8.

36. Russo RN, Crotty M, Miller MD, Murchland S, Flett P, Haan E. Upper-limb botulinum toxin A injection and occupational therapy in children with hemiplegic cerebral palsy identified from a population register: a single-blind, randomized, controlled trial. Pediatrics. 2007;119(5):e1149–58.

37. Sanger TD, Kukke SN, Sherman-Levine S. Botulinum toxin type B improves the speed of reaching in children with cerebral palsy and arm dystonia: an open-label, dose-escalation pilot study. J Child Neurol. 2007;22(1):116–22.

38. Racette BA, Lauryssen C, Perlmutter JS. Preoperative treatment with botulinum toxin to facilitate cervical fusion in dystonic cerebral palsy. Report of two cases. J Neurosurg. 1998;88(2):328–30.

39. Wong C, Pedersen SA, Kristensen BB, Gosvig K, Sonne-Holm S. The effect of botulinum toxin a injections in the spine muscles for cerebral palsy scoliosis, examined in a prospective, randomized triple-blinded study. Spine (Phila Pa 1976). 2015;40(23):E1205–11.
40. Suskind DL, Tilton A. Clinical study of botulinum-A toxin in the treatment of sialorrhea in children with cerebral palsy. Laryngoscope. 2002;112(1):73–81.
41. Jongerius PH, Rotteveel JJ, van Limbeek J, Gabreels FJ, van Hulst K, van den Hoogen FJ. Botulinum toxin effect on salivary flow rate in children with cerebral palsy. Neurology. 2004;63(8):1371–5.
42. Lee ZI, Cho DH, Choi WD, Park DH, Byun SD. Effect of botulinum toxin type a on morphology of salivary glands in patients with cerebral palsy. Ann Rehabil Med. 2011;35(5):636–40.
43. Gonzalez LM, Martinez C, Bori YFI, Suso-Vergara S. Factors in the efficacy, safety, and impact on quality of life for treatment of drooling with botulinum toxin type a in patients with cerebral palsy. Am J Phys Med Rehabil. 2017;96(2):68–76.
44. Basciani M, Di Rienzo F, Fontana A, Copetti M, Pellegrini F, Intiso D. Botulinum toxin type B for sialorrhoea in children with cerebral palsy: a randomized trial comparing three doses. Dev Med Child Neurol. 2011;53(6):559–64.
45. Reddihough D, Erasmus CE, Johnson H, McKellar GM, Jongerius PH. Cereral Palsy I. Botulinum toxin assessment, intervention and aftercare for paediatric and adult drooling: international consensus statement. Eur J Neurol. 2010;17(Suppl 2):109–21.
46. Fortuna R, Vaz MA, Youssef AR, Longino D, Herzog W. Changes in contractile properties of muscles receiving repeat injections of botulinum toxin (Botox). J Biomech. 2011;44(1):39–44.
47. Reddihough D, Graham HK. Botulinum toxin type B for sialorrhea in children with cerebral palsy. Dev Med Child Neurol. 2011;53(6):488–9.
48. Yuan M, Shelton J. Acute sialadenitis secondary to submandibular calculi after botulinum neurotoxin injection for sialorrhea in a child with cerebral palsy. Am J Phys Med Rehabil. 2011;90(12):1064–7.
49. Barwood S, Baillieu C, Boyd R, Brereton K, Low J, Nattrass G, et al. Analgesic effects of botulinum toxin A: a randomized, placebo-controlled clinical trial. Dev Med Child Neurol. 2000;42(2):116–21.
50. Sandahl Michelsen J, Normann G, Wong C. Analgesic effects of botulinum toxin in children with CP. Toxins (Basel). 2018;10(4):162.
51. Jongerius PH, Joosten F, Hoogen FJ, Gabreels FJ, Rotteveel JJ. The treatment of drooling by ultrasound-guided intraglandular injections of botulinum toxin type A into the salivary glands. Laryngoscope. 2003;113(1):107–11.
52. Jost WH, Friedman A, Michel O, Oehlwein C, Slawek J, Bogucki A, et al. SIAXI: Placebo-controlled, randomized, double-blind study of incobotulinumtoxinA for sialorrhea. Neurology. 2019;92(17):e1982–e91.
53. Myobloc package insert/prescribing information. http://wwwmyobloccom/hp_about/pdf. Louisville, KY: Solstice Neurosciences.
54. Chin TY, Nattrass GR, Selber P, Graham HK. Accuracy of intramuscular injection of botulinum toxin A in juvenile cerebral palsy: a comparison between manual needle placement and placement guided by electrical stimulation. J Pediatr Orthop. 2005;25(3):286–91.
55. Berweck S, Schroeder AS, Fietzek UM, Heinen F. Sonography-guided injection of botulinum toxin in children with cerebral palsy. Lancet. 2004;363(9404):249–50.
56. Kaishou X, Tiebin Y, Jianning M. A randomized controlled trial to compare two botulinum toxin injection techniques on the functional improvement of the leg of children with cerebral palsy. Clin Rehabil. 2009;23(9):800–11.
57. Chan AK, Finlayson H, Mills PB. Does the method of botulinum neurotoxin injection for limb spasticity affect outcomes? A systematic review. Clin Rehabil. 2017;31(6):713–21.
58. Grigoriu AI, Dinomais M, Remy-Neris O, Brochard S. Impact of injection-guiding techniques on the effectiveness of botulinum toxin for the treatment of focal spasticity and dystonia: a systematic review. Arch Phys Med Rehabil. 2015;96(11):2067–78 e1.

59. Linder-Lucht M, Kirschner J, Herrmann J, Geth K, Korinthenberg R, Berweck S, et al. Why do children with cerebral palsy discontinue therapy with botulinum toxin A? Dev Med Child Neurol. 2006;48(4):319–20.
60. Montastruc J, Marque P, Moulis F, Bourg V, Lambert V, Durrieu G, et al. Adverse drug reactions of botulinum neurotoxin type A in children with cerebral palsy: a pharmaco-epidemiological study in VigiBase. Dev Med Child Neurol. 2017;59(3):329–34.
61. Naidu K, Smith K, Sheedy M, Adair B, Yu X, Graham HK. Systemic adverse events following botulinum toxin A therapy in children with cerebral palsy. Dev Med Child Neurol. 2010;52(2):139–44.
62. Vles GF, Vles J. Constipation as an adverse event after botulinum toxin A treatment in children with cerebral palsy. Dev Med Child Neurol. 2010;52(10):972; author reply 4.
63. Multani I, Manji J, Tang MJ, Herzog W, Howard JJ, Graham HK. Sarcopenia, cerebral palsy, and botulinum toxin type A. JBJS Rev. 2019;7(8):e4.
64. Eastwood DM, Menelaus MB, Dickens DR, Broughton NS, Cole WG. Idiopathic toe-walking: does treatment alter the natural history? J Pediatr Orthop B. 2000;9(1):47–9.
65. Engstrom P, Gutierrez-Farewik EM, Bartonek A, Tedroff K, Orefelt C, Haglund-Akerlind Y. Does botulinum toxin A improve the walking pattern in children with idiopathic toe-walking? J Child Orthop. 2010;4(4):301–8.
66. Engstrom P, Bartonek A, Tedroff K, Orefelt C, Haglund-Akerlind Y, Gutierrez-Farewik EM. Botulinum toxin A does not improve the results of cast treatment for idiopathic toe-walking: a randomized controlled trial. J Bone Joint Surg Am. 2013;95(5):400–7.
67. Satila H, Beilmann A, Olsen P, Helander H, Eskelinen M, Huhtala H. Does botulinum toxin A treatment enhance the walking pattern in idiopathic toe-walking? Neuropediatrics. 2016;47(3):162–8.
68. Gobets D, Beckerman H, de Groot V, Van Doorn-Loogman MH, Becher JG. Indications and effects of botulinum toxin A for obstetric brachial plexus injury: a systematic literature review. Dev Med Child Neurol. 2010;52(6):517–28.
69. Buchanan PJ, Grossman JAI, Price AE, Reddy C, Chopan M, Chim H. The use of botulinum toxin injection for brachial plexus birth injuries: a systematic review of the literature. Hand (N Y). 2019;14(2):150–4.
70. Pons C, Eddi D, Le Gal G, Garetier M, Ben Salem D, Houx L, et al. Effectiveness and safety of early intramuscular botulinum toxin injections to prevent shoulder deformity in babies with brachial plexus birth injury (POPB-TOX), a randomised controlled trial: study protocol. BMJ Open. 2019;9(9):e032901.
71. Servelhere KR, Faber I, Martinez A, Nickel R, Moro A, Germiniani FMB, et al. Botulinum toxin for hereditary spastic paraplegia: effects on motor and non-motor manifestations. Arq Neuropsiquiatr. 2018;76(3):183–8.
72. van Lith BJH, den Boer J, van de Warrenburg BPC, Weerdesteyn V, Geurts AC. Functional effects of botulinum toxin type A in the hip adductors and subsequent stretching in patients with hereditary spastic paraplegia. J Rehabil Med. 2019;51(6):434–41.
73. Geva-Dayan K, Domenievitz D, Zahalka R, Fattal-Valevski A. Botulinum toxin injections for pediatric patients with hereditary spastic paraparesis. J Child Neurol. 2010;25(8):969–75.
74. Collins A, Jankovic J. Botulinum toxin injection for congenital muscular torticollis presenting in children and adults. Neurology. 2006;67(6):1083–5.
75. Oleszek JL, Chang N, Apkon SD, Wilson PE. Botulinum toxin type a in the treatment of children with congenital muscular torticollis. Am J Phys Med Rehabil. 2005;84(10):813–6.
76. Bouchard M, Chouinard S, Suchowersky O. Adult cases of congenital muscular torticollis successfully treated with botulinum toxin. Mov Disord. 2010;25(14):2453–6.
77. Limpaphayom N, Kohan E, Huser A, Michalska-Flynn M, Stewart S, Dobbs MB. Use of combined botulinum toxin and physical therapy for treatment resistant congenital muscular torticollis. J Pediatr Orthop. 2019;39(5):e343–e8.

78. Jiang B, Zu W, Xu J, Xiong Z, Zhang Y, Gao S, et al. Botulinum toxin type A relieves sternocleidomastoid muscle fibrosis in congenital muscular torticollis. Int J Biol Macromol. 2018;112:1014–20.

79. McDowell DT, Noone D, Tareen F, Waldron M, Quinn F. Urinary incontinence in children: botulinum toxin is a safe and effective treatment option. Pediatr Surg Int. 2012;28(3):315–20.

80. Schulte-Baukloh H, Michael T, Schobert J, Stolze T, Knispel HH. Efficacy of botulinum-a toxin in children with detrusor hyperreflexia due to myelomeningocele: preliminary results. Urology. 2002;59(3):325–7; discussion 7–8.

81. Horst M, Weber DM, Bodmer C, Gobet R. Repeated Botulinum-A toxin injection in the treatment of neuropathic bladder dysfunction and poor bladder compliance in children with myelomeningocele. Neurourol Urodyn. 2011;30(8):1546–9.

82. Zeino M, Becker T, Koen M, Berger C, Riccabona M. Long-term follow-up after botulinum toxin A (BTX-A) injection into the detrusor for treatment of neurogenic detrusor hyperactivity in children. Cent European J Urol. 2012;65(3):156–61.

83. Kim SW, Choi JH, Lee YS, Han SW, Im YJ. Preoperative urodynamic factors predicting outcome of botulinum toxin-A intradetrusor injection in children with neurogenic detrusor overactivity. Urology. 2014;84(6):1480–4.

84. Capitanucci ML, Rivosecchi M, Silveri M, Lucchetti MC, Mosiello G, De Gennaro M. Neurovesical dysfunction due to spinal dysraphism in anorectal anomalies. Eur J Pediatr Surg. 1996;6(3):159–62.

85. Do Ngoc Thanh C, Audry G, Forin V. Botulinum toxin type A for neurogenic detrusor overactivity due to spinal cord lesions in children: a retrospective study of seven cases. J Pediatr Urol. 2009;5(6):430–6.

86. Deshpande AV, Sampang R, Smith GH. Study of botulinum toxin A in neurogenic bladder due to spina bifida in children. ANZ J Surg. 2010;80(4):250–3.

87. Riccabona M, Koen M, Schindler M, Goedele B, Pycha A, Lusuardi L, et al. Botulinum-A toxin injection into the detrusor: a safe alternative in the treatment of children with myelomeningocele with detrusor hyperreflexia. J Urol. 2004;171(2 Pt 1):845–8; discussion 8.

88. Altaweel W, Jednack R, Bilodeau C, Corcos J. Repeated intradetrusor botulinum toxin type A in children with neurogenic bladder due to myelomeningocele. J Urol. 2006;175(3 Pt 1):1102–5.

89. Le Nue R, Harper L, De Seze M, Bouteiller C, Goossens D, Dobremez E. Evolution of the management of acquired neurogenic bladder in children using intradetrusor botulinum toxin type A injections: 5-year experience and perspectives. J Pediatr Urol. 2012;8(5):497–503.

90. Marte A, Borrelli M, Sabatino MD, Balzo BD, Prezioso M, Pintozzi L, et al. Effectiveness of botulinum-A toxin for the treatment of refractory overactive bladder in children. Eur J Pediatr Surg. 2010;20(3):153–7.

91. Blackburn SC, Jones C, Bedoya S, Steinbrecher HA, Malone PS, Griffin SJ. Intravesical botulinum type-A toxin (Dysport(R)) in the treatment of idiopathic detrusor overactivity in children. J Pediatr Urol. 2013;9(6 Pt A):750–3.

92. Hascoet J, Peyronnet B, Forin V, Baron M, Capon G, Prudhomme T, et al. Intradetrusor injections of botulinum toxin type a in children with spina bifida: a multicenter study. Urology. 2018;116:161–7.

93. Schulte-Baukloh H, Michael T, Sturzebecher B, Knispel HH. Botulinum-a toxin detrusor injection as a novel approach in the treatment of bladder spasticity in children with neurogenic bladder. Eur Urol. 2003;44(1):139–43.

94. Pascali MP, Mosiello G, Boldrini R, Salsano ML, Castelli E, De Gennaro M. Effects of botulinum toxin type a in the bladder wall of children with neurogenic bladder dysfunction: a comparison of histological features before and after injections. J Urol. 2011;185(6 Suppl):2552–7.

95. Kajbafzadeh AM, Moosavi S, Tajik P, Arshadi H, Payabvash S, Salmasi AH, et al. Intravesical injection of botulinum toxin type A: management of neuropathic bladder and bowel dysfunction in children with myelomeningocele. Urology. 2006;68(5):1091–6; discussion 6–7.
96. Schulte-Baukloh H, Priefert J, Knispel HH, Lawrence GW, Miller K, Neuhaus J. Botulinum toxin A detrusor injections reduce postsynaptic muscular M2, M3, P2X2, and P2X3 receptors in children and adolescents who have neurogenic detrusor overactivity: a single-blind study. Urology. 2013;81(5):1052–7.
97. Hoebeke P, De Caestecker K, Vande Walle J, Dehoorne J, Raes A, Verleyen P, et al. The effect of botulinum-A toxin in incontinent children with therapy resistant overactive detrusor. J Urol. 2006;176(1):328–30; discussion 30–1.
98. Mokhless I, Gaafar S, Fouda K, Shafik M, Assem A. Botulinum A toxin urethral sphincter injection in children with nonneurogenic neurogenic bladder. J Urol. 2006;176(4 Pt 2):1767–70; discussion 70.
99. Leon P, Jolly C, Binet A, Fiquet C, Vilette C, Lefebvre F, et al. Botulinum toxin injections in the management of non-neurogenic overactive bladders in children. J Pediatr Surg. 2014;49(9):1424–8.
100. Vricella GJ, Campigotto M, Coplen DE, Traxel EJ, Austin PF. Long-term efficacy and durability of botulinum-A toxin for refractory dysfunctional voiding in children. J Urol. 2014;191(5 Suppl):1586–91.
101. Radojicic ZI, Perovic SV, Milic NM. Is it reasonable to treat refractory voiding dysfunction in children with botulinum-A toxin? J Urol. 2006;176(1):332–6; discussion 6.
102. Ladi-Seyedian SS, Sharifi-Rad L, Kajbafzadeh AM. Intravesical electromotive botulinum toxin type "A" administration for management of urinary incontinence secondary to neuropathic detrusor overactivity in children: long-term follow-up. Urology. 2018;114:167–74.
103. Sharifi-Rad L, Ladi-Seyedian SS, Nabavizadeh B, Alijani M, Kajbafzadeh AM. Intravesical electromotive botulinum toxin type A (Dysport) administration in children with myelomeningocele. Urology. 2019;132:210–1.
104. Koh C, Melling CV, Jennings C, Lewis M, Goyal A. Efficacy of electromotive drug administration in delivering botulinum toxin a in children with neuropathic detrusor overactivity-outcomes of a pilot study. J Pediatr Urol. 2019;15(5):552 e1–8.
105. Khoshoo V, LaGarde DC, Udall JN Jr. Intrasphincteric injection of Botulinum toxin for treating achalasia in children. J Pediatr Gastroenterol Nutr. 1997;24(4):439–41.
106. Hurwitz M, Bahar RJ, Ament ME, Tolia V, Molleston J, Reinstein LJ, et al. Evaluation of the use of botulinum toxin in children with achalasia. J Pediatr Gastroenterol Nutr. 2000;30(5):509–14.
107. Ciamarra P, Nurko S, Barksdale E, Fishman S, Di Lorenzo C. Internal anal sphincter achalasia in children: clinical characteristics and treatment with Clostridium botulinum toxin. J Pediatr Gastroenterol Nutr. 2003;37(3):315–9.
108. Scholes MA, McEvoy T, Mousa H, Wiet GJ. Cricopharyngeal achalasia in children: botulinum toxin injection as a tool for diagnosis and treatment. Laryngoscope. 2014;124(6):1475–80.
109. Minkes RK, Langer JC. A prospective study of botulinum toxin for internal anal sphincter hypertonicity in children with Hirschsprung's disease. J Pediatr Surg. 2000;35(12):1733–6.
110. Irani K, Rodriguez L, Doody DP, Goldstein AM. Botulinum toxin for the treatment of chronic constipation in children with internal anal sphincter dysfunction. Pediatr Surg Int. 2008;24(7):779–83.
111. Keshtgar AS, Ward HC, Sanei A, Clayden GS. Botulinum toxin, a new treatment modality for chronic idiopathic constipation in children: long-term follow-up of a double-blind randomized trial. J Pediatr Surg. 2007;42(4):672–80.
112. Chumpitazi BP, Fishman SJ, Nurko S. Long-term clinical outcome after botulinum toxin injection in children with nonrelaxing internal anal sphincter. Am J Gastroenterol. 2009;104(4):976–83.
113. Wester T, Granstrom AL. Botulinum toxin is efficient to treat obstructive symptoms in children with Hirschsprung disease. Pediatr Surg Int. 2015;31(3):255–9.

114. Louis-Borrione C, Faure A, Garnier S, Guys JM, Merrot T, Hery G, et al. Neurostimulation-guided anal Intrasphincteric botulinum toxin injection in children with hirschsprung disease. J Pediatr Gastroenterol Nutr. 2019;68(4):527–32.
115. Husberg B, Malmborg P, Strigard K. Treatment with botulinum toxin in children with chronic anal fissure. Eur J Pediatr Surg. 2009;19(5):290–2.
116. Khout H, Kadi N. Safety of botulinum toxin for the treatment of children with chronic anal fissure. Eur J Pediatr Surg. 2010;20(6):412.
117. Halleran DR, Lu PL, Ahmad H, Paradiso MM, Lehmkuhl H, Akers A, et al. Anal sphincter botulinum toxin injection in children with functional anorectal and colonic disorders: a large institutional study and review of the literature focusing on complications. J Pediatr Surg. 2019;54(11):2305–10.
118. Arbizu RA, Rodriguez L. Use of Clostridium botulinum toxin in gastrointestinal motility disorders in children. World J Gastrointest Endosc. 2015;7(5):433–7.
119. Ahmadi J, Azary S, Ashjaei B, Paragomi P, Khalifeh-Soltani A. Intrasphincteric botulinum toxin injection in treatment of chronic idiopathic constipation in children. Iran J Pediatr. 2013;23(5):574–8.
120. Rodriguez L, Rosen R, Manfredi M, Nurko S. Endoscopic intrapyloric injection of botulinum toxin A in the treatment of children with gastroparesis: a retrospective, open-label study. Gastrointest Endosc. 2012;75(2):302–9.
121. Coutinho dos Santos LH, Gomes AM, Giraldi S, Abagge KT, Marinoni LP. Palmar hyper-hidrosis: long-term follow-up of nine children and adolescents treated with botulinum toxin type A. Pediatr Dermatol. 2009;26(4):439–44.
122. Mirkovic SE, Rystedt A, Balling M, Swartling C. Hyperhidrosis substantially reduces quality of life in children: a retrospective study describing symptoms, consequences and treatment with botulinum toxin. Acta Derm Venereol. 2018;98(1):103–7.

Chapter 12
Botulinum Toxin Treatment in Plastic Surgery

Marie E. Noland and Steven F. Morris

Abstract Injectable botulinum toxin type A is currently the leading plastic surgery procedure and its popularity continues to rise year after year. Botulinum toxin's use within the field of plastic surgery is summarized in this chapter and will outline guidelines for its use on targeting specific rhytides of the face, modification of facial form, improvement of skin quality, scar management, and salivary gland hypertrophy.

Keywords Plastic surgery · Rhytides · Scars · Salivary gland hypertrophy · Facial aesthetics

Injectable botulinum toxin type A is currently the leading plastic surgery procedure and its popularity continues to rise year after year [1]. Its utility spans a broad range of cosmetic concerns beyond botulinum toxin's dramatic benefit in the treatment of rhytides.

The first cosmetic use of botulinum toxin occurred serendipitously in 1987 by the Carruthers family. Dr. Jean Carruthers, an ophthalmologist, and Dr. Alastair Carruthers, a dermatologist, noted softening of patients' frown lines while treating blepharospasm. They published their first clinical study of Botox (onabotulinumtoxinA) for the treatment of glabellar lines in 1992 [2], and a decade later, it was approved by the Food and Drug Administration (FDA) for this limited indication. It was clear that onabotulinumtoxinA showed a distinct benefit in the treatment of glabellar lines and had no major adverse events. Since then, the FDA has expanded onabotulinumtoxinA's indications to also include forehead and lateral canthal lines.

Techniques for injections are constantly evolving as more cosmetic indications become approved and newer neuromodulators come to market. Currently, there are four botulinum toxin type A products (Botox, Dysport, Xeomin, and Nuceiva) and

M. E. Noland (✉)
Division of Plastic Surgery, University of Toronto, Toronto, Canada

S. F. Morris
Division of Plastic Surgery, Dalhousie University, Halifax, Canada
e-mail: sfmorris@dal.ca

© Springer Nature Switzerland AG 2020　　　　　　　　　　　　　　　　247
B. Jabbari (ed.), *Botulinum Toxin Treatment in Surgery, Dentistry, and Veterinary Medicine*, https://doi.org/10.1007/978-3-030-50691-9_12

one type B (Myobloc) available in North America. These neuromodulator products generally function in the same way and differ mainly in their potencies and dilutions. They can be used interchangeably depending on the practitioner's preference. While Botox, Xeomin, and Nuceiva are considered to be equipotent, Dysport dosing is generally believed to be 2.5 to one unit of Botox. Some studies demonstrate Myobloc's efficacy in wrinkle reduction [3]; however, its dosing still needs to be determined. Current conversion theories consider 55 units of Myobloc to be approximately equivalent to one unit of Botox [4].

Understanding the mechanism of action of botulinum toxin grants the practitioner the ability to use the product beyond the official indications. Botulinum neurotoxin works locally by inhibiting acetylcholine transmission from nerves [5]. When injected into muscle, the toxin inhibits the release of acetylcholine at the neuromuscular junction, causing local paralysis. It has been shown to have a dose-dependent effect influenced by injection technique and the size of the muscle [6]. Accurate injections of small volumes of properly concentrated solution is preferred to target specific muscles [7]. Larger volumes favor drug dispersion and should be avoided in small muscles. The effects of botulinum neurotoxin are typically seen within 3–10 days after the injection and last from 3 to 6 months.

Because aesthetic enhancement is not an exact science, the following guides should be used as a starting point. The techniques and doses should be tailored to the individual when determining a treatment plan. Unless otherwise specified, recommended needle size is 30 gauge, 1/2-inch length [8]. The injection needle should be changed regularly to minimize the risk of infection and increased discomfort caused by the use of a blunt needle.

Prior to injections, the skin should be assessed for any dermatologic pathology as injections through inflamed or irritated skin should be avoided [8]. Complications can be minimized by developing a deep understanding of the structure and function of the underlying facial anatomy.

Botulinum toxin's use within the field of plastic surgery will be summarized below and will outline guidelines for its use on targeting specific rhytides of the face, modification of facial form, improvement of skin quality, scar management, and salivary gland hypertrophy.

Rhytides

As demonstrated by Carruthers in 1987, intramuscular botulinum toxin injections result in temporary improvement in wrinkles by inhibiting the contraction of targeted facial muscles. Thus, dynamic lines respond well to neuromodulators, while static lines related to old age, sun damage, and redundant skin are less responsive.

Dynamic rhytides are more easily appreciated in the upper third of the face, as influenced by the function of the frontalis, procerus, corrugator supercilii, and orbicularis oculi. For this reason, the upper third of the face has often been the target of treatment with botulinum toxin type A [7]. Major muscles in the midface include the nasalis, levator labii superioris alaeque nasi, and levator labii superioris. The lower third of the face includes the orbicularis oris, depressor anguli oris, and mentalis muscle. Dosage recommendations are illustrated in Table 12.1. Static rhytides are common in this region and typically do not improve with botulinum treatment. In general, treatment of these areas can result in functional deficits and should be approached with caution [7].

Rhytides form perpendicular to the underlying muscle. Overactive muscles can be partially or entirely chemodenervated to achieve the desired aesthetic outcome. Although clinical trials emphasize the efficacy of botulinum toxin injections at maximum doses, the frozen look is no longer desired by most patients [2]. Physicians commonly tailor their dosing to suit the individual's muscular strength, wrinkle pattern, and asymmetries. As such, it is the physician's responsibility to evaluate the patient at rest and with full movement prior to determining a treatment plan.

Forehead Lines

The frontalis muscle is the only elevator muscle in the upper face [9]. It is responsible for the development of horizontal lines in the forehead. Its function is to elevate the medial and lateral eyebrows. The dosage and injection points for botulinum toxin use in this area depend on the desired aesthetic outcome. It is important to note that it will also have an effect on the positioning of the eyebrows. As the frontalis muscle is inactivated, the brows will naturally rest in a lower position. This effect can be both desirable and unwanted [2]. Injectors should be conservative in this region as the goal is to soften the forehead lines without causing brow ptosis and loss of expressiveness [2].

To assess the degree of muscle activity, the patient is asked to forcefully raise their eyebrows. Any discrepancies between the positioning of the brows are noted both at rest and during maximal contraction. If desired, small dose adjustments can be made between sides to adjust for asymmetries.

Injection sites should stay within the upper to middle third of the forehead to minimize the effects of brow ptosis. The needle should be introduced perpendicular to the skin and injected into the deep frontalis muscle. The injector can follow the creases of the forehead in 4–6 sites for a total of 2–20 onabotulinumtoxinA units [2]

Table 12.1 Recommended onabotulinumtoxinA injections for rhytides

Indications	Dose range	No. of injections
Forehead	2–20	4–6
Glabella	20–30	5
Crow's feet	4–10	2–3 per side
Lip lines	4–6	2–4 upper lip, 2 lower lip

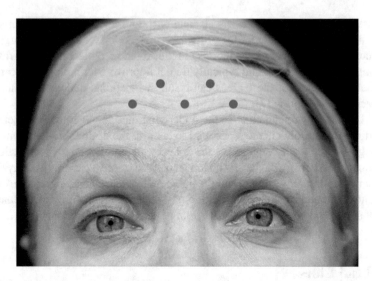

Fig. 12.1 Recommended injection points for the targeted treatment of forehead lines. A total of 2–20 onabotulinumtoxinA units are delivered depending on the severity of the wrinkles and degree of paralysis desired

(Fig.12.1). Avoid injecting lateral to the lateral canthus as this can cause an undesirable brow shape.

To avoid depression of the eyebrows medially, the glabella should also be treated to avoid the unopposed pull of these depressor muscles. Overtreatment of the medial forehead can result in a "Spock" appearance of the brows which are unnaturally elevated laterally. This can be corrected or prevented with a small injection of botulinum toxin 2 cm above the orbital rim in line with the lateral limbus [8]. Keep injections 2 cm above the orbital rim to avoid inadvertent diffusion into the levator palpebrae superioris muscle which could result in eyelid ptosis. If eyelid ptosis does occur, this can be temporarily treated by activating Muller's muscle with 0.5% apraclonidine three times daily until the effects of the botulinum toxin wear off [8].

Glabellar Lines

The glabella refers to the region between the eyebrows. It is the original cosmetic treatment site for botulinum toxin [2]. The muscles responsible for depression of the medial eyebrows when frowning are the corrugator supercilii, depressor supercilii, procerus, and orbicularis oculi. Repeated contraction of the corrugator muscles is what causes the two vertical creases, commonly referred to as the "11s." Contraction of the procerus muscles pulls the brows downward, resulting in a horizontal crease [10]. This region was once considered an independent indication but is now considered an important component of brow harmonization. The total dosage can be decreased significantly to allow for movement and expression as desired [2].

The glabella is assessed for the location, orientation, and severity of rhytides. The degree of muscle activity is determined by asking the patient to forcefully frown. Once again, the positioning and shape of the eyebrows is noted and any asymmetries are recorded.

The glabella typically involves five injection sites for a total of 20–30 units of onabotulinumtoxinA. The sites include one point into the procerus muscle, and two sites into each medial and lateral corrugator muscle [8] (Fig. 12.2). To guide the injection placement, the patient is asked to frown as the skin and muscle are gently pinched by the injector's finger. The patient is then asked to relax and the injection is made deep into the muscle. The two lateral injection points can be made by inserting the needle to one-third of its depth, just below the skin, while angling upward due to the lateral corrugator's more superficial location [8].

If the glabellar region is treated without the frontalis, there may be unwanted medial elevation of the eyebrows from the unopposed pull of the forehead elevator muscle. Inadvertent diffusion of botulin toxin may result in eyelid ptosis if the injection sites are placed too laterally [8].

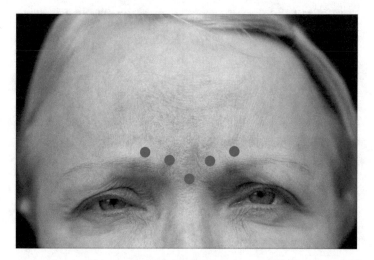

Fig. 12.2 Recommended injection points for the targeted treatment of glabellar lines. A total of 20–30 onabotulinumtoxinA units are delivered across five injection points into the procerus and corrugator muscles

Crow's Feet Lines

Lateral canthal lines, also referred to as crow's feet, are one of the earliest signs of aging. As the skin changes with age and becomes more photodamaged, these dynamic lines can become static. They are caused by repeated contraction of the muscles involved in squinting and smiling. The muscle that has the most effect on these lines is the orbicularis oculi. Its function is to close the eyelid. As a consequence, it also has a downward pull on the eyebrow. This area becomes less responsive to botulinum toxin in older patients with static wrinkling.

The patient's lateral canthal lines should be assessed both at rest and with active contraction. They should be asked to squint while smiling to determine the degree and extent of muscle activity. Note any asymmetries of the eyebrows.

The orbicularis oculi muscle is more superficial than most facial muscles. Injection of botulinum toxin should therefore be very superficial, just below the skin, producing a visible bleb [8]. These lines are typically treated with 2–3 injections sites of 2–4 onabotulinumtoxinA units into each horizontal rhytid (Fig. 12.3). Keep the injection sites 1 cm lateral to the orbital rim to avoid inadvertent diffusion into the palpebral portion of the orbicularis oculi or into the levator palpebrae muscle. The patient's eyes should be kept closed during the injection [2]. If no lifting of the lateral eyebrow is desired, then avoid injecting the superior-most lateral canthal line.

This area is prone to bruising due to its high vascularity. Keep pressure on the skin after injection and avoid injecting into visible superficial veins. Inadvertent

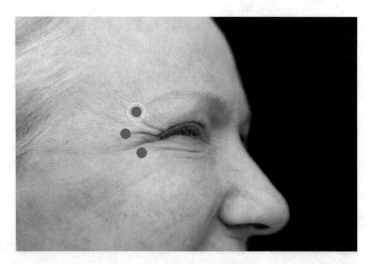

Fig. 12.3 Recommended injection points for the targeted treatment of lateral canthal lines. A total of 2–5 onabotulinumtoxinA units are delivered intradermally across 2 injection points. Additionally, the superior-most injection point may be made to achieve a slight brow lift with 3–5 extra units

injection into the zygomatic muscle can weaken a patient's smile and result in asymmetries. Avoid chasing lateral canthal lines inferior to the zygoma to avoid this potential problem [2].

Lip Lines

The main muscle found in the lips is the orbicularis oris [11]. It is a circular muscle surrounding the oral aperture and it acts as a sphincter to close the lips and keep food inside the mouth. The orbicularis is also involved in puckering the lips, as would be important in speech production and sucking [12]. With age and photodamage, the lip tends to thin and elongate, leading to loss of the Cupid's bow and flatness of the vermillion border. Vertical perioral rhytides become evident with repeated contraction of the perioral musculature, as well as soft tissue volume loss and bony resorption of the mandible and maxilla [13]. Botulinum toxin injection can have a secondary benefit of everting the lips.

Assessment of the lips should be made at rest and during animation. The patient should be asked to smile and pucker. Assess for the presence of dynamic and static vertical perioral rhytids. Make note of any loss of lip and perioral volume, as well as the projection of the lips on profile view.

Perioral lip lines can be treated at one to two sites per side along the upper lip and at one site per side along the lower lip [11]. The injection is made at the vermillion border and can be placed deep to the bevel of the needle. A total of 4–6 units of onabotulinumtoxinA can be used [14] (Fig. 12.4).

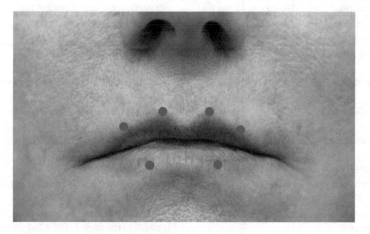

Fig. 12.4 Recommended injection points for the targeted treatment of lip lines. A total of 4–6 onabotulinumtoxinA units are delivered deep into the vermillion border

Administering high doses can result in difficulty drinking out of straws and lip pursing. This can affect speech and the pronunciation of the letter "p." Drooling can also become an issue [11]. This can be avoided by keeping the injection dosages conservative and injection sites further away from the oral aperture.

Facial Sculpting

Beyond the immediate benefit of injectable neuromodulators on wrinkle reduction, they can also be used to improve the shape and position of various facial landmarks. Facial expression is achieved by activation of muscles that either elevate or depress the features of the face. This balance of muscles can be altered strategically by weakening the muscles that alter the face undesirably. For instance, denervating a depressor muscle leaves an unopposed action of the elevator muscles resulting in a lifted appearance of a given facial structure. Furthermore, muscles that are inactive undergo atrophy over time resulting in a slimming effect. This can be desirable when the targeted muscle is hypertrophic or contributing to an unaesthetic appearance. Dosage recommendations are illustrated in Table 12.2.

Table 12.2 Recommended onabotulinumtoxinA injections for facial sculpting

Indications	Total dose range	No. of injections	Injection sites
Eyebrow lift	6–10	1 per side	Superior-most lateral canthal line
Eye aperture widening	2–4	1 per side	Lower eyelid midpupil
Gummy smile	6–10	3 if moderate, 5 if severe	Inferior to columella; lateral to ala
Lateral lip lift	4–8	1 per side	1 cm lateral to oral commissure along mandibular border
Mentalis muscle	4–8	1–2	1 cm from mandibular border, at least 1.5 cm inferior to the vermillion
Masseter hypertrophy	24–48	3 per side	Inverted triangle centered on the masseter body
Platysmal bands	25–30	3–4 per band	Vertically along each band
Parotid hypertrophy	60–80	2–9 per side	Posterior to the masseter, midway between the tragus and mandibular angle
Submandibular gland hypertrophy	24–30	2 per side	Ultrasound guided or 1 finger breadth medial to the midpoint of a line from mandibular angle to chin

Eyebrow Lift

Botulinum toxin can be used to achieve a more desirable eyebrow shape by manipulating the vectors of pull from the muscles of the upper face. The frontalis muscle is the only elevator muscle in the upper face and it is responsible for lifting both the medial and lateral eyebrows [9]. The glabellar muscle complex is responsible for depressing the medial eyebrows, while the lateral orbicularis oculi are responsible for depressing the lateral eyebrows. Achieving more eyebrow lift laterally can be achieved by deactivating either the lateral orbicularis oculi or the medial frontalis muscle. The ideal eyebrow shape has varied over the years with the coming of various trends; however, a classic youthful aesthetic shape always remains. An aesthetically desirable female eyebrow should rest at the supraorbital margin medially and the lateral tail should rest slightly above the inferior aspect of the medial brow [8]. The peak of the brow should be positioned somewhere between the lateral limbus and the lateral canthus extending superiorly to the level of the supraorbital ridge. The male eyebrow follows a similar shape but is lower and flatter than in a female [8]. With age, in some patients, the medial eyebrows will lift and separate, while the lateral eyebrows depress [15].

Assessment of the eyebrows should be made with the patient looking forward with their eyes open. Many patients will compensate for eyelid ptosis or blepharochalasia by overactivating their frontalis. This can result in a surprised appearance and asymmetry of the eyebrows. Ask the patient to then close their eyes and note the positioning of the eyebrows. Determine the positioning of the medial and lateral eyebrows relative to the supraorbital rim and note the vertical positioning of the tail of the brow relative to the medial head. The patient should be asked to squint and the superior-most lateral canthal line should be marked.

A single injection point of botulin toxin is made into the orbicularis oculi muscle at the superior-most lateral canthal line (Fig. 12.3). This point should be 1 cm lateral to the orbital rim to avoid inadvertent diffusion into the palpebral portion of the orbicularis oculi or into the levator palpebrae muscle. Injections should be made intradermally forming a visible bleb due to the superficial location of the orbicularis oculi muscle. A total of 3–5 onabotulinumtoxinA units can be injected per side. To avoid a "Spock" appearance, it is recommended to also place 1 unit of onabotulinumtoxinA into the frontalis muscle 2 cm above the superior orbital rim in line with the midpupil [8]. This keeps the lift isolated to the lateral aspect of the brow only and produces a more aesthetically pleasing result. Injection of several units of botulin toxin can also be made into the medial rhytides of the forehead and this can result in a compensatory hyperactivation of the lateral frontalis leading to a lateral eyebrow lift as well.

Keep in mind that if the medial eyebrow is lowered to prevent hyperactivation of the frontalis, the patient may complain of "heaviness" of their eyelids. If ptosis is a significant issue, it should be corrected surgically. The injector should also be mindful that paralyzing the glabellar complex will result in separation and elevation of the medial eyebrows. This may not be a desirable effect aesthetically and may be mitigated by deactivating the frontalis muscle medially.

Eye-Aperture Widening

The orbicularis oculi muscle is a sphincter muscle that functions to close the eyelids. It can be separated into orbital and palpebral sections. The palpebral section can be further subdivided into the preseptal and pretarsal portions [16]. The orbital section of the orbicularis oculi is more involved in voluntary squeezing and winking of the eyelid while the palpebral section has a greater role in involuntary blink closure as well as keeping the eyelids closed during sleep [16]. With age, the preseptal fibers are responsible for narrowing of the palpebral aperture [8]. Botulinum injection into the preseptal orbicularis oculi can improve the appearance of a narrowed palpebral aperture as well as correct congenital and senile entropion [17].

With the patient looking straight, assess the patient's palpebral aperture bilaterally noting any asymmetries. Perform a snap test before injection to verify lower lid functional recovery. Identify the presence of any ectropion, entropion, and lower lid show.

A single injection site in the lower eyelid 3–4 mm below the eyelash margin in line with the midpupil is required. Have the patient close their eyes and inject superficially into the dermis 1–2 onabotulinumtoxinA units per side [8] (Fig. 12.5). Keep the needle parallel to the skin to avoid injury to the eye.

This area should not be treated if the patient has scleral show, ectropion, or a poor snap test as botulinum toxin injections can worsen these conditions [8].

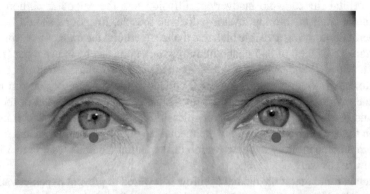

Fig. 12.5 Recommended injection points to achieve widening of the eye aperture. A single injection of 1–2 onabotulinumtoxinA units per side is made into the lower eyelid 3–4 mm below the eyelash margin

Gummy Smile

A gummy smile refers to the showing of excess gum while smiling [13]. In certain individuals, hyperactivity of the muscles responsible for smiling can result in this problem, specifically the levator labii superioris alaeque nasi muscle which elevates and everts the upper lip and the depressor septi nasi muscle which draws the nasal tip downward. In severe cases, the levator labii superioris and zygomaticus minor muscles are also hyperactive [10].

Assess the lips and amount of teeth and gum show both at rest and with smiling. Make note of any depression of the nasal tip with smiling, as well as the length of the upper lip. Identify any asymmetries.

Injection of botulin toxin can be made at three sites if the gummy smile is moderate and at five sites if it is severe [13]. Botulinum toxin is injected deep into the muscles at full depth. One injection site per side, lateral to the ala, targets the levator labii superioris alaeque nasi, while one central injection, inferior the nasal columella, targets the depressor septi nasi muscle. A second injection site in line with the ala and the pupil can be made to target the levator labii superioris and zygomaticus minor muscles. Two onabotulinumtoxinA units per injection site can be used for a total of 6–10 units.

Overinjection with botulinum toxin may lead to elongation of the upper lip. Patients with long upper lips may not be ideal candidates for this procedure [13].

Lateral Lip Lift

The depressor anguli oris muscle is involved in frowning and functions to draw the corners of the mouth downwards. It originates on the mandible and inserts at the angle of the mouth onto the modiolus [11]. Excessive contraction of this muscle and soft tissue depletion leads to a sullen appearance and contributes to the creation of marionette lines, forming downwards from the lateral oral commissure [18].

The patient's mouth should be assessed at rest and with activity. Note the direction of the oral commissure at rest. They should be asked to frown to determine the strength and location of the depressor anguli oris muscle. As always, note any asymmetries between each side.

To achieve a subtle lift of the oral commissures, a single injection site per side is made (Fig. 12.6). A dose of 2–4 onabotulinumtoxinA units is injected deep into the muscle at full depth of the needle. The injection site should be 1 cm lateral to the oral commissure along the base of the muscle at the mandibular border [18].

This area is prone to asymmetries. Diffusion medially can result in inadvertent paralysis of the depressor labii inferioris muscle leading to an asymmetrical smile. This unwanted effect can be minimized by avoiding excessive dosing and keeping injections lateral to the marionette lines [13].

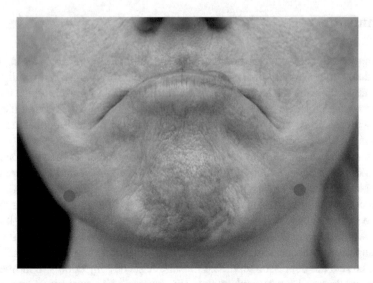

Fig. 12.6 Recommended injection points to achieve a lateral lip lift. A dose of 2–4 onabotulinumtoxinA units is injected deep into the depressor anguli oris muscle, 1 cm lateral to the oral commissure at the mandibular border

Mentalis Muscle

The mentalis muscle is a paired muscle located at the center of the mandible. It is the only elevator muscle of the lower lip [19]. It functions to maintain oral competence and support the lower lip. It also serves to elevate the overlying skin via its thick fibrous septa [20]. A hyperdynamic mentalis muscle can accentuate the mentolabial crease, as well as create unwanted dimpling of the mental area with speech and mouth closure [11]. This can take on the appearance of peau d'orange or cobblestone.

The chin should be assessed before injection. The patient is asked to pull the lower lip up over the upper lip to determine the outline of the mentalis muscle and identify areas of contour irregularities [20].

Injection sites should be at least 1.5 cm inferior to the border of the lower lip and approximately 5–10 mm above the lower border of the mandible [18]. The injections should be aimed at the superficial fibers of the muscle to preserve the function of the deep mentalis [20]. The needle should therefore be aiming parallel to the skin. The total dosage is 4–8 onabotulinumtoxinA units [13]. The injection sites can be spread out over 1–2 points (Fig. 12.7). However, care must be taken not to inject too laterally as this can result in unwanted spread to the depressor labii inferioris muscle, resulting in an asymmetrical smile [11].

Overinjection of the mentalis can have significantly undesirable consequences ranging from lower incisor show to oral incompetence and drooling [19]. If after botulinum toxin injection, the lower lip rests too low, it may be of benefit to also

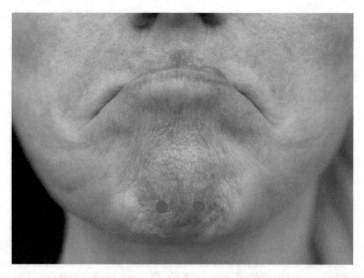

Fig. 12.7 Recommended injection points to treat chin dimpling. Injection sites should be at least 1.5 cm inferior to the border of the lower lip and approximately 5–10 mm above the lower border of the mandible. A total dose of 4–8 onabotulinumtoxinA units are delivered over 1–2 injection sites superficially

inject the depressor anguli oris muscles to balance the lip position [20]. This can be a challenging muscle to inject for this reason. Avoidance deep injection into the mentalis muscle can also be of major benefit.

Masseter Hypertrophy

The masseter muscle is a thick quadrangular muscle that rests superficial to the angle of the mandible. It has an important functional role in chewing. It functions to elevate the mandible [11]. It can become enlarged with repeated clenching of the jaw resulting in a widened or squaring of the lower face. Hypertrophy of the masseter can be aesthetically displeasing in a female [11].

The patient should be assessed from the front view to determine the width of the lower face. Assess the strength, size, and location of the masseter muscle by asking the patient to clench their jaw. Mark out the anterior border of the muscle. Furthermore, patients should also be assessed for parotid hypertrophy as this can also contribute to the impression of enlarged mandibular angles [21]. Parotid enlargement can be identified by the presence of diffuse swelling that extends beyond the posterior border of the mandible. Luckily, this too can be treated with botulinum toxin.

Treatment of masseter hypertrophy is made at three sites on each side of the face [13]. Four to eight onabotulinumtoxinA units should be administered at each

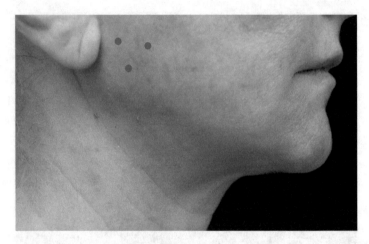

Fig. 12.8 Treatment of masseter hypertrophy is made at three sites on each side of the face. Four to eight onabotulinumtoxinA units should be administered at each injection site deep to the masseter muscle with the needle injected to its full depth. The three injection sites should be 1 cm apart from one another and form an inverted triangle centered on the masseter body

injection site deep to the muscle with the needle injected to its full depth. Palpate the point of maximum muscle contraction as well as the anterior margin of the muscle by asking the patient to clench their jaw. The three injection sites should be 1 cm apart from one another and form an inverted triangle centered on the masseter body [11] (Fig. 12.8). The average initial total dose of onabotulinumtoxinA is 12–24 units into each muscle. This can be repeated at 1-month intervals until no palpable movement of the muscle is felt with clenching. This can take up to three or four treatments. Maintenance dosing is typically 20 units total once or twice a year [21].

Several unwanted consequences of botulinum toxin injection into the masseter may occur including asymmetries, hematomas [13], and jowling due to volume reduction and sagging of the skin [21]. Avoid unwanted diffusion into the risorius, zygomaticus major, and levator anguli oris by keeping the volume of injection less than 1.5 mL at a time [21] and remaining inferior and lateral along the muscle [11]. Furthermore, diffusion through the coronoid notch can affect the lateral and medial pterygoid muscles, thereby weakening chewing. Although the lateral and medial pterygoids and temporalis muscles can typically compensate adequately for the loss of masseter function in mastication, it is still possible for some patients to report weakness with wide mouth opening and aching sensation with chewing [21]. Patients may also notice fasciculations temporarily [21].

Platysmal Bands

The platysma muscle acts as a major depressor of the lower face, drawing down the mandible and corners of the mouth [18]. It appears as two superficial thin sheets of muscle that run down the lateral neck below the subcutaneous tissue [18]. The platysma originates on the pectoralis and deltoid fascia and inserts partially onto the mandible and partially extending up to the muscles of the lower lip and the superficial musculoaponeurotic system (SMAS) [22]. These superior extensions allow the platysma to have a downward pulling effect on the cheek and the corners of the mouth.

One of the first signs of aging is prominent vertical platysmal bands in the neck [23]. This is generally believed to be the result of hyperactivity of the platysma as well as generalized skin laxity [24]. Patients with less skin laxity are better candidates for botulinum treatment, as relaxation of the bands may worsen the appearance of saggy skin [13].

Prior to injection, assess the patient's neck at rest and with maximum frown. Assess the presence of platysmal bands medially and laterally and mark out their trajectory. Note any skin excess.

Treatment of each band is made at four sites laterally and three sites medially [13]. Ask the patient to contract their neck and pinch the band to help guide the injection [18]. Inject 2 onabotulinumtoxinA units at each site. Insert the needle to one-third of its depth. Since injections along the medial band are more challenging and associated with more complications, keep the doses to a minimum and begin by treating the lateral bands first [13].

Dysphagia and dysphonia have been reported as potential complications of botulinum toxin in the neck [13]. To mitigate this, avoid injecting more than 50 onabotulinumtoxinA units at one time, keep injections along the medial bands to a minimum, and avoid injecting too deep [25]. This area is also prone to bruising.

Microbotox

The microbotox technique is a relatively new method of delivery that was first described by Wu in 2015 as a means of improving the overall appearance of the skin. Although it has been used throughout the whole face, it has now become popularized for the use in the neck. With this technique, multiple microdroplets of diluted botulinum toxin are injected superficially into the dermis to target the sebaceous glands, sweat glands, and superficial fibers of the facial muscles [26]. Patients report an overall improvement in their skin texture, mandibular definition, and the cervicomental contour [26]. It remains a simple nonsurgical solution for those patients seeking improvement in mild neck laxity, jowling, horizontal neck lines, and rough crepey skin and is a useful adjunct to earlier mentioned techniques.

By affecting the sebaceous and sweat glands, the skin takes on a characteristic sheen that is desirable by many patients and the appearance of rhytides can be softened due to relaxation of superficial muscular dermal attachments [27]. Muscle function is mostly preserved by sparing their deeper surfaces, conferring a more natural dynamic appearance. A secondary effect of microbotox is improvement in jawline definition due to Wu's theory of improved platysmal apposition. The theory is that the cylindrically shaped platysma muscle will exert a pulling action due to the contraction of only the deep surface of the muscle, creating a more defined cervicomental angle and jowl improvement [27]. Also, by staying superficial with the injections, unwanted diffusion into the deep neck structures can be avoided mitigating adverse events such as dysphonia and dysphagia [26].

To prepare the solution, 100 units of onabotulinumtoxinA is diluted in four to five milliliters of saline to obtain a concentration of 20–25 U/mL. A total of two or three milliliters of the solution can be used throughout the entire anterior neck. Using 31- or 32-gauge needles, 100–150 equally spaced injections are made into the neck. The injections should be made superficially into the dermis producing a small blanched bleb. The injections should span the width of the platysma muscle defined by a line parallel to the mandibular border 3 fingerbreadths above, a vertical line 1 fingerbreadth posterior to the depressor anguli oris medially, the clavicle inferiorly, and the sternocleidomastoid posteriorly [27] (Fig. 12.9).

Although this technique has a soft improvement on vertical platysmal bands with contraction, it has limited improvement at rest [26]. For this reason, this technique is best for those seeking improvements in skin laxity and soft tissue ptosis with minimal platysmal banding.

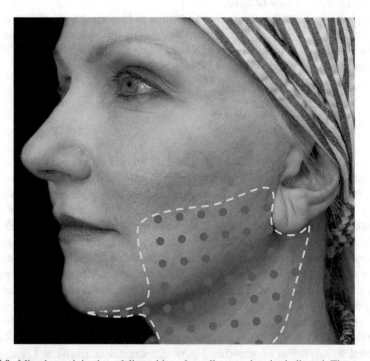

Fig. 12.9 Microbotox injections delivered intradermally at each point indicated. The margins of the area to be injected correspond to the extent of the platysma. The anatomical landmarks are defined by a line parallel to the mandibular border 3 fingerbreadths above, a vertical line 1 finger-breadth posterior to the depressor anguli oris medially, the clavicle inferiorly, and the sternocleido-mastoid posteriorly

Scar Management

Recent studies have shown that botulinum toxin has a positive effect on the prevention and treatment of scars including hypertrophic and keloid scars. It can be a helpful adjunct to other treatment modalities including microneedling and corticosteroid injection [28]. Improvements have been reported in both the appearance of scars and subjective negative symptoms of pruritus and pain [29]. Significant changes were noted in scar vascularity, pigmentation, pliability, and height when comparing to injections with saline in multiple studies [30]. Furthermore, collagen production and organization was found to be significantly improved with intralesional botulinum toxin injections leading to faster vascularization and reepithelialization of wounds [31].

The exact mechanism is not completely understood; however, several mechanisms proposed from in vivo human and animal studies have been demonstrated. Firstly, by immobilizing local muscles acting on a wound, tension is reduced during healing, minimizing inflammation and overproduction of collagen [29]. Studies have also shown that botulinum toxin inhibits fibroblast proliferation as well as fibroblast-to-myofibroblast differentiation in hypertrophic scars [30] by downregulating the expression of α-smooth muscle actin and myosin II proteins [32]. Additionally, botulinum toxin was further found to mediate cutaneous inflammation by inhibiting local cytokines including TGF-β1 and connective tissue growth factor [31, 33], as well as substance P, glutamate, and calcitonin gene-related peptide (CGRP) [34]. This could account for the improved effect on scar tenderness and itch by relieving trapped nerve fibers within keloids [35]. Of note, these effects of botulinum toxin were not observed in fibroblasts isolated from normal skin [33].

The exact injection protocol and timing for botulinum toxin has not been confirmed and injection technique varies greatly in the literature; however, timing the botulinum toxin injection at the time of surgery is a common practice [30]. A common injection practice is to inject intradermally within five millimeters of the scar along its length at a dose of 1.5–10 onabotulinumtoxinA U/cm [36]. Concentrations of botulinum toxin should not exceed 20 onabotulinumtoxinA U/mL, as they have been shown to inhibit angiogenesis and thus affect wound healing [37].

In general, botulinum toxin injections are a safe and effective method for the management and prevention of scarring; however, the exact efficacy and injection method still needs to be supported by larger high-quality studies.

Salivary Gland Hypertrophy

Certain patients will present with hypertrophy of the salivary glands. Although this may not necessarily be clinically problematic, it may lead to an undesired aesthetic appearance by widening the face or neck or blunting the jaw line. Salivary gland enlargement can be minimized with intraglandular injections of botulinum toxin [5].

Because botulinum toxin blocks all cholinergic transmission, it therefore also blocks acetylcholine release from postganglionic parasympathetic fibers to the muscarinic receptors of the salivary glands [5]. As a result, botulinum toxin injection is commonly used for the treatment of sialorrhea. It has also been reported to induce gland atrophy without affecting saliva production [21, 38]. With repeated injections, this reduction in gland size can be longstanding [5].

Two major salivary glands including the parotid and submandibular glands can be targeted with botulinum toxin. The parotid is the largest of the major glands [39]. It is located bilaterally in the preauricular region along the posterior surface of the mandible, superficial to the masseter muscles. The submandibular glands are located in the neck, just inferior to the border of the mandible, between the two bellies of the digastric muscles bilaterally [39]. They can be found deep to the platysma muscle.

Hypertrophy of the salivary glands can have a broad range of etiologies ranging from familial, drug-induced, autoimmune, infectious, and malignant to obstructive causes [40]. When suspecting parotid gland enlargement, the practitioner must first exclude the presence of a solid mass or other disorders [5]. This is accomplished with a thorough clinical history and physical exam. Imaging with a CT of the head is also helpful.

Patients with parotid gland hypertrophy often present with the appearance of a "bull neck" and may have lateral rotation of their ear lobules [5]. Palpation will identify diffuse swelling that extends beyond the posterior border of the mandibular angle. Also, note any asymmetries as this should prompt further investigations. Ask the patient to clench their jaw to distinguish between hypertrophy of the masseters which would be palpable with contraction. This can also be treated with botulinum toxin injections.

The exact technique for botulinum toxin injections in the treatment of salivary gland hypertrophy as well as sialorrhea is still evolving and a subject of debate [39]. Although use of anatomic markers is an acceptable approach, ultrasound-guided injections are recommended, particularly when targeting the submandibular glands.

To target the parotid gland, the masseter muscle is identified with forced clenching of the jaw, and two vertically placed injection sites are made just posterior to the masseter. A 29-gauge tuberculin syringe can be used at a depth of 1 cm from the skin [39]. The injection sites should center around the midpoint along a line that is made from the tragus to the mandibular angle (Fig. 12.10). The total botulinum toxin dose is 30–40 onabotulinumtoxinA units per parotid. The total dose can be spread out between 2 and 9 injection sites if desired [39].

The landmark for the submandibular gland is one fingerbreadth medial to the midpoint of a line that is made from the mandibular angle to the chin (Fig. 12.10). The injections are made subcutaneously with a 30-gauge, half-inch needle [39]. Two injection points are made for a total dose of 12–15 units per side.

Injections can be repeated up to four times separated by 1–2 months until the desired aesthetic result is achieved [5, 21]. Maintenance injections can be made every 6–12 months thereafter, though the exact doses and optimal treatment intervals have yet to be determined [5].

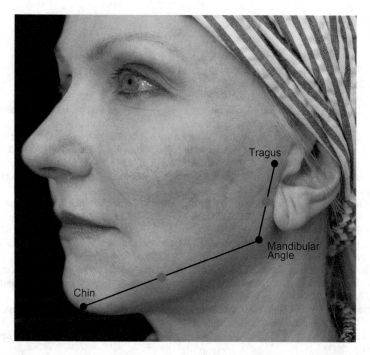

Fig. 12.10 Recommended injection points for the targeted treatment of parotid and submandibular gland hypertrophy. To target the parotid gland, 2–9 injection sites are made posterior to the masseter at the midpoint along a line that is made from the tragus to the mandibular angle. To target the submandibular gland, two injection sites are made at a point one fingerbreadth medial to the midpoint of a line that is made from the mandibular angle to the chin

In general, side effects are mild and few [39]; however, some patients have reported problems with increased saliva thickness, dysphagia, and xerostomia. These effects typically resolve within a few weeks and can be mitigated by keeping treatment doses below 50 onabotulinumtoxinA units [39].Other possible side effects include infection, hematoma, and diffusion into neighboring muscles. No studies have yet been conducted to determine the long-term effects of this treatment [5].

Conclusion

Botulinum neurotoxins have become a staple product in a plastic surgeon's armamentarium. Although they are best known for their role in wrinkle reduction, their efficacy in other applications should not be understated. Facial features can be strategically altered through selective muscular chemodenervation resulting in improved facial balance and form. Furthermore, botulinum toxin also has a role in improving skin texture and scar quality in addition to its effect on salivary gland hypertrophy. This remains an active area for research as new applications for this powerful drug are identified and more specific injection protocols are developed.

References

1. ASPS. Plastic surgery statistics report 2018.
2. Monheit G. Neurotoxins: current concepts in cosmetic use on the face and neck-upper face (glabella, forehead, and crow's feet). Plast Reconstr Surg. 2015;136(5):72S–5S. https://doi.org/10.1097/PRS.0000000000001771.
3. Sposito M. New indications for botulinum toxin type a in cosmetics: mouth and neck. Plast Reconstr Surg. 2002;110(2):601–11.
4. Matarasso A, Matarasso SL, Brandt FS, Bellman B. Botulinum A exotoxin for the management of platysma bands. Plast Reconstr Surg. 1999;103:645–52; discussion 653–655.
5. Bae GY, Yune YM, Seo K, Il HS. Botulinum toxin injection for salivary gland enlargement evaluated using computed tomographic volumetry. Dermatologic Surg. 2013;39(9):1404–7. https://doi.org/10.1111/dsu.12247.
6. Hui JI, Lee WW. Efficacy of fresh versus refrigerated botulinum toxin in the treatment of lateral periorbital rhytids. Ophthal Plast Reconstr Surg. 2007;23(6):433–8. https://doi.org/10.1097/IOP.0b013e31815793b7.
7. Noland ME, Lalonde DH, Yee GJ, Rohrich RJ. Current uses of botulinum neurotoxins in plastic surgery. Plast Reconstr Surg. 2016;138(3):519e–30e.
8. de Maio M, Swift A, Signorini M, Fagien S. Facial assessment and injection guide for botulinum toxin and injectable hyaluronic acid fillers: focus on the upper face. Plast Reconstr Surg. 2017;140(2):265e–76e.
9. Jaspers G, Pijpe J, Jansma J. The use of botulinum toxin type A in cosmetic facial procedures. Int J Oral Maxillofac Surg. 2011;40:127–33.
10. de Maio M, Rzany B. Botulinum toxin in aesthetic medicine. Berlin/Heidelberg: Springer-Verlag; 2009.
11. Wu DC, Fabi SG, Goldman MP. Neurotoxins: current concepts in cosmetic use on the face and neck-lower face. Plast Reconstr Surg. 2015;136(5):76S–9S.
12. Jain P, Rathee M. Anatomy, head and neck, orbicularis oris muscle. StatPearls. 2019.
13. de Maio M, Wu WTL, Goodman GJ, Monheit G. Facial assessment and injection guide for botulinum toxin and injectable hyaluronic acid fillers: focus on the lower face. Plast Reconstr Surg. 2017;140(3):393e–404e.
14. Cohen J, Dayan S, Cox S. OnabotulinumtoxinA dose-ranging study for hyperdynamic perioral lines. Dermatol Surg. 2012;38:1497–505.
15. Yun S, Son D, Yeo H, et al. Changes of eyebrow muscle activity with aging: functional analysis revealed by electromyography. Plast Reconstr Surg. 2014;133(4):455–63.
16. Tong J, BC Patel. Anatomy, head and neck, eye orbicularis oculi muscle. StatPearls. 2019.
17. Deka A, Saikia SP. Botulinum toxin for lower lid entropion correction. Orbit. 2011;30(1):40–2.
18. Carruthers JD, Glogau RG, Blitzer A, Facial Aesthetics Consensus Group Faculty. Advances in facial rejuvenation: botulinum toxin type a, hyaluronic acid dermal fillers, and combination therapies. Consensus recommendations. Plast Reconstr Surg. 2008;121(5):5S–30S.
19. Hur MS, Kim HJ, Choi BY, Hu KS, Kim HJ, Lee KS. Morphology of the mentalis muscle and its relationship with the orbicularis oris and incisivus labii inferioris muscles. J Craniofac Surg. 2013;24(2):602–4.
20. Kane MAC. The functional anatomy of the lower face as it applies to rejuvenation via chemodenervation. Facial Plast Surg. 2005;21(1):55–64.
21. Wu WT. Botox facial slimming/facial sculpting: the role of botulinum toxin-a in the treatment of hypertophic masseteric muscle and parotid enlargement to narrow the lower facial width. Facial Plast Surg Clin N Am. 2010;18:133–40.
22. Levy PM. Neurotoxins: current concepts in cosmetic use on the face and neck-jawline contouring/platysma bands/necklace lines. Plast Reconstr Surg. 2015;136(5):80S–3S.
23. Sandulescu T, Stoltenberg F, Buechner H, et al. Platysma and the cervical superficial musculoaponeurotic system — comparative analysis of facial crease and platysmal band development. Ann Anat. 2019;227:151414.

24. Trévidic P, Criollo-Lamilla G. Platysma bands: is a change needed in the surgical paradigm? Plast Reconstr Surg. 2017;139(1):41–7.
25. Carruthers J, Carruthers A. Aesthetic botulinum A toxin in the mid and lower face and neck. Dermatol Surg. 2003;29:468–76.
26. Awaida CJ, Jabbour SF, Rayess YA, El Khoury JS, Kechichian EG, Nasr MW. Evaluation of the microbotox technique: an algorithmic approach for lower face and neck rejuvenation and a crossover clinical trial. Plast Reconstr Surg. 2018;142(3):640–9.
27. Wu W. Microbotox of the lower face and neck: evolution of a personal technique and its clinical effects. Plast Reconstr Surg. 2015;136(5 Suppl):92S–100S.
28. El ME, Hussien TM, Maksoud OMA. Needling combined with intralesional corticosteroid injections compared to Intralesional botulinum toxin a injections in the treatment of hypertrophic scars and. J Dermatology Plast Surg. 2019;3(1):1–6.
29. Scala J, Vojvodic A, Vojvodic P, et al. Botulin toxin use in scars/keloids treatment botulin toxin use in scars/keloids treatment. Maced J Med Sci. 2019;7(18):2979.
30. Yang W, Li G. The safety and efficacy of botulinum toxin type A injection for postoperative scar prevention: a systematic review and meta-analysis. J Cosmet Dermatol. 2020;19(4):799–808.
31. Xiao Z, Zhang F, Lin W, Zhang M, Liu Y. Effect of botulinum toxin type A on transforming growth factor beta1 in fibroblasts derived from hypertrophic scar: a preliminary report. Aesthet Plast Surg. 2010;34(4):424–7.
32. Jeong HS, Lee BH, Sung HM, et al. Effect of botulinum toxin type A on differentiation of fibroblasts derived from scar tissue. Plast Reconstr Surg. 2015;136(2):171e–8e.
33. Huang C, Akaishi S, Hyakusoku H, Ogawa R. Are keloid and hypertrophic scar different forms of the same disorder? A fibroproliferative skin disorder hypothesis based on keloid findings. Int Wound J. 2014;11(5):517–22.
34. Kellogg D, Pergola P, Piest K, et al. Cutaneous active vasodilation in humans is mediated by cholinergic nerve cotransmission. Circ Res. 1995;77:1222–8.
35. Uyesugi B, Lippincott B, Dave S. Treatment of painful keloid with botulinum toxin type A. Am J Phys Med Rehabil. 2010;89:153–5.
36. Li Y, Yang J, Liu J, et al. A randomized, placebo-controlled, double-blind, prospective clinical trial of botulinum toxin type A in prevention of hypertrophic scar development in median sternotomy wound. Aesthet Plast Surg. 2018;42:1364–9.
37. Gugerell A, Kober J, Schmid M. Botulinum toxin A: dose- dependent effect on reepithelialization and angiogenesis. Plast Reconstrive Surg Glob Open. 2016;4:e837.
38. Teymoortash A, Sommer F, Mandic R, Schulz S, Teymoortash A, Sommer F, Mandic R, Schulz S, et al. Intraglandular application of botulinum toxin leads to structural and functional changes in rat acinar cells. Br J Pharmacol. 2007;152:161–7.
39. Lakraj AA, Moghimi N, Jabbari B. Sialorrhea: Anatomy, pathophysiology and treatment with emphasis on the role of botulinum toxins. Toxins (Basel). 2013;5(5):1010–31. https://doi.org/10.3390/toxins5051010.
40. Chen S, Paul BC, Myssiorek D. An algorithm approach to diagnosing bilateral parotid enlargement. Otolaryngol – Head Neck Surg. 2013;148(5):732–9.

Chapter 13
Botulinum Toxin Treatment in Ophthalmology and Ophthalmic Surgery

Keya Jafari and Saurabh Jain

Abstract This chapter explores the clinical use of botulinum toxin therapy in ophthalmology and ophthalmic surgery. Ophthalmic conditions that can benefit from botulinum toxin therapy include blepharospasm, strabismus, nystagmus, lacrimal hypersecretion syndromes, eyelid retraction and spastic entropion among others. Since its first use in blepharospasm in 1983, toxin therapy has become the treatment of choice for blepharospasm with successful outcomes. This chapter also explores the techniques of injection, application and complications of toxin therapy in these conditions. Whilst generally considered safe, some of the complications of ophthalmic toxin therapy include ptosis, diplopia, dry eyes and epiphora.

Keywords Botulinum Toxin therapy · Ophthalmology · Strabismus

Introduction

Clinical use of botulinum toxin as medical therapy was first established in the treatment of strabismus by Alan Scott in 1980 [1]. Following successful clinical trials, botulinum toxin type A was approved by the U.S. Food and Drug Administration (FDA) for the treatment of strabismus, blepharospasm and hemifacial spasm in patients over 12 years of age in 1989. The early success of botulinum toxin therapy in treating strabismus bolstered research into additional therapeutic uses within the field of ophthalmology. Early botulinum toxin therapy within ophthalmology pioneered the expansion of its clinical application to the wide range of medical therapies we see today in multiple medical and surgical specialities.

K. Jafari (✉)
Luton & Dunstable Hospital NHS Trust, University College London, London, UK
e-mail: Keya.jafari.13@ucl.ac.uk

S. Jain
Royal Free Hospital, London, UK
e-mail: Saurabh.jain@nhs.net

Table 13.1 Ophthalmic conditions that can benefit from botulinum toxin therapy

Periocular and eyelid	Blepharospasm
	Hemifacial spasm
	Myokymia
	Exposure keratopathy
	Thyroid eye disease
	Spastic entropion
Strabismus	Infantile esotropia
	Intermittent exotropia
	Nerve palsies
	Thyroid eye disease
	Nystagmus
Cosmetic	Glabellar furrows
	Lateral periocular rhytids ("crow's feet")
Other	Dry eye
	Lacrimal hypersecretion

The current application of toxin therapy within ophthalmology is extensive, as shown in the Table 13.1 below. Ophthalmic conditions that can benefit from botulinum toxin therapy include blepharospasm, strabismus, nystagmus, lacrimal hypersecretion syndromes, eyelid retraction and spastic entropion among others.

Periocular

Blepharospasm (Image 13.1)

Benign essential blepharospasm is a distressing idiopathic dystonia involving the orbicularis oculi and upper facial muscles. It is characterised by involuntary muscle contraction resulting in the appearance of forceful, prolonged bilateral blinking. In severe cases, the increased force and frequency of blinking can render the patient functionally blind. This is a lifelong condition with significant impact on quality of life. Whilst the cause is not yet well understood, spasms can be triggered by activities that put strain on the eyes – reading, driving, stress and bright lights.

Botulinum toxin has been well established as in the treatment of blepharospasm, first shown to be effective in 1983. It has since become the treatment of choice, with very successful results [2–14].

Technique

Figure 13.1 illustrates the recommended injection sites for the treatment of blepharospasm. Care must be taken to direct the injecting needle away from the central region of the eyelid to avoid the *levator palpebrae superioris*, damage to which might result in ptosis.

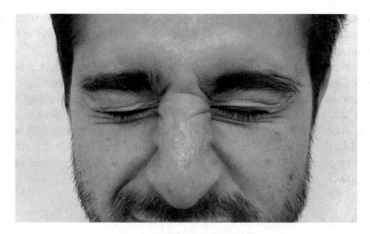

Image 13.1 Essential blepharospasm involving the orbicularis and upper facial muscles

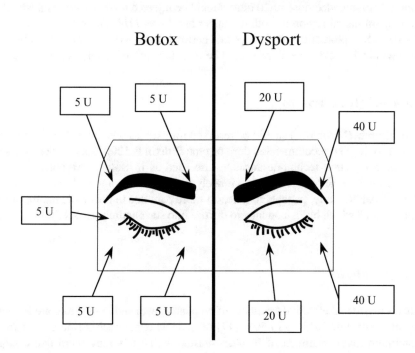

Fig. 13.1 Recommended injection sites for toxin therapy in blepharospasm

Botox® (Botulinum Toxin Type A)

The initial recommended dose is 2.5 to 5 U injected into the medial and lateral pre-tarsal orbicularis oculi of the upper lid and the later pre-tarsal orbicularis oculi of the lower lid. The injections are given subcutaneously to ensure maximal effectiveness and safety. It is prudent to remain outside the orbital rim whilst inject-ing to avoid inadvertent weakening of the levator palpebrae superioris or the extra-ocular muscles.

The initial effect of the injections is seen within 72 hours and peaks at 1–2 weeks post injection. The effects last for approximately 13 weeks. The procedure can then be repeated indefinitely, with increasing doses if necessary. If the initial treatment does not last longer than 2 months, then a twofold increase in dosage is recom-mended. There have been some reports of decreasing effectiveness with prolonged use [15, 16], though this is rare and there is no evidence of any adverse effects with prolonged treatment. The cumulative dose of Botox® in a 30-day period should not exceed 200 U.

Dysport®

Initial recommended dose of 20 units should be injected medially 40 units laterally into the pre-tarsal region of both the upper and lower *orbicularis oculi* muscles of each eye. Symptomatic relief is expected between 2 and 4 days with maximal effect seen within 2 weeks. Injections should be repeated approximately every 8 weeks.

Myobloc® (Toxin Type B)

Type B toxin (Myobloc®) should be reserved for patients who develop resistance to type A toxin. The recommended dose of type B toxin is 1200–2500 U per eye, and the same injection technique and sites are used as in Botox®. Myobloc ® has a shorter duration of action of approximately 8–10 weeks, compared to 13 weeks in Botox®. Additionally, patients may report more pain due to the acidic nature of the preparations which has a tendency to diffuse into surrounding tissues (Table 13.2).

Complications

This is a safe and effective treatment of blepharospasm and is well tolerated. Some reports have described up to 30% [17] of patients experiencing side effects from botulinum toxin treatment of blepharospasm. Whilst this may seem like a large proportion, the side effects are often mild, transient and reversible, with symptoms subsiding with gradual recovery of muscle function. Table 13.3 lists some of the potential adverse effects following periocular botulinum toxin injection. The most common complication is ptosis, seen in around 13% of cases [18], and this risk significantly increases both with number of treatments [5] and dose [19]. Patients may not be able to distinguish the difference between eyelid closure secondary to ptosis or blepharospasm and thus may report ptosis as a failure of botulinum toxin treatment. It is therefore the clinician's responsibility to determine the difference

Table 13.2 Recommended dosage at relevant injection sites in the treatment of blepharospasm

Toxin	Upper lid (U)	Lower lid (U)			Other	Recommended dosage per eye (U)
	Medial	Lateral	Medial	Lateral	External angle	
Toxin type A						
Botox ®	1.25–5	1.25–5	1.25–5	1.25–5	1.25–5	12.5–25
Dysport ®	20	40	20	40		100–120
Xeomin ®	5	5	5	5		25
Toxin type B						
Myobloc ®	150	150	150	150		1200–2500

Table 13.3 Side effect profile for toxin therapy in blepharospasm

Side effect	Mean incidence (%) [18]	Reported range (%) [18]
Ptosis	13.4	0–52.3
Keratitis	4.1	0–46.2
Epiphora	3.5	0–20.0
Dry eyes	2.5	0–18.2
Diplopia	2.1	0–17.2
Lid oedema	1.6	0–30.4
Facial weakness	0.9	0–4.6
Lagophthalmos	3.0	0–63.6
Ecchymosis	0.3	0–9.0
Ectropion/entropion	0.3	0–6.7
Local pain	0.2	0–100
Blurred vision	0.2	0–2.1
Facial numbness	0.1	0–4.0

and identify the complication of ptosis where it occurs and avoid unnecessary early re-treatment and potential exacerbation of the ptosis.

Injecting botulinum toxin into the orbicularis muscle can result in a weakened blink as well as lagophthalmos. This can result in dry eyes, another commonly reported side effect of toxin therapy in blepharospasm. This can be overcome by using artificial tears routinely during toxin therapy.

Strabismus (Image 13.2)

The first therapeutic use of botulinum toxin in humans was for the treatment of strabismus. Strabismus is a common condition where there is an imbalance in extra-ocular muscle function, leading to misalignment of the eyes. The commonest strabismus causes are congenital whilst others may be acquired in adulthood, such as cranial nerve palsies. This deviation of ocular alignment may be intermittent or constant. Strabismus can also be subdivided into groups based on the direction of deviation: esotropia (inturning deviation), exotropia (out-turning deviation), hypertropia (upturning deviation), hypotropia (downturning deviation) or cyclotropia (rotatory deviation). Strabismus can be caused by pathologies affecting the extraocular muscles, the nerves that control these muscles or the central processing that directs eye movements at a cortical level. Toxin might be used as a diagnostic or a therapeutic tool in the management of strabismus.

Diagnostic

Botulinum toxin can be used preoperatively to detect whether fusion is present once the deviation is corrected. It may also help aid the prediction of surgical outcomes for incomitant deviations and to rule out the incidence of postoperative diplopia. It can also be used to investigate a possible postoperative slipped muscle and gauge the power of a paretic one.

Therapeutic

Strabismus treatment is targeted at aligning the visual axes. Conservative options include the use of prisms and orthoptic exercises to help establish binocular control of ocular alignment. Invasive options such as surgery are used to weaken or strengthen extraocular muscles and permanently change ocular alignment. Botulinum toxin therapy can be used to temporarily paralyse individual extraocular

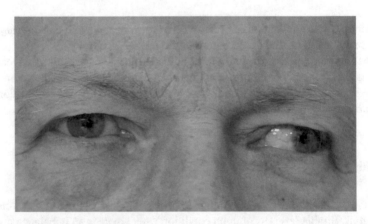

Image 13.2 Left divergent strabismus

muscles in attempt to establish better ocular alignment. This effect may be permanent in children with neuroplasticity.

Botulinum toxin acts by weakening the muscle of interest that leads to a reduction, or in some cases complete correction, of the angle of deviation of strabismus. For example, to correct convergent squint caused by a sixth nerve palsy, the toxin would be injected into the medial rectus of the affected eye.

Once toxin is injected, paralysis sets in within 72 hours; the maximal effect of the toxin is usually seen around 14 days after injection and lasts for approximately 3 months. It is important to use electromyographic guidance to ensure the toxin is placed in the correct location and to use a small volume to prevent inadvertent involvement of other extraocular muscles or the levator muscle.

As the effect of the toxin sets in, it can cause an initial overcorrection of the deviation (a divergent deviation in the example of injection into the medial rectus in a sixth nerve palsy), but this effect is usually transient. It is important to monitor for unexpected vertical or horizontal deviations and ptosis which may occur if the solution extravasates during injection, affecting adjoining structures.

Aside from its use as primary treatment for strabismus, botulinum toxin can also be used as an adjunct to correct residual symptoms postoperatively in large-angle strabismus [20, 21]. It has also been used intraoperatively for large-angle strabismus, though this has not yet shown to improve outcomes over surgery alone [22].

Infantile Esotropia

Whilst botulinum toxin use in adults is a well-established alternative treatment option to surgical correction, it is not as well studied in children. It has been shown that early intervention with botulinum toxin therapy can re-establish motor and sensory fusion with good long-term results [23]. However, studies show varying results depending on the age of the patients and pattern of injection. The image below illustrates the injection of botulinum toxin into the medial rectus of a child under general anaesthetic (Image 13.3).

Sixth Nerve Palsy

Botulinum toxin has also been trialled in the treatment of acquired sixth nerve palsy. Injecting the medial rectus muscle has been shown to improve the rate of recovery. It also helps improve the deviation in the short term, lessening the need to use prisms or occlusion of the affected eye. However, the long-term outcomes are uncertain with many studies reporting equal efficacy between botulinum toxin therapy and conservative management of sixth nerve palsy.

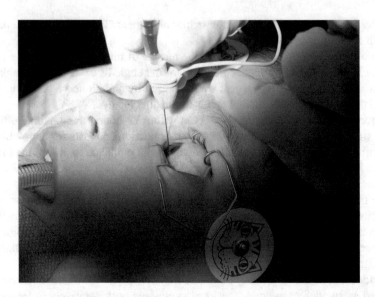

Image 13.3 Botulinum toxin injection into the medial rectus muscle under general anaesthesia

Technique

To achieve paralysis of the muscle, botulinum toxin must be injected directly into the belly of an extraocular muscle. In order to correctly isolate the muscle in question, electromyography (EMG) is used (Image 13.4). One end of the EMG machine is connected to the base of the injecting needle and the other is connected to the patient's forehead to complete the circuit. Topical anaesthesia is used to anaesthetise the conjunctiva. The needle is then passed through the conjunctiva posterior to the muscle insertion site on the sclera, staying superficial to the sclera to avoid penetration of the globe. The patient is first asked to look in the opposite direction to the action of the muscle being injected. When the needle is deemed to be in the muscle belly, the patient is then asked to look in the direction of action of the extraocular muscle being injected. This will result in an increased signal output from the EMG, confirming the correct location of the needle. The toxin is then slowly injected.

Different techniques for injecting botulinum toxin in strabismus:

1. EMG-guided injection.
2. Injection without EMG guidance.
3. Injection under direct vision of the muscle during squint surgery.
4. Injection through a conjunctival incision to visualise the muscle.
5. Injection via a sub-Tenon's lacrimal cannula alongside a muscle.
6. Transconjunctival injection after grasping the muscle with forceps.

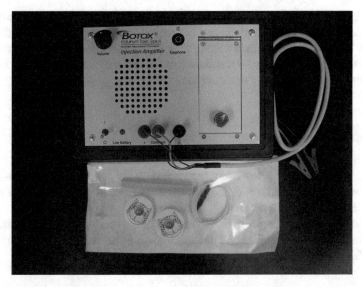

Image 13.4 Electromyographic equipment for extraocular muscle toxin injection including an injection amplifier, needle electrodes and adhesive skin electrodes

Indication	Botox® dose	Dysport
Strabismus of less than 20 prism diopters	1.25–2.5 U	5–10 U
Strabismus of 20–50 prism diopter	2.5–5 U	10–20 U
VI nerve palsy	1.25–2 U	

Myokymia

Eyelid myokymia is the involuntary contraction of the orbicularis muscle. It predominantly affects the lower eyelid and upper eyelid involvement is rare. It is a benign, non-progressive disorder that is often self-limiting and the underlying pathology is not fully understood. It can be triggered by stress, anxiety, fatigue, caffeine or alcohol. Botulinum toxin can be injected into the twitching orbicularis to temporarily paralyse and relax the muscle until spontaneous resolution is achieved. The recommended dose and technique is similar to that for the treatment of blepharospasm but only the upper or lower lid may need to be treated.

Chronic Dry Eyes

The aqueous component of the tear film is produced by the lacrimal gland and drained by the lacrimal pump. The lacrimal pump is located in the medial canthus and it is regulated by the orbicularis oculi. Thus, conditions causing an excess of blinking, such as blepharospasm or hemifacial spasm, can lead to a chronic dry eye state. Botulinum toxin injections can be used to reduce the blink rate and consequently improve ocular surface wetting [24]. Injecting the medial region of the orbicularis muscle of the lower lid has shown to reduce lacrimal pump action, increase tear output and improve dry eye symptoms [25].

Acquired Nystagmus

Acquired nystagmus is a rare condition caused by involuntary repetitive to-and-fro eye movements, leading to visual disturbances such as oscillopsia and blurred vision. Studies have shown success in treating nystagmus by injecting botulinum toxin directly into the rectus muscles [26–28]. However, the treatment should only be attempted in wheelchair-bound patients if all muscles are to be blocked as it may also inhibit the vestibular reflex or the ocular tilt reaction.

Cosmetic

Patients with blepharospasm treated with botulinum toxin were noted to have a stress-free appearance. This observation inspired research on the potential cosmetic applications of the toxin.

Botulinum toxin has revolutionised the cosmetic industry in recent years. The first cosmetically approved use for Botox® was for the treatment of glabellar furrows in 2002 and its cosmetic application has since expanded to treat lateral periocular rhytids ("crow's feet"), perioral rhytids ("smoker's lines"), mesolabial folds ("marionette lines"), transverse brow and forehead furrows and platysmal bands.

The safety profile for cosmetic Botox® is very promising, with no serious adverse events reported. Mild side effects include local pain and bruising, infection, brow and eyelid ptosis.

Complications

Botulinum toxin therapy is generally considered a safe and well-tolerated procedure.

Whilst side effects can occur, they are usually transient and rarely sight threatening.

Side effects secondary to the technique of administration are common to most procedures involving an injection. These include oedema, bruising, haemorrhage and mild pain. Bruising and haemorrhage can be minimised by stopping any anticoagulant medications 2 weeks prior to the injection. Additionally, use of ice packs prior to injection, careful placement of the needle and immediate gentle local pressure to the injection site can help prevent bruising.

The most common complication secondary to the chemodenervation associated with botulinum toxin therapy is ptosis. Diffusion of the neurotoxin into the orbital septum can result in impairment of the levator muscle. This can occur as early as 48 hours post injection and can last up to 12 weeks. Techniques to avoid the levator muscle such as avoiding the central portion of the upper lid are recommended to reduce the risk of ptosis.

Diplopia can occur, most commonly due inadvertent paralysis of the inferior oblique muscle, though this is rare. Additionally, unwanted horizontal deviation can occur, though uncommon.

Other common side effects of botulinum toxin therapy include dry eye and epiphora. Patients can develop lagophthalmos and impaired blinking due to orbicularis muscle weakening. This can lead to characteristic dry eye symptoms of burning, photophobia and redness. Conversely, toxin therapy can also result in epiphora by means of impaired lacrimal pump function secondary to reduced lower lid tone.

More severe reported side effects include incidences of acute angle-closure glaucoma [29, 30] and retinal detachment secondary to globe penetration associated with botulinum toxin injection [31]. However, these are very rare and often avoidable.

Bibliography

1. Scott AB. Botulinum toxin injection into extraocular muscles as an alternative to strabismus surgery. Ophthalmology. 1980;87(10):1044–9. https://doi.org/10.1016/s0161-6420(80)35127-0.
2. Taylor JD, Kraft SP, Kazdan MS, Flanders M, Cadera W, Orton RB. Treatment of blepharospasm and hemifacial spasm with botulinum A toxin: a Canadian multicentre study. Can J Ophthalmol. 1991;26(3):133–8. http://www.ncbi.nlm.nih.gov/pubmed/2054723. Accessed December 1, 2019
3. Scott AB, Stubbs HA, Kennedy RA. Botulinum a toxin injection as a treatment for blepharospasm. Arch Ophthalmol. 1985;103(3):347–50. https://doi.org/10.1001/archopht.1985.01050030043017.
4. Tsoy EA, Buckley EG, Dutton JJ. Treatment of Blepharospasm with botulinum toxin. Am J Ophthalmol. 1985;99(2):176–9. https://doi.org/10.1016/0002-9394(85)90228-4.
5. Dutton JJ, Buckley EG. Long-term results and complications of botulinum A toxin in the treatment of blepharospasm. Ophthalmology. 1988;95(11):1529–34. https://doi.org/10.1016/s0161-6420(88)32977-5.
6. Calace P, Cortese G, Piscopo R, et al. Treatment of Blepharospasm with botulinum neurotoxin type A: long-term results. Eur J Ophthalmol. 2003;13(4):331–6. https://doi.org/10.1177/112067210301300401.
7. Osako M, Keltner JL. Botulinum A toxin (Oculinum) in ophthalmology. Surv Ophthalmol. 1991;36(1):28–46. https://doi.org/10.1016/0039-6257(91)90207-v.
8. Kraft SP, Lang AE. Botulinum toxin injections in the treatment of blepharospasm, hemifacial spasm, and eyelid fasciculations. Can J Neurol Sci. 1988;15(3):276–80. https://doi.org/10.1017/s0317167100027748.
9. Mauriello JA Jr. Blepharospasm, Meige syndrome, and hemifacial spasm: treatment with botulinum toxin. Neurology. 1985;35(0028-3878 (Print)):1499–500.

10. Jitpimolmard S, Tiamkao S, Laopaiboon M. Long term results of botulinum toxin type A (Dysport) in the treatment of hemifacial spasm: a report of 175 cases. J Neurol Neurosurg Psychiatry. 1998;64(6):751–7. https://doi.org/10.1136/jnnp.64.6.751.
11. Grandas F, Elston J, Quinn N, Marsden CD. Blepharospasm: a review of 264 patients. J Neurol Neurosurg Psychiatry. 1988;51(6):767–72. https://doi.org/10.1136/jnnp.51.6.767.
12. Cillino S, Raimondi G, Guépratte N, et al. Long-term efficacy of botulinum toxin A for treatment of blepharospasm, hemifacial spasm, and spastic entropion: a multicentre study using two drug-dose escalation indexes. Eye. 2010;24(4):600–7. https://doi.org/10.1038/eye.2009.192.
13. Elston JS. Long-term results of treatment of idiopathic blepharospasm with botulinum toxin injections. Br J Ophthalmol. 1987;71(9):664–8. https://doi.org/10.1136/bjo.71.9.664.
14. Grandas F, Elston J, Quinn JN, Marsden CD, Quinn N. Blepharospasm: a review of 264 patients. J Neurol Neurosurg Psychiatry. 1988;51:767–72. https://doi.org/10.1136/jnnp.51.6.767.
15. Engstrom PF, Arnoult JB, Mazow ML, et al. Effectiveness of botulinum toxin therapy for essential Blepharospasm. Ophthalmology. 1987;94(8):971–5. https://doi.org/10.1016/S0161-6420(87)33338-X.
16. Frueh BR, Musch DC. Treatment of facial spasm with botulinum toxin. An interim report. Ophthalmology. 1986;93(7):917–23. https://doi.org/10.1016/s0161-6420(86)33641-8.
17. Dutton JJ. Botulinum-A toxin in the treatment of craniocervical muscle spasms: short- and long-term, local and systemic effects. Surv Ophthalmol. 1996;41(1):51–65. https://doi.org/10.1016/s0039-6257(97)81995-9.
18. Dutton JJ, Fowler AM. Botulinum toxin in ophthalmology. Surv Ophthalmol. 2007;52(1):13–31. https://doi.org/10.1016/j.survophthal.2006.10.003.
19. Carruthers J, Stubbs HA. Botulinum toxin for benign essential blepharospasm, hemifacial spasm and age-related lower eyelid entropion. Can J Neurol Sci. 1987;14(1):42–5. https://doi.org/10.1017/s0317167100026159.
20. Owens PL, Strominger MB, Rubin PA, Veronneau-Troutman S. Large-angle exotropia corrected by intraoperative botulinum toxin a and monocular recession resection surgery. J AAPOS Off Publ Am Assoc Pediatr Ophthalmol Strabismus. 1998;2(3):144–6. https://doi.org/10.1016/s1091-8531(98)90004-0.
21. Khan AO. Two horizontal rectus eye muscle surgery combined with botulinum toxin for the treatment of very large angle esotropia. A pilot study. Binocul Vis Strabismus Q. 2005;20(1):15–20. http://www.ncbi.nlm.nih.gov/pubmed/15828866. Accessed December 4, 2019
22. Jain S, Anand SS, Jones A. Intraoperative botulinum toxin in large angle strabismus. J Am Assoc Pediatr Ophthalmol Strabismus. 2015;19(4):e12. https://doi.org/10.1016/j.jaapos.2015.07.007.
23. McNeer KW, Tucker MG, Guerry CH, Spencer RF. Incidence of stereopsis after treatment of infantile esotropia with botulinum toxin A. J Pediatr Ophthalmol Strabismus. 2003;40(5):288–92. http://www.ncbi.nlm.nih.gov/pubmed/14560837. Accessed December 4, 2019
24. de Oliveira FC, de Oliveira GC, Cariello AJ, Felberg S, Osaki MH. Botulinum toxin type A influence on the lacrimal function of patients with facial dystonia. Arq Bras Oftalmol. 2010;73(5):405–8. https://doi.org/10.1590/s0004-27492010000500003.
25. Sahlin S, Chen E, Kaugesaar T, Almqvist H, Kjellberg K, Lennerstrand G. Effect of eyelid botulinum toxin injection on lacrimal drainage. Am J Ophthalmol. 2000;129(4):481–6. https://doi.org/10.1016/s0002-9394(99)00408-0.
26. Carruthers J. The treatment of congenital nystagmus with Botox. J Pediatr Ophthalmol Strabismus. 1995;32(5):306–8. https://doi.org/10.3928/0191-3913-19950901-09.
27. Leigh RJ, Tomsak RL, Grant MP, et al. Effectiveness of botulinum toxin administered to abolish acquired nystagmus. Ann Neurol. 1992;32(5):633–42. https://doi.org/10.1002/ana.410320506.

28. Repka MX, Savino PJ, Reinecke RD. Treatment of acquired nystagmus with botulinum neurotoxin A. Arch Ophthalmol. 1994;112(10):1320–4. https://doi.org/10.1001/archo pht.1994.01090220070025.
29. Corridan P, Nightingale S, Mashoudi N, Williams AC. Acute angle-closure glaucoma following botulinum toxin injection for blepharospasm. Br J Ophthalmol. 1990;74(5):309–10. https://doi.org/10.1136/bjo.74.5.309.
30. Zheng L, Azar D. Angle-closure glaucoma following periorbital botulinum toxin injection. Clin Exp Ophthalmol. 2014;42(7):690–3. https://doi.org/10.1111/ceo.12293.
31. Liu M, Lee HC, Hertle RW, Ho AC. Retinal detachment from inadvertent intraocular injection of botulinum toxin A. Am J Ophthalmol. 2004;137(1):201–2. https://doi.org/10.1016/s0002-9394(03)00837-7.

Chapter 14
Botulinum Toxin Treatment in Gastrointestinal Disorders

Ammar Nassri, Kaveh Sharzehi, and Ron Schey

Abstract Botulinum toxin is used extensively for the management of gastrointestinal smooth muscle disorders. This chapter is a summary of the current status of this therapy. Botulinum toxin appears to be beneficial for achalasia, hypertensive esophageal disorders, and anal fissure and unclear utility in gastroparesis, upper esophageal sphincter dysfunction, and sphincter of Oddi dysfunction. Very few placebo-controlled trials have been performed despite widespread use of toxin for the past 25 years. Botulinum toxin appears to be safe and side effects are uncommon. Despite uncontrolled data, botulinum toxin is now used for a variety of spastic disorders of GI smooth muscle. In some instances, this therapy may preclude the need for more invasive treatments. Controlled trials are needed.

Keywords Botulinum toxin · Achalasia · Gastroparesis · Hypertensive esophageal disorders · Anal fissure · Sphincter of Oddi dysfunction

Introduction

The toxin of *Clostridium botulinum* inhibits the release of acetylcholine from nerve terminals and causes paralysis of skeletal muscle. Botulinum toxin (Botox) injection was first described in 1977 in children with strabismus, and since then it has been utilized in a multitude of clinical indications, ranging from conditions such as focal dystonia, urinary incontinence, hemifacial spasm, and cervical dystonia to a variety of cosmetic procedures [1–3]. In 1993, it was hypothesized that Botox may have a similar effect on gastrointestinal smooth muscle. This was tested by injecting Botox into the lower esophageal sphincter of five piglets and comparing the effect with the injection of normal saline [4]. A reduction of about 60% was observed

A. Nassri (✉) · R. Schey
University of Florida, Miami, FL, USA
e-mail: ammar.nassri@jax.ufl.edu

K. Sharzehi
Oregon Health and Science University, Portland, OR, USA

© Springer Nature Switzerland AG 2020
B. Jabbari (ed.), *Botulinum Toxin Treatment in Surgery, Dentistry, and Veterinary Medicine*, https://doi.org/10.1007/978-3-030-50691-9_14

without evidence of toxicity [4]. In a pilot trial, Pasricha et al. demonstrated that intra-sphincteric injection of botulinum toxin in humans had the potential to be useful in the treatment of achalasia [5] and these findings were followed by a seminal randomized trial [6]. Since then, Botox has been used in the GI tract in various applications described below.

Upper Esophageal Sphincter

Oropharyngeal dysphagia and aspiration can be caused by spasticity, hypertonus, or delayed relaxation of the upper esophageal sphincter (UES). UES dysfunction during swallowing has been reported in numerous acute and progressive neurological conditions including, but not limited to, brainstem stroke, motor neuron disease, Parkinson's disease, myasthenia gravis, and inclusion body myositis [7–11]. Management of impaired UES varies across individuals and intervention can be pharmacological, compensatory, rehabilitative, or surgical in nature [12]. In cases where patients have demonstrated minimal benefit from a trial of compensatory and rehabilitation programs, they may be considered for surgical or pharmacological interventions. Surgical intervention includes cricopharyngeal myotomy and upper esophageal dilatation. Pharmacological intervention consists of injection of Botox into the cricopharyngeus.

The first use of Botox in this setting was described in 1994 in a series of 7 patients. Conventional therapy (i.e., lateral cricopharyngotomy and laser dissection of the UES) was replaced by Botox injection with complete resolution of symptoms in 5 of 7 patients [13]. Since this initial 1994 study, cricopharyngeal Botox injection has been reported in over 30 studies with a mean success rate of 76% (43–100%) [14], although endoscopic myotomy is considered superior and had the highest success rate. Patients with Botox need repeat injections due to a higher risk of recurrence, but its use has a role in the elderly and in patients with comorbidities [15].

Achalasia

Achalasia is a disorder characterized by a failure of the lower esophageal sphincter to relax with swallowing as well as a lack of esophageal peristalsis. It was first described in 1674 by Sir Thomas Willis, who postulated that the disease is due to the loss of normal inhibition in the distal esophagus [16].

Although the etiology is largely unknown, the pathophysiology is well described, with pathology revealing a loss of esophageal nitric oxide-releasing inhibitory neurons, which leads to an imbalance between the excitatory and inhibitory neurons in the myenteric plexus, thus resulting in a failure of relaxation of the LES and an increased residual pressure. Esophageal motor innervation is through the vagus nerve via the myenteric plexus. Neural innervation differs in the proximal and distal esophagus. The striated muscle of the proximal esophagus is innervated by the somatic efferent fibers of the vagus nerve. The cell bodies for these fibers originate in the nucleus ambiguous and terminate on the motor end plate directly via cholinergic receptors [17, 18]. The smooth muscle of the distal esophagus is innervated by the preganglionic vagus nerve fibers with cell bodies located in the dorsal motor nucleus [19]. The postganglionic excitatory neurons release acetylcholine while the inhibitory neurons release nitric oxide and vasoactive intestinal polypeptide resulting in esophageal and LES contractions and relaxations, respectively [20, 21]. The inhibitory neurons also play a role in normal peristalsis. At baseline, the esophageal muscle is in a contractile state. With swallowing, the inhibitory neurons are excited, which results in esophageal relaxation. A coordinated series of relaxation followed by contraction in a cephalic-caudal direction results in peristalsis [22]. In patients with achalasia, there is loss of the inhibitory neurons. This results in failure of LES relaxation as well as loss of esophageal peristalsis [23].

Achalasia is characterized manometrically by insufficient relaxation of the lower esophageal sphincter (LES) and loss of esophageal peristalsis; radiographically by aperistalsis, esophageal dilation, with minimal LES opening, "bird-beak" appearance, and poor emptying of barium; and endoscopically by a dilated esophagus with retained saliva, liquid, and undigested food particles in the absence of mucosal stricturing or tumor [24].

Idiopathic achalasia is rare, with mean incidences of 0.3–1.63 per 100 000 people per year in adults [25, 26]. Achalasia has an insidious onset, and disease progression is gradual. Patients typically experience symptoms for years prior to seeking medical attention. The mean duration of symptoms is 4.7 years prior to diagnosis [27]. In one series dysphagia to solids (91%) and liquids (85%), regurgitation (76%), heartburn (52%), chest pain (41%), and weight loss (35%) were the most frequent symptoms in patients with achalasia [28]. In the early stages of the disease, dysphagia may be very subtle and can be misinterpreted as dyspepsia, poor gastric emptying, or stress.

Achalasia is a chronic condition without cure. Current treatment options in achalasia are aimed at reducing the hypertonicity of the LES by pharmacologic, endoscopic, or surgical means.

For patients who are at low surgical risk, pneumatic dilation or surgical myotomy should be performed to treat achalasia. Per-oral endoscopic myotomy (POEM) is a promising new endoscopic technique for performing myotomy. Pneumatic dilation involves the forceful dilation of the LES with a pneumatic balloon to weaken the LES by tearing its muscle fibers and appears to be the most cost-effective treatment for achalasia [29]. Initial success rates are high with either modality (85% for pneumatic dilation and 90% for surgical myotomy); however, about one-third of patients have recurrence of symptoms in 4–6 years [30]. The two most often used pharmacological drugs are nitrates and calcium channel blockers. Medical therapy is the least effective treatment option in patients with achalasia and should be considered in patients who are unwilling or unable to tolerate invasive therapy and for patients who have failed Botox injections [31].

Botox therapy is strongly considered in patients who are not good candidates for more definitive therapy with pneumatic dilation or surgical myotomy. Botulinum toxin A, which blocks the release of acetylcholine from the nerve terminals, is directly injected into the LES during upper endoscopy. The lower esophageal sphincter is visualized endoscopically by identification of the sphincteric rosette, seen at the squamocolumnar junction. Botox is injected into the region of the lower esophageal sphincter. Aliquots of 1 ml each (20–25 units of botulinum toxin per milliliter of saline) are injected into quadrants, for a total of 80–100 units [32].

More than 80% of cases have a clinical response by 1 month, but response fades rapidly, with less than 60% of patients in remission at 1 year [33]. At least a second treatment is needed in 46.6% of patients [34]. In general, there is almost universal symptom relapse by 2 years, although some studies have shown continued efficacy in up to 34% of patients at 2 years [35].

Findings from six randomized trials comparing Botox with pneumatic dilatation and laparoscopic myotomy are shown in Table 14.1. These studies demonstrated comparable relief from dysphagia, but a rapid deterioration in patients treated with Botox after 6–12 months compared to the other modalities [35–40].

Botox injection is less invasive compared with surgery and can be easily performed with endoscopy. As seen in Table 14.1, initial success rates with Botox are comparable to pneumatic dilation and surgical myotomy [34]. However, patients treated with Botox have more frequent relapses and a shorter time to relapse, and repeated Botox injections can negatively impact the outcome of subsequent myotomy [41]. Despite this, Botox therapy has an important role to play in elderly patients with comorbidities and as salvage therapy.

Table 14.1 Randomized trials comparing Botox injection to balloon dilation and myotomy for treatment of achalasia

Author	Compared to	N	Response rate (30 day) Botox group vs non-Botox group	Recurrence rate (12–24 months) Botox group vs non-Botox group
Zaninotto	Surgical myotomy	80	66% vs 82% ($P < 0.05$)	87.5% vs 34% ($p < 0.05$)
Zhu	Balloon dilation and balloon dilation + Botox	90	75% vs 85% vs 93%	84% vs 64% vs 43%
Mikaeli	Balloon dilation	40	Not available	85% vs 47% ($p < 0.05$)
Ghoshal	Balloon dilation	17	86% vs 80% ($p = NS$)	71% vs 25% ($p = 0.027$)
Vaezi	Balloon dilation	42	Not available	68% vs 30% ($p < 0.01$)
Muehldorfer	Balloon dilation	24	75% vs 83% ($p = NS$)	100% vs 40% ($p < 0.05$)

Hypertensive Esophageal Disorders

This group of esophageal motility disorders are a somewhat rare but troublesome group of disorders that can lead to severe symptoms including nausea, regurgitation, dysphagia, and chest pain [42]. Since the introduction of Botox for the treatment of achalasia in 1995, its utility has been expanded to a spectrum of esophageal motility diseases, most importantly diffuse esophageal spasm (DES), nutcracker esophagus, and hypertensive lower esophageal sphincter. These conditions are also collectively called hypercontractile esophageal disorders.

There are limited data on the prevalence of hypercontractile esophageal disorders. The prevalence of these conditions among individuals with atypical chest pain appears to be between 4% and 13% [43]. The underlying pathophysiology for these conditions is relatively unknown. DES has been associated with an impairment of inhibitory innervation and malfunction in endogenous nitric oxide synthesis [44]. Nutcracker esophagus and hypertensive LES are due to overactivity of excitatory innervation or asynchrony of the smooth muscle response due to a hypercholinergic state [45].

The typical symptoms of patients with DES are dysphagia associated with retrosternal chest pain. Many of the patients with nutcracker esophagus or hypertensive LES have no symptoms. The diagnosis of these patients is often made through esophageal manometry after a normal endoscopic examination. Each of these conditions have distinct manometric findings, and diagnosis is often made once manometric criteria are met.

Multiple therapies have been used to treat diffuse DES, nutcracker esophagus, and hypertensive LES, and the most effective treatment has not been defined. Calcium channel blockers and tricyclic antidepressants have been shown to be effective in the treatment of dysphagia and chest pain, respectively, and they have been considered first-line treatment for them [46–48].

For patients who do not respond to the first-line treatment, injection of Botox or oral nitrates (isosorbide 10 mg or sildenafil 50 mg on an as-needed basis for pain) is considered as the next treatment option [49, 50]. Unlike in achalasia, Botox therapy in these patients has not been as well studied in non-achalasia esophageal motor disorders, with the majority of data from open label series [51]. Typically, 100 units of Botox is diluted in 4 mL saline. During the EGD, aliquots of 0.5 mL Botox is injected in the 4 quadrants at 2 cm above the gastroesophageal junction and 5 cm more proximally into the esophagus.

In one series, 29 patients with non-achalasia esophageal motor disorders with chest pain as the major complaint were treated with 5 injections of 20 U BTX at the EGJ [52]. There was a 62% reduction in the chest pain score 1 month after treatment, with a mean duration of response of 6 months, regardless of the underlying motility disorder. Dysphagia scores were reduced by 54%, although the mean preinjection dysphagia score was low owing to the selection of the patients based on chest pain. A subsequent randomized trial included 22 patients with dysphagia-predominant, manometry-confirmed DES or NE [51]. Patients in the study group had decreases in total dysphagia and chest pain symptom scores, as well as a reduction of unintentional weight loss. Fifty percent of patients had a response compared to 10% on placebo ($p = 0.04$) and 30% had a response at 1 year.

Gastroparesis

Normal gastric motility is a complex series of events that requires coordination of the sympathetic and parasympathetic nervous systems, neurons, and pacemaker cells of Cajal within the stomach and the smooth muscle cells. Abnormalities of this process can lead to a delay in gastric emptying [53]. Gastroparesis is defined by delayed gastric emptying in the absence of a mechanical obstruction. The etiology of over half of the patients with gastroparesis is unknown and is classified as idiopathic gastroparesis. Both long-standing diabetes mellitus and hyperglycemia are associated with delayed gastric emptying. In the former, this occurs through diabetic neuropathy, which causes abnormal postprandial proximal gastric accommodation and difficulties with antral motor function [54, 55]. Various medications including narcotics and dopamine agonists have also been shown to delay gastric emptying [56]. Previous gastric and thoracic surgery can result in gastroparesis due to intentional or accidental injury to the vagus nerves [57]. Several common neurologic disorders are associated with gastroparesis, which include multiple sclerosis and Parkinson's disease [58].

The management of gastroparesis can be very challenging, and treatment options include dietary changes, prokinetic drugs, antiemetics, jejunal feeding, parenteral nutrition, gastric neurostimulation therapy, and surgery [59, 60].

Since the late 1990s, there has been conflicting evidence behind the efficacy of intrapyloric botulinum toxin on gastroparesis. The first data on the intrapyloric application of Botox in patients with gastroparesis was published in 2002. Injection of 100 units of Botox into the pylorus in patients with diabetic gastroparesis showed 50% improvement in their symptoms and gastric emptying tests [61]. Further, open-labeled trials showed promising evidence of improvement of gastric emptying tests, symptoms, and SF-36 scores with intrapyloric injection of 200 units Botox [72]. Miller et al. demonstrated effectiveness of repeat injection but at the same time raised a question regarding long-term outcomes of the procedure [73]. The largest study published to date was a retrospective study of 179 patients including 81 with diabetic gastroparesis and 76 idiopathic gastroparesis cases. Overall, there was a decrease in symptoms in 51.4% of patients at 1–4 months, 73.4% of patients that had a second injection had a response [62]. The only randomized trials came from two subsequent studies which each had less than 20 patients in their study arm. They failed to report improvement in symptom scores or gastric emptying scans in patients who received Botox compared to placebo although there was improvement in the treatment arm compared to baseline [63, 64].

Some authors have emphasized that improvement in gastric emptying has not been shown to correlate with symptom improvement in this patient population, and the discrepancy between the results of the randomized trials and the open label trials may also be secondary to suboptimal dosing of Botox in the randomized trial as well as the small sample sizes [65].

Thus, despite the fact that it is currently not recommended by the ACG Gastroparesis Guidelines [66], due to the limited availability of treatment options, many gastroenterologists consider Botox as a trial therapy before directing patient with refractory gastroparesis for more aggressive surgical interventions.

Sphincter of Oddi Dysfunction

Sphincter of Oddi dysfunction (SOD) refers to a clinical syndrome that occurs because of abnormal sphincter of Oddi (SO) contractility. Elevated pressure in the sphincter can lead to pancreatitis, chronic right upper quadrant pain, and elevated liver function tests. Historically, it was split into three groups, with SOD type III as one of the subgroups having only biliary-type pain in the absence of abnormal liver enzymes of biliary dilation. Pilot studies showed substantial decrease in the SO pressure with the use of Botox injection [67], but there are no placebo-controlled studies available formally evaluating the effect of Botox injection on SOD type III. One study has shown that 50% of patients receiving Botox for SOD type III had some improvement of their pain. It has also served as a predictor to who may respond to endoscopic sphincterotomy [68]. However, long-term follow-up on patients with SOD type III has shown no benefit from ERCP and sphincterotomy to the extent that this subgroup has been discarded from GI functional gastrointestinal disorders in the most recent guidelines, the Rome IV criteria [69]. This undermines the usefulness of any intervention of the SO (sphincterotomy or Botox) in patients with type III SOD.

Prevention of Pancreatic Fistula

Recently, Botox has been successfully used to temporarily reduce the SO pressure after distal pancreatectomy to prevent pancreatic fistula formation. Postoperative pancreatic fistula is one of the most common complication after distal pancreatectomy which can occur up to 50% of procedures [70]. Improved drainage of the Vater appears to prevent pressure-induced leakage from the pancreatic stump. Previously, studies have shown successful prophylaxis by placing a pancreatic stent [71]. In a prospective Phase I/II trial, 29 patients had preoperative Botox injection into the SOD and had a reduced incidence of fistula formation compared to controls (0% vs 33%, $p < 0.004$) without any major or minor side effects [72], although these findings have not yet been replicated [73].

Anorectal Disorders

Botox injection has been used for a variety of conditions involving the anal sphincter including Hirschsprung disease, internal anal sphincter achalasia, severe functional constipation, fecal incontinence, and chronic anal fissure.

Hirschsprung disease (HD) is a congenital birth defect in which there is a lack of ganglion cells in the myenteric and submucosal plexus due to a failure of neural crest cell migration [74]. The aganglionosis always involves the anus and extends proximally a variable distance. It can cause constipation, enterocolitis, bowel obstruction, and intestinal perforation and is commonly treated with a pull-through surgical procedure which involves surgically removing the affected bowel segment. Persistent symptoms of bowel obstruction such as fecal incontinence and enterocolitis can develop in patients with HD after a pull-through procedure which is thought to be due to a failure of the internal anal sphincter (IAS) to relax. For this patient population, IAS myectomy has been the surgical treatment of choice for the past several decades, but carries the risk of permanent injury to the IAS, possible fecal incontinence, and lack of universal efficacy [75]. In 1997, Langer et al. introduced Botox injection into the IAS as a treatment for persistent obstructive symptoms after pull-through surgery in patients with HD, avoiding damage to the IAS [76].

A recent meta-analysis of small poor-quality studies revealed heterogeneity in the amounts of BT used, ranging from 3–12 IU/kg to a maximum of 200 IU. There was a short-term response of 77.3% (68.2–85.2) (I2 = 38.2%; $p = 0.13$) and overall long-term response of 43.0% (26.9–59.9) (I2 = 78.4%; $p = 0.0001$) [77].

Internal anal sphincter achalasia (IASA) is a disease with similar symptomology for which Botox therapy has been investigated. Although there is also a failure of relaxation of the IAS, in contrast to Hirschsprung's rectal biopsies, it does not reveal aganglionosis. Despite the paucity of data, this approach is well accepted and studies have shown favorable results. However, IAS myectomy remains more effective, with a meta-analysis revealing that Botox injection had a higher rate of primary nonresponse, high relapse rate, and need for subsequent surgery compared to IAS myectomy [78].

Dyssynergic defecation, previously termed anismus, paradoxical puborectalis contraction, or pelvic outlet obstruction, is a functional anorectal disorder with several subtypes and can be present in up to half of patients with chronic constipation [79]. It stems from the inability to coordinate the abdominal and pelvic floor muscles to evacuate stools, and this lack of recto-anal coordination may consist of inadequate propulsive force, paradoxical anal contraction, or inadequate anal relaxation [79]. The first-line treatment is biofeedback therapy, which can have efficacy rates of over 70% in well-motivated patients [80]. Injection of Botox into the anal sphincter has been tried in several studies but is considered inferior to biofeedback due to high rates of symptomatic relapse [81]; however, it does have a role in children [80] and may have a role patients with inadequate response to biofeedback therapy. For example, one study recruited patients diagnosed with dyssynergia who had successfully completed a course of biofeedback therapy with unsatisfactory results. They were then treated with 100u of ultrasound-guided Botox injection in the puborectalis and external anal sphincter and were given another course of biofeedback therapy. The patients were found to have improved clinical and anorectal manometric scores after treatment; however, there was transient fecal incontinence and lack of overall subjective patient satisfaction at follow-up [82].

The role of Botox in fecal incontinence has not been well studied. One group recruited a heterogenous group of patients ($n = 26$) with fecal incontinence from a variety of causes [83]. Botox injection into the rectum or neo-reservoir (in patients that had a proctectomy for rectal cancer) was performed. Median scores on standardized quality of life and continence scoring system improved significantly; duration of response for first injection lasted a median of 4.5 months and 46.1% of patients required repeat injection due to symptom recurrence. Overall, 69.2% of patients expressed satisfaction at 3 months follow-up.

Botox injection of the internal anal sphincter is a well-established therapy for chronic anal fissures. An anal fissure is a painful linear ulcer or tear situated in the anal canal and extending from just below the dentate line to the margin of the anus [84]. If patients fail dietary modifications and topical pharmacological ointments such as nitroglycerin or calcium channel blockers, Botox is an option. By blocking the inhibitory extrinsic cholinergic innervation to the IAS, Botox relaxes the hypertonic sphincter and facilitates healing, with resolution rates of up to 60–80% reported, although the treatment effect only lasts 2–3 months, necessitating retreatment [84].

References

1. Carruthers ACJ. Botulinum toxin products overview. Skin Therapy Lett. 2008;13(6):1–4.
2. Dressler D. Clinical applications of botulinum toxin. Curr Opin Microbiol. 2012;15(3):325–36.
3. Walker TJ, Dayan SH. Comparison and overview of currently available neurotoxins. J Clin Aesthet Dermatol. 2014;7(2):31–9.
4. Pasricha PJ, Ravich WJ, Kalloo AN. Effects of intrasphincteric botulinum toxin on the lower esophageal sphincter in piglets. Gastroenterology. 1993;105(4):1045–9.
5. Pasricha PJ, Ravich WJ, Hendrix TR, Sostre S, Jones B, Kalloo AN. Treatment of achalasia with intrasphincteric injection of botulinum toxin. A pilot trial. Ann Intern Med. 1994;121(8):590–1.
6. Pasricha PJ, Ravich WJ, Hendrix TR, Sostre S, Jones B, Kalloo AN. Intrasphincteric botulinum toxin for the treatment of achalasia. N Engl J Med. 1995;332(12):774–8.
7. Bian RX, Choi IS, Kim JH, Han JY, Lee SG. Impaired opening of the upper esophageal sphincter in patients with medullary infarctions. Dysphagia. 2009;24(2):238–45.
8. Colton-Hudson A, Koopman WJ, Moosa T, Smith D, Bach D, Nicolle M. A prospective assessment of the characteristics of dysphagia in myasthenia gravis. Dysphagia. 2002;17(2):147–51.
9. Higo R, Tayama N, Watanabe T, Nitou T. Videomanofluorometric study in amyotrophic lateral sclerosis. Laryngoscope. 2002;112(5):911–7.
10. Oh TH, Brumfield KA, Hoskin TL, Kasperbauer JL, Basford JR. Dysphagia in inclusion body myositis: clinical features, management, and clinical outcome. Am J Phys Med Rehabil. 2008;87(11):883–9.

11. Restivo DA, Palmeri A, Marchese-Ragona R. Botulinum toxin for cricopharyngeal dysfunction in Parkinson's disease. N Engl J Med. 2002;346(15):1174–5.
12. Regan J, Murphy A, Chiang M, McMahon BP, Coughlan T, Walshe M. Botulinum toxin for upper oesophageal sphincter dysfunction in neurological swallowing disorders. Cochrane Database Syst Rev. 2014;5:CD009968.
13. Schneider I, Thumfart WF, Pototschnig C, Eckel HE. Treatment of dysfunction of the cricopharyngeal muscle with botulinum A toxin: introduction of a new, noninvasive method. Ann Otol Rhinol Laryngol. 1994;103(1):31–5.
14. Kocdor P, Siegel ER, Tulunay-Ugur OE. Cricopharyngeal dysfunction: a systematic review comparing outcomes of dilatation, botulinum toxin injection, and myotomy. Laryngoscope. 2016;126(1):135–41.
15. Ashman A, Dale OT, Baldwin DL. Management of isolated cricopharyngeal dysfunction: systematic review. J Laryngol Otol. 2016;130(7):611–5.
16. Birgisson S, Richter JE. Achalasia: what's new in diagnosis and treatment? Dig Dis (Basel, Switzerland). 1997;15(Suppl 1):1–27.
17. Bieger D, Hopkins DA. Viscerotopic representation of the upper alimentary tract in the medulla oblongata in the rat: the nucleus ambiguus. J Comp Neurol. 1987;262(4):546–62.
18. Toyama T, Yokoyama I, Nishi K. Effects of hexamethonium and other ganglionic blocking agents on electrical activity of the esophagus induced by vagal stimulation in the dog. Eur J Pharmacol. 1975;31(1):63–71.
19. Collman PI, Tremblay L, Diamant NE. The central vagal efferent supply to the esophagus and lower esophageal sphincter of the cat. Gastroenterology. 1993;104(5):1430–8.
20. Goyal RK, Rattan S, Said SI. VIP as a possible neurotransmitter of non-cholinergic non-adrenergic inhibitory neurones. Nature. 1980;288(5789):378–80.
21. Yamato S, Spechler SJ, Goyal RK. Role of nitric oxide in esophageal peristalsis in the opossum. Gastroenterology. 1992;103(1):197–204.
22. Crist J, Gidda JS, Goyal RK. Intramural mechanism of esophageal peristalsis: roles of cholinergic and noncholinergic nerves. Proc Natl Acad Sci U S A. 1984;81(11):3595–9.
23. Mearin F, Mourelle M, Guarner F, et al. Patients with achalasia lack nitric oxide synthase in the gastro-oesophageal junction. Eur J Clin Investig. 1993;23(11):724–8.
24. Ates F, Vaezi MF. The pathogenesis and management of achalasia: current status and future directions. Gut Liver. 2015;9(4):449–63.
25. Farrukh A, DeCaestecker J, Mayberry JF. An epidemiological study of achalasia among the South Asian population of Leicester, 1986–2005. Dysphagia. 2008;23(2):161–4.
26. Sadowski DC, Ackah F, Jiang B, Svenson LW. Achalasia: incidence, prevalence and survival. A population-based study. Neurogastroenterol Motil. 2010;22(9):e256–61.
27. Eckardt VF, Kohne U, Junginger T, Westermeier T. Risk factors for diagnostic delay in achalasia. Dig Dis Sci. 1997;42(3):580–5.
28. Fisichella PM, Raz D, Palazzo F, Niponmick I, Patti MG. Clinical, radiological, and manometric profile in 145 patients with untreated achalasia. World J Surg. 2008;32(9):1974–9.
29. Kostic S, Johnsson E, Kjellin A, et al. Health economic evaluation of therapeutic strategies in patients with idiopathic achalasia: results of a randomized trial comparing pneumatic dilatation with laparoscopic cardiomyotomy. Surg Endosc. 2007;21(7):1184–9.
30. Boeckxstaens GE, Annese V, des Varannes SB, et al. Pneumatic dilation versus laparoscopic Heller's myotomy for idiopathic achalasia. N Engl J Med. 2011;364(19):1807–16.
31. Boeckxstaens GE, Zaninotto G, Richter JE. Achalasia. Lancet (London, England). 2014;383(9911):83–93.
32. Annese V, Bassotti G, Coccia G, et al. A multicentre randomised study of intrasphincteric botulinum toxin in patients with oesophageal achalasia. GISMAD Achalasia Study Group. Gut. 2000;46(5):597–600.
33. Leyden JE, Moss AC, MacMathuna P. Endoscopic pneumatic dilation versus botulinum toxin injection in the management of primary achalasia. Cochrane Database Syst Rev. 2006;4:CD005046.

34. Campos GM, Vittinghoff E, Rabl C, et al. Endoscopic and surgical treatments for achalasia: a systematic review and meta-analysis. Ann Surg. 2009;249(1):45–57.
35. Zaninotto G, Annese V, Costantini M, et al. Randomized controlled trial of botulinum toxin versus laparoscopic heller myotomy for esophageal achalasia. Ann Surg. 2004;239(3):364–70.
36. Muehldorfer SM, Schneider TH, Hochberger J, Martus P, Hahn EG, Ell C. Esophageal achalasia: intrasphincteric injection of botulinum toxin A versus balloon dilation. Endoscopy. 1999;31(7):517–21.
37. Vaezi MF, Richter JE, Wilcox CM, et al. Botulinum toxin versus pneumatic dilatation in the treatment of achalasia: a randomised trial. Gut. 1999;44(2):231–9.
38. Ghoshal UC, Chaudhuri S, Pal BB, Dhar K, Ray G, Banerjee PK. Randomized controlled trial of intrasphincteric botulinum toxin A injection versus balloon dilatation in treatment of achalasia cardia. Dis Esophagus. 2001;14(3–4):227–31.
39. Mikaeli J, Fazel A, Montazeri G, Yaghoobi M, Malekzadeh R. Randomized controlled trial comparing botulinum toxin injection to pneumatic dilatation for the treatment of achalasia. Aliment Pharmacol Ther. 2001;15(9):1389–96.
40. Zhu Q, Liu J, Yang C. Clinical study on combined therapy of botulinum toxin injection and small balloon dilation in patients with esophageal achalasia. Dig Surg. 2009;26(6):493–8.
41. Bonavina L, Incarbone R, Reitano M, Antoniazzi L, Peracchia A. Does previous endoscopic treatment affect the outcome of laparoscopic Heller myotomy? Ann Chir. 2000;125(1):45–9.
42. Amarasinghe G, Sifrim D. Functional esophageal disorders: pharmacological options. Drugs. 2014;74(12):1335–44.
43. Dalton CB, Castell DO, Hewson EG, Wu WC, Richter JE. Diffuse esophageal spasm. A rare motility disorder not characterized by high-amplitude contractions. Dig Dis Sci. 1991;36(8):1025–8.
44. Konturek JW, Gillessen A, Domschke W. Diffuse esophageal spasm: a malfunction that involves nitric oxide? Scand J Gastroenterol. 1995;30(11):1041–5.
45. Korsapati H, Bhargava V, Mittal RK. Reversal of asynchrony between circular and longitudinal muscle contraction in nutcracker esophagus by atropine. Gastroenterology. 2008;135(3):796–802.
46. Cattau EL Jr, Castell DO, Johnson DA, et al. Diltiazem therapy for symptoms associated with nutcracker esophagus. Am J Gastroenterol. 1991;86(3):272–6.
47. Clouse RE, Lustman PJ, Eckert TC, Ferney DM, Griffith LS. Low-dose trazodone for symptomatic patients with esophageal contraction abnormalities. A double-blind, placebo-controlled trial. Gastroenterology. 1987;92(4):1027–36.
48. Cannon RO 3rd, Quyyumi AA, Mincemoyer R, et al. Imipramine in patients with chest pain despite normal coronary angiograms. N Engl J Med. 1994;330(20):1411–7.
49. Eherer AJ, Schwetz I, Hammer HF, et al. Effect of sildenafil on oesophageal motor function in healthy subjects and patients with oesophageal motor disorders. Gut. 2002;50(6):758–64.
50. Miller LS, Parkman HP, Schiano TD, et al. Treatment of symptomatic nonachalasia esophageal motor disorders with botulinum toxin injection at the lower esophageal sphincter. Dig Dis Sci. 1996;41(10):2025–31.
51. Vanuytsel T, Bisschops R, Farre R, et al. Botulinum toxin reduces dysphagia in patients with nonachalasia primary esophageal motility disorders. Clin Gastroenterol Hepatol. 2013;11(9):1115–1121.e1112.
52. Miller LS, Pullela SV, Parkman HP, et al. Treatment of chest pain in patients with noncardiac, nonreflux, nonachalasia spastic esophageal motor disorders using botulinum toxin injection into the gastroesophageal junction. Am J Gastroenterol. 2002;97(7):1640–6.
53. Camilleri M. Clinical practice. Diabetic gastroparesis. N Engl J Med. 2007;356(8):820–9.
54. Forster J, Damjanov I, Lin Z, Sarosiek I, Wetzel P, McCallum RW. Absence of the interstitial cells of Cajal in patients with gastroparesis and correlation with clinical findings. J Gastrointest Surg. 2005;9(1):102–8.

55. Vittal H, Farrugia G, Gomez G, Pasricha PJ. Mechanisms of disease: the pathological basis of gastroparesis–a review of experimental and clinical studies. Nat Clin Pract Gastroenterol Hepatol. 2007;4(6):336–46.
56. Jeong ID, Camilleri M, Shin A, et al. A randomised, placebo-controlled trial comparing the effects of tapentadol and oxycodone on gastrointestinal and colonic transit in healthy humans. Aliment Pharmacol Ther. 2012;35(9):1088–96.
57. Fich A, Neri M, Camilleri M, Kelly KA, Phillips SF. Stasis syndromes following gastric surgery: clinical and motility features of 60 symptomatic patients. J Clin Gastroenterol. 1990;12(5):505–12.
58. Jost WH. Gastrointestinal dysfunction in Parkinson's disease. J Neurol Sci. 2010;289(1–2):69–73.
59. Langworthy J, Parkman HP, Schey R. Emerging strategies for the treatment of gastroparesis. Expert Rev Gastroenterol Hepatol. 2016;10(7):817–25.
60. Malamood M, Parkman H, Schey R. Current advances in treatment of gastroparesis. Expert Opin Pharmacother. 2015;16(13):1997–2008.
61. Ezzeddine D, Jit R, Katz N, Gopalswamy N, Bhutani MS. Pyloric injection of botulinum toxin for treatment of diabetic gastroparesis. Gastrointest Endosc. 2002;55(7):920–3.
62. Coleski R, Anderson MA, Hasler WL. Factors associated with symptom response to pyloric injection of botulinum toxin in a large series of gastroparesis patients. Dig Dis Sci. 2009;54(12):2634–42.
63. Friedenberg FK, Palit A, Parkman HP, Hanlon A, Nelson DB. Botulinum toxin A for the treatment of delayed gastric emptying. Am J Gastroenterol. 2008;103(2):416–23.
64. Arts J, Holvoet L, Caenepeel P, et al. Clinical trial: a randomized-controlled crossover study of intrapyloric injection of botulinum toxin in gastroparesis. Aliment Pharmacol Ther. 2007;26(9):1251–8.
65. Ukleja A, Tandon K, Shah K, Alvarez A. Endoscopic botox injections in therapy of refractory gastroparesis. World J Gastrointest Endosc. 2015;7(8):790–8.
66. Camilleri M, Parkman HP, Shafi MA, Abell TL, Gerson L. Clinical guideline: management of gastroparesis. Am J Gastroenterol. 2013;108(1):18–37. quiz 38
67. Pasricha PJ, Miskovsky EP, Kalloo AN. Intrasphincteric injection of botulinum toxin for suspected sphincter of Oddi dysfunction. Gut. 1994;35(9):1319–21.
68. Wehrmann T, Seifert H, Seipp M, Lembcke B, Caspary WF. Endoscopic injection of botulinum toxin for biliary sphincter of Oddi dysfunction. Endoscopy. 1998;30(8):702–7.
69. Cotton PB, Elta GH, Carter CR, Pasricha PJ, Corazziari ES, Rome IV. Gallbladder and sphincter of Oddi disorders. Gastroenterology. 2016;S0016-5085(16)00224-9.
70. Bassi C, Dervenis C, Butturini G, et al. Postoperative pancreatic fistula: an international study group (ISGPF) definition. Surgery. 2005;138(1):8–13.
71. Rieder B, Krampulz D, Adolf J, Pfeiffer A. Endoscopic pancreatic sphincterotomy and stenting for preoperative prophylaxis of pancreatic fistula after distal pancreatectomy. Gastrointest Endosc. 2010;72(3):536–42.
72. Hackert T, Klaiber U, Hinz U, et al. Sphincter of Oddi botulinum toxin injection to prevent pancreatic fistula after distal pancreatectomy. Surgery. 2016;S0016-5085(16)00224-9.
73. Volk A, Distler M, Mussle B, et al. Reproducibility of preoperative endoscopic injection of botulinum toxin into the sphincter of Oddi to prevent postoperative pancreatic fistula. Innovat Surg Sci. 2018;3(1):69–75.
74. Swenson O. Hirschsprung's disease: a review. Pediatrics. 2002;109(5):914–8.
75. Youn JK, Han JW, Oh C, Kim SY, Jung SE, Kim HY. Botulinum toxin injection for internal anal sphincter achalasia after pull-through surgery in Hirschsprung disease. Medicine. 2019;98(45):e17855.
76. Langer JC, Birnbaum E. Preliminary experience with intrasphincteric botulinum toxin for persistent constipation after pull-through for Hirschsprung's disease. J Pediatr Surg. 1997;32(7):1059–61; discussion 1061–1052

77. Soh HJ, Nataraja RM, Pacilli M. Prevention and management of recurrent postoperative Hirschsprung's disease obstructive symptoms and enterocolitis: systematic review and meta-analysis. J Pediatr Surg. 2018;53(12):2423–9.
78. Friedmacher F, Puri P. Comparison of posterior internal anal sphincter myectomy and intra-sphincteric botulinum toxin injection for treatment of internal anal sphincter achalasia: a meta-analysis. Pediatr Surg Int. 2012;28(8):765–71.
79. Rao SS, Patcharatrakul T. Diagnosis and treatment of dyssynergic defecation. J Neurogastroenterol Motil. 2016;22(3):423–35.
80. Rao SS, Benninga MA, Bharucha AE, Chiarioni G, Di Lorenzo C, Whitehead WE. ANMS-ESNM position paper and consensus guidelines on biofeedback therapy for anorectal disorders. Neurogastroenterol Motil. 2015;27(5):594–609.
81. Emile SH, Elfeki HA, Elbanna HG, et al. Efficacy and safety of botulinum toxin in treatment of anismus: a systematic review. World J Gastrointest Pharmacol Ther. 2016;7(3):453–62.
82. Zhang Y, Wang ZN, He L, et al. Botulinum toxin type-A injection to treat patients with intractable anismus unresponsive to simple biofeedback training. World J Gastroenterol. 2014;20(35):12602–7.
83. Gourcerol G, Benard C, Melchior C, et al. Botulinum toxin: an endoscopic approach for treating fecal incontinence. Endoscopy. 2016;48(5):484–8.
84. Mathur N, Qureshi W. Anal fissure management by the gastroenterologist. Curr Opin Gastroenterol. 2020;36(1):19–24.

Chapter 15
Botulinum Toxin Treatment in Urological Disorders

Christopher P. Smith and Michael B. Chancellor

Abstract Botulinum toxin (BoNT) injection has been widely accepted by the urology and urogynecology medical communities as a safe and effective treatment for refractory urinary incontinence based on two decades of published literature. Currently, there are two approved genitourinary indications for botulinum toxin within the United States. OnabotulinumtoxinA (onaBoNTA) 200 units for the treatment of urinary incontinence due to detrusor overactivity associated with a neurologic condition (e.g., spinal cord injury, multiple sclerosis) in adults who have an inadequate response to or are intolerant to an anticholinergic medication was approved by the FDA in 2011. In addition, onaBoNTA 100 units for the treatment of overactive bladder with symptoms of urinary incontinence, urgency, and frequency, in adult patients who have an inadequate response to or are intolerant to an anticholinergic medication was approved by the FDA in 2013. We will update the reader on the latest application of botulinum toxin for urologic indications with a focus on bladder injections as well as on potential uses of BoNT in the prostate and pelvic floor.

Keywords Neurogenic detrusor overactivity · Overactive bladder · Benign prostatic hyperplasia · Interstitial cystitis · OnabotulinumtoxinA · AbobotulinumtoxinA

C. P. Smith (✉)
Scott Department of Urology, Baylor College of Medicine, Houston, TX, USA
e-mail: cps@bcm.edu

M. B. Chancellor
Aikens Center for Neurourology Research, Department of Urology, Beaumont Health System and Oakland University William Beaumont School of Medicine, Rochester Hills, MI, USA

© Springer Nature Switzerland AG 2020   297
B. Jabbari (ed.), *Botulinum Toxin Treatment in Surgery, Dentistry, and Veterinary Medicine*, https://doi.org/10.1007/978-3-030-50691-9_15

Introduction

The first application of botulinum toxin (BoNT) within the genitourinary system was not into the bladder but rather the external urethral sphincter. In 1988, Dyskstra and colleagues injected BoNT into the skeletal muscle urethral sphincter of spinal cord-injured (SCI) patients to treat detrusor sphincter dyssynergia [14]. Just over a decade later, Schurch and colleagues revolutionized the care of SCI patients through their novel application of BoNT into bladder smooth muscle to treat neurogenic detrusor overactivity in 21 SCI patients that failed high-dose anticholinergic medications [29, 30]. Their clinical success was confirmed by basic science experiments by Smith and colleagues that demonstrated that BoNT impaired electrically evoked neurotransmitter release from bladder tissue that resulted in diminished bladder contractile activity [31, 32]. These early results of exciting and promising initial off-label use of BoNT led to a registry trial and two Phase III multicenter, double-blind, placebo-controlled trials that led to the 2011 regulatory approval of onabotulinumtoxinA (onaBoNTA), at 100 and 200 units, for the treatment of urge incontinence due to NDO [11, 17]. Subsequently, phase III multicenter trials led to the 2013 regulatory approval of onaBoNTA for the treatment of idiopathic overactive bladder (OAB) without neurological diseases and refractory to anticholinergics [9, 27].

Other applications for BoNT include benign prostatic hyperplasia (BPH) and interstitial cystitis/bladder pain syndrome (IC/BPS). McVary et al. [26] reported on a phase 2 randomized clinical trial comparing onaBoNTA 200 U to placebo for the treatment of BPH, but no differences were seen in the primary and majority of secondary outcome parameters. For the treatment of IC/BPS, Kuo and Chancellor [24] reported a signal of efficacy in the off-label use of BoNT in the bladder pain score in IC/BPS patients. BoNT is currently listed as a fourth-line treatment in the American Urological Association guideline for the treatment of IC/BPS [19].

Neurogenic Detrusor Overactivity

Clinical Trials

Neurogenic detrusor overactivity (NDO), most common in MS and SCI, but also seen in other neurological diseases including stroke and Parkinson's disease, is characterized by the presence of involuntary detrusor contractions (IDC) during filling cystometry [7]. NDO, particularly in the presence of detrusor sphincter dyssynergia, can lead to high-pressure obstructed voiding patterns that can place a patient's upper tracts at risk. In addition, incontinence and reduced functional bladder capacity can greatly impair quality of life (QoL). Current frontline treatments for NDO using anticholinergic medications are of only modest benefit and fraught with intolerable side effects such as dry mouth and constipation as well as concerns on cognitive function [6].

Cruz et al. [11] published the first regulatory study examining the effect of ona-BoNTA for NDO. A total of 275 multiple sclerosis (MS) or SCI patients who had inadequate response to or were intolerant to ≥ 1 anticholinergic medication were enrolled. These patients were randomized to receive onaBoNTA 200 U ($n = 92$), onaBoNTA 300 U ($n = 91$), or placebo ($n = 92$). Results are presented comparing onaBoNTA 200 U to placebo since FDA regulatory approval was given for 200 U dose. By week 6, mean weekly urge incontinent episodes had decreased by 21.8 in the onaBoNTA 200 U group compared to a decrease of 13.2 in the placebo group ($p < 0.05$). The proportion of patients with a $\geq 50\%$ reduction in weekly urge incontinence symptoms (i.e., clinically significant change) was significantly greater in patients receiving 200 U onaBoNTA vs. placebo (77.2% vs. 39.1%, respectively). In addition, full continence ("dry") was achieved in 38% of patients in the 200 U group compared to only 7.6% of placebo-treated patients ($p < 0.05$). Median duration of effect was 9–10 months in the onaBoNTA-treated group vs. 3 months in placebo-treated patients. No significant difference in efficacy was observed between 200 U and 300 U onaBoNTA groups. The main adverse events were urinary tract infections (UTIs) and urinary retention resulting in the need for clean intermittent catheterization (CIC). Urinary tract infection rates were similar across all treatment groups in SCI patients in whom 91.6% were using CIC at baseline. However, UTI rates in MS patients were linked not only with onaBoNTA dose but also with the need for CIC suggesting that initiation of CIC and not necessarily onaBoNTA itself was more responsible for the risk of developing a UTI. Overall, CIC was initiated in 12% of placebo patients, 29.5% of 200 U onaBoNTA, and 42.2% of 300 U onaBoNTA-injected patients.

Ginsberg and colleagues reported on the second large phase 3 trial in MS and SCI patients with NDO who received either placebo ($n = 149$), onaBoNTA 200 U ($n = 135$), or onaBoNTA 300 U ($n = 132$) [17]. Mean weekly urinary incontinence (UI) episodes decreased by 21 in the onaBoNTA 200 U group compared to a decrease of 9 in the placebo group ($p < 0.05$). In addition, 75% of onaBoNTA 200 U group achieved a 50% or greater reduction in weekly UI episodes compared to 38% in the placebo group. Moreover, a significantly larger proportion of onaBoNTA 200 U-treated patients were fully continent following treatment compared to placebo-injected patients (i.e., 36% vs. 10%, respectively). The mean increase in maximum cystometric capacity was 151 ml in the onaBoNTA 200 U group compared to an increase of 16 ml in placebo patients. Maximum detrusor pressures were reduced by 69% in the onaBoNTA 200 U group vs. 9.5% in the placebo-treated patients. The median duration of effect was similar to the earlier trial of Cruz and colleagues (i.e., 8–9 months in the onaBoNTA 200 U group vs. 3 months in the placebo group). The main adverse events were UTIs and the need for CIC. CIC rates showed a dose-dependent response to onaBoNTA injection (i.e., placebo 10%, ona-BoNTA 200 U 35%, onaBoNTA 300 U 42%). However, the need for CIC did not negatively impact clinical outcomes as improvements in quality of life (I-QoL) scores were similar in patients with or without the need for CIC. UTI rates were similar in all SCI groups but were higher in MS patients treated with onaBoNTA and presumably related to the concurrent increased need for CIC with onaBoNTA injection. Muscle weakness was seen in 7 patients treated with onaBoNTA 300 U and 4 patients each in placebo and onaBoNTA 200 U groups. No neutralizing antibodies against onaBoNTA were observed after treatment.

Denys et al. [12] reported the efficacy and safety of two administration modes of bladder injection of abobotulinumtoxinA (aboBoNTA) 750 U in patients suffering from refractory NDO in a randomized placebo-controlled phase 2 study. Forty-seven MS or SCI patients were treated with 15 or 30 bladder injections of aboBoNTA 750 U or placebo. The primary end point was the change from baseline in the mean number of daily incontinence episode frequency (IEF) at 12 weeks. In both injection groups, the mean decrease in IEF was greater in the aboBoNTA-treated vs. placebo groups but it did not reach statistical significance ($p > 0.05$). However, increases in maximum cystometric capacity and reduction in maximum detrusor pressure were significantly greater in both aboBoNTA groups compared to their respective placebo groups. No difference in effect was observed between the two injection groups of aboBoNTA. Thus, the authors concluded that reduction to 15 injection sites did not appear to be associated with any impact on efficacy.

Repeated Injections

Kennelly and colleagues reported on the results of an open-label 3-year extension of the phase III trial of onaBoNTA for NDO [22]. Three hundred ninety-six patients entered the extension study, and 68 patients received six injections over a 4-year period. The authors showed persistent benefits of onaBoNTA 200 U with time. The mean reduction in UI episodes/day ranged from 3.2 to 4.1 over all six injections. Between 83.2% and 91.3% of patients demonstrated ≥50% reduction in UI episodes and between 43.4% and 55.6% of patients were totally continent after treatment 1–6. The incidence of UTIs ranged from 14.3% to 27.6% and the finding of urinary retention varied between none and 20.2%. Both UTI and urinary retention risk decreased with each treatment cycle. In addition, onaBoNTA was shown to be a durable treatment as the duration of response remained steady at 9 months following injection. Table 15.1 summarizes the results of NDO trials using onaBoNTA.

Table 15.1 Effect of OnaBoNTA in reducing urinary incontinence in NDO patients

Author	Trial type	≥50% reduction in UI episodes	100% reduction in UI episodes
Cruz et al. [11]	Phase III	77%	38%
Ginsberg et al. [17]	Phase III	75%	36%
Kennelly et al. [22]	Open-label 3-year extension	83–91%	43–56%

OnaBoNTA onabotulinumtoxinA, *UI* urinary incontinence, *NDO* neurogenic detrusor overactivity

Overactive Bladder

Overactive bladder (OAB) is defined as urinary urgency, with or without urge urinary incontinence (UUI), usually accompanied with urinary frequency and nocturia [3]. The prevalence of OAB in the general population is 12–17%, and about half of OAB patients have incontinence [35]. The current guidelines for the management of OAB lists first- and second-line therapies as behavioral therapies and pharmacotherapy, respectively [18]. A meta-analysis of several RCTs of different anticholinergic drugs used for the treatment of OAB demonstrated improvements in both symptoms and QOL [8]. Unfortunately, most individuals discontinue anticholinergic therapy because of either inadequate long-term efficacy and/or intolerable side effects.

Nitti and colleagues presented results from the first phase 3 trial in 557 patients with refractory idiopathic OAB randomized to receive either onaBoNTA 100 U or placebo bladder injections [27]. At 12-week follow-up, the investigators found that patients receiving onaBoNTA had a 47.9% reduction in mean daily urge incontinence episodes vs. a 12.5% reduction in placebo-treated patients. Moreover, 57.9% of patients injected with onaBoNTA had ≥50% reduction in their urge incontinence symptoms and 22.9% were totally continent, compared to 28.9% and 6.5%, respectively, in the placebo group. The most common adverse events were UTIs (15.5% in the onaBoNTA group vs. 5.9% in the placebo group) and incomplete emptying resulting in the need for CIC (6.1% in the onaBoNTA group vs. 0% in the placebo group). The duration of CIC was less than or equal to 6 weeks in 59% of patients.

Improvements in other symptoms of overactive bladder, daily frequency of urination, and the amount of urine voided also occurred with onaBoNTA treatment compared to placebo at week 12. A second European-based randomized clinical trial in 548 patients comparing onaBoNTA 100 U to placebo showed comparable results [9]. At 12 weeks following injection, onaBoNTA-treated patients had a significantly greater reduction in daily incontinence episodes compared to the placebo group (53.1% vs. 16.8%). The most common adverse events were UTIs and the need for CIC demonstrated in 20.4% and 6.9% of onaBoNTA patients, respectively, compared to 5.2% and 0.7% of placebo-treated patients, respectively (Table 15.2).

Table 15.2 Incidence of most frequent adverse events in NDO and OAB randomized trials

Author	Patient type	Dose of onaBoNTA(U)	UTI (%)	CIC (%)
Cruz et al. [11]	NDO	200	28	30
Ginsberg et al. [17]	NDO	200	28	35
Nitti et al. [27]	OAB	100	16	6
Chapple et al. [9]	OAB	100	20	7

OnaBoNTA onabotulinumtoxinA, *UTI* urinary tract infection, *CIC* clean intermittent catheterization, *NDO* neurogenic detrusor overactivity, *OAB* overactive bladder

Repeated Injections

Durable efficacy and safety of onaBoNTA was demonstrated in a 3-year open label extension trial of two initial phase 3 randomized trials [28]. Four hundred thirty patients completed the 3-year extension study, and 33 patients received 6 treatments with onaBoNTA 100 U. The decrease in mean daily urge incontinence episodes ranged from 3.1 to 3.8 after each treatment with a median duration of effect of 7.6 months. Treatment duration greater than 12 months was seen in 28.5% of patients. The need for CIC was 4% after the first treatment cycle but this number decreased with each subsequent treatment cycle. No patient experienced seroconversion after receiving the 100 U dose. Patients with diabetes mellitus treated with onaBoNTA were twice as likely to develop urinary retention and require CIC. The most frequent adverse events of NDO and OAB trials using onaBoNTA are summarized in Table 15.2.

Comparative Trial

The U.S. National Institute of Health sponsored a comparative study between onaBoNTA vs. neuromodulation [4]. For this study, conducted at nine centers, only women with refractory urgency urinary incontinence were randomized to an injection of onaBoNTA ($n = 192$) or sacral neuromodulation ($n = 189$). Of the 364 women, mean age 63 years, the onaBoNTA group had a statistically significant greater reduction in a 6-month average number of episodes of urgency incontinence per day than did the sacral neuromodulation group (−3.9 vs. −3.3 episodes per day). There were no cases of urinary retention with sacral neuromodulation while onaBoNTA increased the risk of UTI, retention, and need for self-catheterization. Although subjects treated with onaBoNTA noted greater improvement for symptom bother and treatment satisfaction than neuromodulation, there was no significant difference for quality of life or for measures of treatment preference, convenience, or adverse effects. A more recent publication compared economic costs between these two treatment modalities at a primary time point of 2 years and secondary time point at 5 years [20]. In both cases, onaBoNTA 200 U was a more cost-effective treatment than sacral neuromodulation for urge urinary incontinence (Table 15.3).

Table 15.3 Economic costs of onaBoNTA 200 U vs. two-stage neuromodulation in patients enrolled in ROSETTA trial [20]

Treatment	2-year economic cost	5-year economic cost
OnaBoNTA	$35,680	$7460
Sacral neuromodulation	$36,550	$12,020

OnaBoNTA onabotulinumtoxinA, *ROSETTA* Refractory overactive bladder: Sacral NEuromodulation vs. BoTulinum Toxin Assessment

Pediatric Uses

Spina Bifida

The most common use of BoNTA in pediatrics is in patients with spinal dysraphism. A recent multicenter study detailed results of onaBoNTA (98%) or aboBoNTA (2%) injections in 53 patients with spina bifida [21]. The investigators found improvements in compliance (9.9 cm/H_2O to 16.3 cm/H_2O) and maximum cystometric capacity following BoNTA treatment although maximum detrusor pressure was not significantly reduced. One subcategory (poor bladder compliance without detrusor overactivity) showed no significant improvement in any urodynamic parameter following BoNTA treatment suggesting that the bladder dysfunction may be related to bladder fibrosis and more appropriately treated with bladder augmentation surgery.

Non-neurogenic DO

Recent interest in use of onaBoNTA in the pediatric population has extended to non-neurogenic patients. Bayrak and colleagues demonstrated reductions in urinary frequency, urge incontinence, and increases in bladder capacity in patients with non-neurogenic detrusor overactivity [5]. Moreover, vesicoureteral reflux disappeared in 50% of patients and was reduced in 30% of patients following onaBoNTA injection. Patients with VUR had higher pretreatment detrusor contractile pressures and poorer compliance compared to patients without VUR.

External Urinary Sphincter

There are one Class I and two Class II studies of BoNT in detrusor sphincter dyssynergia (DSD) [13–15]. In the Class I study, the effects of BoNT vs. placebo was studied on DSD in 86 patients with multiple sclerosis (MS) [15]. The study employed a single transperineal injection of onaBoNTA, 100 U in 4 mL normal saline, or placebo, into the striated sphincter with EMG guidance. A single injection of BoNT did not decrease residual urine volume in this group of MS patients. These findings differ from those in patients with spinal cord injury and may be due to lower detrusor pressures observed in patients with MS. The American Academy of Neurology recommends BoNT to be considered for DSD but recognizes the limited head-to-head comparisons of treatment options in DSD. Kuo [23] evaluated the effects of onaBoNTA urethral injection in 27 patients with idiopathic low detrusor contractility. Detrusor contractility recovered in 48% of those treated. Patients with normal bladder sensation combined with poor relaxation or hyperactive urethral sphincter activity were most likely to respond to urethral injections with ona-BoNTA. Complications of BoNT injection into the external sphincter are rare except for transient stress urinary incontinence. In 38% of patients, the therapeutic effect of restoring detrusor contractility lasted over 1 year.

Pelvic Floor Injections

Ghazizadeh and Nikzad [16] injected 150–400 U of aboBoNTA into the levator ani of 24 women with refractory vaginismus. Symptoms significantly improved such that 75% of patients could have satisfactory intercourse. In contrast, a double-blind randomized clinical trial of onaBoNTA vs. saline in 60 patients with 2 years or more of chronic pelvic pain that received either onaBoNTA 80 U (20 U/ml) or normal saline injections into the puborectalis and pubococcygeus muscles [1] showed mixed results. After 26 weeks of follow-up, quality of life measures were improved in both the onaBoNTA and placebo groups, but the difference between onaBoNTA and placebo groups did not reach statistical significance.

However, the authors found a reduction in resting pelvic muscle tone in women injected with onaBoNTA compared to placebo ($p < 0.001$), and this translated into significant improvements in both dyspareunia ($p < 0.001$) and nonmenstrual pelvic pain ($p = 0.009$). Adelowo et al. [2] reported on their experience using onaBoNTA (100 U–300 U) in 29 women with chronic myofascial pelvic pain. In this retrospective study, the authors placed several onaBoNTA 10 U injections (total 300 U) into the pelvic floor muscles. Pain improvement was seen in 79% of patients at <6 weeks postinjection. After a median of 4 months from the first injection, 52% requested repeat onaBoNTA. Urinary retention (defined by PVR > 100 ml) and fecal incontinence resulted in 3 patients and 2 patients, respectively, and these AEs completely resolved. Larger placebo-controlled RCTs and patient-reported outcomes are needed to support the use of onaBoNTA for women with myofascial pelvic pain refractory to standard pelvic floor physical therapy.

Benign Prostatic Hyperplasia (BPH)

Application of BoNT to treat BPH was reported by Maria et al. [25]. Thirty men with symptomatic BPH were randomized to receive either 200 U of onaBoNTA (n-15) or placebo saline injection ($n = 5$). OnaBoNTA 100 U in 2 ml of saline or saline alone in the placebo arm was injected into each lobe of the prostate through the perineum via a 22-gauge spinal needle with transrectal ultrasound guidance. Clinical improvement was evident after 1 month. The investigators noted that the American Urological Association symptom score, a common index for the assessment of BPH, decreased by 65% compared to baseline in the onaBoNTA patients ($p = 0.00001$). Also, maximum flow rate increased from 8.1 to 14.9 mL/sec with onaBoNTA ($p = 0.00001$). There was no significant improvement in patients injected with saline alone. No urinary incontinence or systemic side effects were reported over the 18-month follow-up.

Chuang et al. [10] stratified drug treatment refractory BPH with either prostate size <30 grams or >30 grams and injected them with either 100 U onaBoNTA or 200 U onaBoNTA, respectively, via ultrasound-guided perineal injection. At 12 months, the percent improvements in International Prostate Symptom Score (IPSS), maximum flow rate, and post void residual urine volume were similar to those of Maria et al. [25], except that the percent shrinkage of prostate size was substantially smaller (13–19% vs. 61%). In 29% of men there was no change in prostate volume, yet 58% of these men still had a >30% improvement in IPSS, maximum flow rate, and post void residual urine volume, suggesting that ona-BoNTA may relieve BPH symptoms by an effect on sensory nerve pathways rather than reducing the prostate size alone.

McVary et al. [26] performed a phase 2 multicenter, placebo-controlled, randomized clinical trial using a onaBoNTA 200 U to treat men with BPH and moderate lower urinary tract symptoms. The men had an IPSS of 14 or >, a maximum flow rate of 4–5 mL/sec, and a post void residual urine volume ≤200 ml; 315 men were randomized to either onaBoNTA 200 U ($n = 158$) or placebo ($n = 157$). The primary end point was the change from baseline in IPSS at week 12. Although a significant decrease from baseline in IPSS was seen with both onaBoNTA (−6.3 points) and placebo (−5.6 points), there was no difference between the groups; however, ona-BoNTA showed efficacy over placebo in improving maximum flow rate at week 6 postinjection ($p \leq 0.01$). The most common adverse events in both groups were hematuria and hematospermia. The authors concluded that intraprostatic injection of onaBoNTA was not more efficacious compared to placebo in improving lower urinary tract symptoms and the commercial development of onaBoNTA for BPH indication was subsequently stopped at this time.

Bladder Pain

Interstitial cystitis/bladder pain syndrome (IC/BPS) is defined as pain perceived to be related to the urinary bladder, associated with lower urinary tract symptoms greater than a 6-month duration, in the absence of infection or other identifiable causes [24]. The first report using BoNT as a therapeutic was a case series of 13 women with NIDDK-defined IC [33]. The patients underwent submucosal transurethral injections of 100–200 U of abobotulinumtoxinA (7 patients) or onaBoNTA 100 U (6 patients) into 20–30 sites in the trigone and bladder base. Validated questionnaire (Interstitial Cystitis Symptom Index, Interstitial Cystitis Problem Index) or voiding charts and a visual analog pain scale were evaluated at baseline, 1-month, and subsequently at 3-month intervals. Statistically significant improvements in frequency, nocturia, and pain were observed 1 month following treatment, with improvements in first desire to void and cystometric capacity in those patients so evaluated. Onset of symptom relief was 5–7 days following treatment, and mean duration of symptom relief was 3.7 months. These results were supported by basic science experiments demonstrating that onaBoNTA reduces urothelial release of ATP in chronic bladder inflammation [34].

Kuo and Chancellor [24] performed a randomized trial in IC/BPS patients comparing bladder hydrodistention (HD) with either 100 U or 200 U doses of onaBoNTA vs. hydrodistention alone. At 3 months, the bladder pain visual analog scale, functional bladder capacity, cystometric bladder capacity, and global response assessment significantly improved only in the onaBoNTA groups vs. the control group. The 200 U dose did not provide better efficacy compared to 100 U, and there were more side effects, including urinary retention, with using 200 U onaBoNTA. These studies suggest a potential promising effect of botulinum toxin for treating bladder pain.

Conclusion

The use of botulinum toxin for the treatment of neurogenic and refractory idiopathic overactive bladder has resulted in improved continence and quality of life. The intraprostatic injection of botulinum toxin for benign prostatic hypertrophy to date has not shown efficacy in improving lower urinary tract symptoms. Treating detrusor sphincter dyssynergia, myofacial pain, and interstitial cystitis/bladder pain syndrome with botulinum toxin have showed some promising results in controlled trials but they are currently an off-label use of the product. Application of botulinum toxin for lower urinary tract dysfunction is exciting, expanding, and evolving. We believe there will be further exciting advances in the application of botulinum toxin in the genitourinary system in the near future.

References

1. Abbott JA, Jarvis SK, Lyons SD, et al. Botulinum toxin type A for chronic pain and pelvic floor spasm in women. Obstet Gynecol. 2006;108:915–23.
2. Adelowo A, Hacker MR, Shapiro A, et al. Botulinum Toxin Type A (BOTOX) for refractory myofascial pelvic pain. Female Pelvic Med Reconstr Surg. 2013;19:288–92.
3. Abrams P, Cardozo L, Fall M, et al. The standardization of terminology of lower urinary tract function: report from the Standardisation Sub-committee of the International Continence Society. Neurourol Urodynam. 2002;21:167–78.
4. Amundsen CL, Richter HE, Menefee SA, et al. OnabotulinumtoxinA vs sacral neuromodulation on refractory urgency urinary incontinence in women: a randomized clinical trial. JAMA. 2016;316:1366–74.
5. Bayrak O, Sadioglu E, Sen H, Dogan K, Erturhan S, Seckiner I. Efficacy of onabotulinum toxin A injection in pediatric patients with non-neurogenic detrusor overactivity. Neurourol Urodyn. 2017;36(8):2078–82.

6. Chancellor MB, Anderson RU, Boone TB. Pharmacotherapy for neurogenic detrusor overactivity. Am J Phys Med Rehabil. 2006;85:536–45.
7. Chancellor MB, Smith CP: Botulinum toxin in urology, 2011, Springers, http://www.springer.com/medicine/urology/book/978-3-642-03579-1?changeHeader.
8. Chapple CR, Khullar V, Gabriel Z, et al. The effects of antimuscarinic treatments in overactive bladder: an update of a systematic review and meta-analysis. Eur Urol. 2008;54:543–62.
9. Chapple C, Sievert K-D, MacDiarmid S, et al. OnabotulinumtoxinA 100 u significantly improves all idiopathic overactive bladder symptoms and quality of life in patients with overactive bladder and urinary incontinence: a randomized, double-blind, placebo-controlled trial. Eur Urol. 2013;64:249–56.
10. Chuang YC, Chiang PH, Yoshimura N, De Miguel F, Chancellor MB. Sustained beneficial effects of intraprostatic botulinum toxin type A on lower urinary tract symptoms and quality of life in men with benign prostatic hyperplasia. BJU Int. 2006;98(5):1033–7.
11. Cruz F, Herschorn S, Aliotta P, et al. Efficacy and safety of onabotulinumtoxinA in patients with urinary incontinence due to neurogenic detrusor overactivity: a randomized, double-blind, placebo-controlled trial. Eur Urol. 2011;60:742–50.
12. Denys P, Del Popolo G, Amarenco G, et al. Dysport Study Group. Efficacy and safety of two administration modes of an intra-detrusor injection of 750 units dysport® (abobotulinumtoxinA) in patients suffering from refractory neurogenic detrusor overactivity (NDO): A randomised placebo-controlled phase IIa study. Neurourol Urodyn. 2016; https://doi.org/10.1002/nau.22954.
13. de Seze M, Petit H, Gallien P, et al. Botulinum A toxin and detrusor-sphincter-dyssynergia: a double-blind lidocaine-controlled study in 13 patients with spinal cord disease. Eur Urol. 2002;42:56–62.
14. Dykstra D, Sidi A, Scott A, et al. Effects of botulinum A toxin on detrusor-sphincter dyssynergia in spinal cord injury patients. J Urol. 1988;139:919–22.
15. Gallien P, Reymann J-M, Amarenco G, et al. Placebo controlled, randomized, double blind study of the effects of botulinum A toxin on detrusor sphincter dyssynergia in multiple sclerosis patients. J Neurol Neurosurg Psychiatry. 2005;76:1670–6.
16. Ghazizadeh S, Nikzad M. Botulinum toxin in the treatment of refractory vaginismus. Obstet Gynecol. 2004;104:922–5.
17. Ginsberg D, Gousse A, Keppenne V, et al. Phase 3 efficacy and tolerability study of onabotulinumtoxinA for urinary incontinence from neurogenic detrusor overactivity. J Urol. 2012;187:2131–9.
18. Gormley EA, Lightner DJ, Faraday M, et al. Diagnosis and treatment of overactive bladder (non-neurogenic) in adults: AUA/SUFU guideline amendment. J Urol. 2015;193:1572–80.
19. Hanno PM, Erickson D, Moldwin R, et al. Diagnosis and treatment of interstitial cystitis/bladder pain syndrome: AUA guideline amendment. J Urol. 2015;193:1545–53.
20. Harvie HS, Amundsen CL, Neuwahl SJ, Honeycutt AA, Lukacz ES, Sung VW, Rogers RG, Ellington D, Ferrando CA, Chermansky CJ, Mazloomdoost D, Thomas S, NICHD Pelvic Floor Disorders Network. Cost effectiveness of sacral neuromodulation versus OnabotulinumtoxinA for refractory urgency urinary incontinence: results of the ROSETTA randomized trial. J Urol. 2019;18:101097JU0000000000000656.   https://doi.org/10.1097/JU.0000000000000656. [Epub ahead of print]
21. Hascoet J, Peyronnet B, Forin V, Baron M, Capon G, Prudhomme T, Allenet C, Tournier S, Maurin C, Cornu JN, Bouali O, Peycelon M, Arnaud A, Renaux-Petel M, Liard A, Karsenty G, Manunta A, Game X. Intradetrusor injections of botulinum toxin type A in children with spina bifida: a multicenter study. Urology. 2018;116:161–7.
22. Kennelly M, Dmochowski R, Ethans K, et al. Efficacy and safety of OnabotulinumtoxinA therapy are sustained over 4 years of treatment in patients with neurogenic detrusor overactivity: final results of a long-term extension study. Neurourol Urodynam. 2015; https://doi.org/10.1002/nau.22934.

23. Kuo HC. Recovery of detrusor function after urethral botulinum A toxin injection in patients with idiopathic low detrusor contractility and voiding dysfunction. Urology. 2007;69:57–61; discussion 61–52

24. Kuo HC, Chancellor MB. Comparison of intravesical botulinum toxin type A injections plus hydrodistention with hydrodistention alone for the treatment of refractory interstitial cystitis/ painful bladder syndrome. BJU Int. 2009;104:657–61.

25. Maria G, Brisinda G, Civello IM, et al. Relief by botulinum toxin of voiding dysfunction due to benign prostatic hyperplasia; results of a randomized, placebo-controlled study. Urology. 2003;62:259–64.

26. McVary KT, Roehrborn CG, Chartier-Kastler E, et al. A multicenter, randomized, double-blind, placebo controlled study of onabotulinumtoxinA 200 U to treat lower urinary tract symptoms in men with benign prostatic hyperplasia. J Urol. 2014;192:150–6.

27. Nitti VW, Dmochowski R, Herschorn S, et al. OnabotulinumtoxinA for the treatment of patients with overactive bladder and urinary incontinence: results of a phase 3, randomized, placebo controlled trial. J Urol. 2013;189:2186–93.

28. Nitti VW, Ginsberg D, Sievert KD, Sussman D, Radomski S, Sand P, De Ridder D, Jenkins B, Magyar A, Chapple C, 191622-096 Investigators. Durable efficacy and safety of long-term OnabotulinumtoxinA treatment in patients with overactive bladder syndrome: final results of a 3.5-year study. J Urol. 2016;196(3):791–800.

29. Schurch B, Schmid D, Stohrer M, et al. Treatment of neurogenic incontinence with botulinum toxin. N Engl J Med. 2000;342:665.

30. Schurch B, de Seze M, Denys P, et al. Botulinum toxin type A is a safe and effective treatment for neurogenic urinary incontinence: results of a single treatment, randomized, placebo controlled 6-month study. J Urol. 2005;174:196–200.

31. Smith CP, Boone TB, de Groat WC, Chancellor MB, Somogyi GT. Effect of stimulation intensity and botulinum toxin isoform on rat bladder strip contractions. Brain Res Bull. 2003a;61:165–71.

32. Smith CP, Franks ME, McNeil BK, Ghosh R, de Groat WC, Chancellor MB, Somogyi GT. Effect of botulinum toxin A on the autonomic nervous system of the rat lower urinary tract. J Urol. 2003b;169(5):1896–900.

33. Smith CP, Radziszewski P, Borkowski A, et al. Botulinum toxin A has antinociceptive effects in treating interstitial cystitis. Urology. 2004;64(5):871–5.

34. Smith CP, Vemulakonda VM, Kiss S, Boone TB, Somogyi GT. Enhanced ATP release from rat bladder urothelium during chronic bladder inflammation: effect of botulinum toxin A. Neurochem Int. 2005 Sep;47(4):291–7.

35. Stewart WF, Van Rooyen JB, Cundiff GW, et al. Prevalence and burden of overactive bladder in the United States. World J Urol. 2003;20:327–36.

Chapter 16
Botulinum Toxin Treatment in Dentistry

Victor Ricardo Manuel Muñoz Lora and Altair Antoninha Del Bel Cury

Abstract In dentistry, botulinum toxin type A (BoNT/A) is already approved for the treatment of sialorrhea by the US Food and Drug Administration (FDA) and European Union (EU). However, following the American Academy of Neurology guidelines, BoNT/A can be considered as an effective treatment for trigeminal neuralgia and as a probably effective approach for temporomandibular disorders and bruxism. In this chapter, we described all the possible evidence-based applications of BoNT/A in dentistry and presented a clinical guide for the use of the neurotoxin in each condition according to high-quality studies found in literature.

Keywords Botulinum toxins · Temporomandibular joint disorders · Bruxism · Trigeminal neuralgia · Sialorrhea

Similar to other medical fields, the use of botulinum toxins (BoNTs) in dentistry is widely increasing, with numerous practitioners offering BoNTs as a treatment for different conditions [1]. Historically, British Columbia dentists were among the first to appreciate the therapeutic properties of BoNTs and integrate its use in dental practice. Up to now, sialorrhea is the only condition in the field of dentistry, for which the use of BoNT type A (BoNT/A) has been approved by the US Food and Drug Administration and European Union [2]. Although the legal status of BoNT/A utilization in other countries is less known, the toxin is frequently employed *off-label* (e.g., the use of a pharmaceutical drug in a manner not specified in the packaging label – not approved by the regulatory agencies) for diverse chronic conditions [3].

Currently, several studies have proven the muscular, analgesic, and anticholinergic effects of BoNT/A. In addition, clinical trials and reviews [3–6] have suggested the efficacy of BoNT/A on the control or treatment of temporomandibular disorders, bruxism, trigeminal neuropathic pain, and the already registered sialorrhea (see Table 16.1). It is noteworthy that the therapeutic action of BoNT/A in the trigeminal region is of major interest in dentistry due to the high prevalence of the

V. R. M. M. Lora (✉) · A. A. D. B. Cury
Department of Prosthodontics and Periodontology, Piracicaba School of Dentistry,
University of Campinas, Campinas, Brazil
e-mail: altair@unicamp.br

© Springer Nature Switzerland AG 2020
B. Jabbari (ed.), *Botulinum Toxin Treatment in Surgery, Dentistry, and Veterinary Medicine*, https://doi.org/10.1007/978-3-030-50691-9_16

aforementioned conditions and the limited success rate of the currently existing therapies [7].

Considering that the reason to not recommend a treatment is supported on its ineffectiveness, harmfulness, or just the lack of well-designed and well-powered evidence-based studies [8, 9], in this chapter we describe all the possible benefits of the therapeutic usage of BoNT/A on chronic conditions related to dental medicine, as well as an evidence-based clinical guide for the application of the toxin. Also, we relate the possible side/adverse effects associated to single or continuous applications of BoNT/A in the orofacial area.

Botulinum Toxin Type A and Temporomandibular Disorders

Temporomandibular disorders (TMDs) represent a set of different conditions involving the temporomandibular joint (TMJ), masticatory muscles, and/or associated structures. The prevalence of TMD varies widely among the general population and studies have reported that almost 33% of individuals present at least one symptom of these conditions, including tenderness of the masticatory muscles, TMJ sounds, functional limitation of jaw opening, and pain of the masticatory muscles or TMJ [10, 11]. Furthermore, TMDs are also associated with high levels of psychosocial impairments and a high prevalence of psychosocial disorders (e.g., anxiety, depression, stress, etc.) [12–14].

The etiology of TMDs is complex and multifactorial, with different systemic and local risk factors reflected in the fluctuating and self-limiting nature of the disorder. Also, positive comorbid relationships between TMDs and cervical spine dysfunction, headaches, fibromyalgia, and other conditions are not uncommon, complicating the diagnosis, treatment, and prognosis of the disorder [15]. For all these reasons, a multidisciplinary approach comprising conservative and less invasive treatments is always suggested.

Currently, the available treatments for TMDs aim to control pain symptomatology and recover lost jaw functions. Existing therapies include the use of oral splints, counseling, physical therapy, laser therapy, and pharmacotherapy with muscle relaxants, benzodiazepines, and antidepressants. However, although all these approaches have been extensively studied, a moderate success rate with limited outcomes is frequently reported, leading to the necessity of novel long-lasting and efficient therapeutic modalities [16, 17].

Table 16.1 High-quality studies[a] on the use of BoNTs for dentistry-related conditions

Author	Patients, n	Diagnosis	Dose, total U	BoNT	Place	Side effects	Outcomes
Patel 2017	21 crossover	TMD (no specific)	170	Xeomin	Masseter Temporalis Lateral pterygoid	No adverse effects noted	Reduction of pain
Ernberg 2011	10 BoNT/A 10 placebo	Myofascial pain	100	Botox	Masseter	Not related to the drug, resolved after 1 mo	Clinically significant reduction of pain. No differences with placebo
Kurtoglu 2008	12 BoNT/A 12 placebo	Myofascial pain	100	Botox	Masseter Temporalis	No evident side effects	Reduction of pain
De la Torre 2019	60 BoNT/A 20 placebo 20 oral splint	Masticatory muscle pain	80 140 200	Botox	Masseter Temporalis	Dose-related side effects Reduction of masticatory efficacy and bone atrophy	Reduction of pain comparable to oral splint
Ondo 2018	13 BoNT/A 10 placebo	Sleep bruxism	100	Botox	Masseter Temporalis	No muscle weakness reported	Reduction of bruxism events Increase of total sleep time Reduction of associated pain
Zhang 2014	54 BoNT/A 26 placebo	Trigeminal neuralgia	25 75	Botox	Subdermal/ epidermal at painful sites	Transient edema, short-term facial asymmetry	Reduction of pain Reduction in number of paroxysms No dose–effect relation found
Wu 2012	22 BoNT/A 20 placebo	Trigeminal neuralgia	75	Botox	Intradermal/ submucosal at painful sites	Transient edema, short-term facial asymmetry	Reduction of pain Reduction of the number of attacks

(continued)

Table 16.1 (continued)

Author	Patients, n	Diagnosis	Dose, total U	BoNT	Place	Side effects	Outcomes
Jost 2019	148 BoNT/A 36 placebo	Sialorrhea	75 100	Xeomin	Intraglandular into parotid and submandibular, guided by ultrasound	Dry mouth Dysphagia	Reduction on unstimulated salivary flow Improvement of patient's Global Impression of Change score
Jackson 2009	11 BoNT/B 9 placebo	Sialorrhea	500 750	Myobloc	Intraglandular into parotid and submandibular, guided by electromyography	Dry mouth	90% efficiency after 4 weeks

[a]High-quality studies were selected according to the American Academy of Neurology Evaluation of Evidence Classification

Preclinical Evidence and Mechanism of Action

A variety of animal models reproducing TMJ pain are frequently employed to study the effects of BoNT/A in TMDs. In a rat model of intra-articular application of complete Freund's adjuvant to provoke inflammatory pain in the TMJ, BoNT/A decreased the evoked allodynia after intra-articular and ganglion injections, proving its effectiveness on pain related to the TMJ [18]. A model of inflammatory arthritis-induced nociception in the TMJ of rats was used in another experimental study [19], and the affected TMJ was treated with different doses of BoNT/A (3.5, 7, and 14 U/kg), which reduced the pain-like behaviors evoked by the induced persistent pain. The outcomes of this study also demonstrated that the toxin diminished the levels of substance P, calcitonin gene-related peptide, and interleukin-1β, all of which are partially associated with pain and inflammation.

Collectively, these findings led to the suggestion that the effectiveness of BoNT/A for TMDs is based on an analgesic activity produced by the decrease of different neuromodulators (e.g., substance P, glutamate, calcitonin gene related peptide, pro-inflammatory cytokines, among others). Nevertheless, a neuromuscular action of the toxin due to the inhibition of acetylcholine release from nerve endings may also contribute to pain relief when a muscle hyperactivity is associated with the TMD (e.g., bruxism) [4].

Evidence-Based Clinical Effectiveness

Over the past several years, BoNT/A has been widely studied and used for the treatment of TMDs, especially when it is associated with masticatory muscle pain (MMP). Although the neuroparalytic effect of BoNT/A was considered to be the responsible factor for its clinical efficacy in the control of TMDs, current data mainly associates its therapeutic effectiveness to an independent analgesic activity [20].

To date, published investigations about the management of myogenic TMDs using BoNT/A have shown inconsistent results. Administration of the toxin into masticatory muscles (i.e., masseter, temporalis, and external pterygoid) has been used in patients diagnosed with TMDs related to MMP [21, 22]. In these cases, a decrease of the electromyographic activity of the treated muscles, reduction of associated pain, and a notable improvement of the psychological status were reported. These studies concluded that, based on the obtained results, BoNT/A can be considered as a valid therapeutic approach for the treatment of myogenic TMDs. Conversely, in a multicenter investigation involving patients diagnosed with persistent MMP [23], a clinically significant reduction of pain (i.e., 30% less pain) was obtained after BoNT/A injections; however, this analgesic effect was also achieved by a placebo solution containing sterile saline. In this particular study, the results were considered insufficient to contemplate the toxin as an effective treatment for

TMDs, and the reduction of pain was explained as a placebo effect attributed to the needling during application of the treatments. However, it is important to mention that the treatment of just one of the masticatory muscles (masseter) instead of two (masseter and temporalis) and the small sample size were considered as limitations of the investigation and possibly influenced the outcomes of the study.

Since most of the shortcomings found in research frequently include a low number of participants and the lack of delivery protocols and standardized doses, a large randomized, double-blind, controlled clinical trial assessing the efficacy of different doses of BoNT/A on persistent MMP was recently conducted [24]. This study showed that BoNT/A was at least as effective as an oral splint (considered as the gold standard treatment for myogenic TMDs) and more effective than a placebo (injection of saline solution) to relieve the pain associated with TMDs. The side effects following BoNT/A injections were also evaluated throughout the study and are described in Section "Adverse Effects/Reactions of BoNT/A Application on Dentistry-Related Conditions" of this chapter.

Considering all the available information regarding the use of BoNT/A for TMDs, it seems like the toxin can be contemplated as a promising alternative to control the associated chronic pain in these disorders. However, more high-quality and well-designed studies still have to be conducted to corroborate the effectiveness of BoNT/A and investigate its possible side effects.

Clinical Guide for the Application of BoNT/A for TMDs

Most of the randomized, controlled, clinical trials using BoNT/A for the treatment of TMDs have reported administration of diverse doses and delivery protocols. Doses of BoNT/A have ranged from 50 to 300 U in different studies and injections into one, two, or even three masticatory muscles have been suggested [3, 25, 26]. Recently, a large study conducted by a Brazilian group in a population diagnosed with chronic myogenic TMDs [24] employed different doses of BoNT/A (low, medium, and high dose) to evaluate its efficacy on pain reduction and to assess its possible adverse effects. The results showed that lower doses of BoNT/A injected into two muscles (30 U masseter and 10 U temporalis) were as effective as higher doses (75 U masseter and 25 U temporalis) and similar to oral splints (used as a positive control) to reduce pain. This research suggests that the analgesic activity of BoNT/A is not dose-dependent, opposite to its neuromuscular action. Indeed, more studies are needed to explain the dose–response relationship and the longer durability of the effects on sensory nerves.

So far, no studies have compared the effectiveness of BoNT/A using single vs multiple injections on masticatory muscles for the treatment of TMDs. However, injections into the masseter and anterior temporalis are recommended, as they are considered two of the main masticatory muscles and are frequently affected in myogenic TMDs. Although applications of BoNT/A on pterygoid muscles have also been reported using electromyographic guidance, its complex anatomical position makes it difficult to properly place the needle, increasing the possibility of reaching nearby structures and developing undesirable side effects. Furthermore, bilateral applications are recommended to avoid facial asymmetry due to the neuromuscular paralysis effect of the toxin (Figs. 16.1, 16.2 and 16.3).

It is also important to consider that after injection, the toxin is primarily distributed within the muscle by convection (i.e., the fluid volume and the force of injection determine the bulk movement of the solution) rather than by diffusion (i.e., spread of the solution from the initial site) [27]. For this reason, it is suggested that injections be administered into 4–5 different points, evenly distributed within each muscle with approximately 10-mm separation between each point so that they cover the majority of the muscular area.

In brief, based on scientific evidence, when BoNT/A is contemplated for the treatment of TMDs, we recommend a bilateral application of low doses of the toxin, i.e., 30 U masseter/10 U temporalis, evenly distributed within 4 to 5 points on each treated muscle (Table 16.2 and Fig. 16.1).

Botulinum Toxin Type A and Bruxism

Bruxism is "a repetitive masticatory muscle activity characterized by clenching or grinding of the teeth and/or bracing or thrusting of the mandible," as defined during the last international consensus meeting on the assessment of bruxism [28]. During this meeting, a grading system to diagnose bruxism as "possible," "probable," or "definitive" was also suggested. Additionally, bruxism was divided according to two different circadian manifestations into sleep bruxism (SB), which is associated

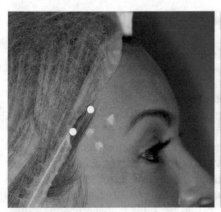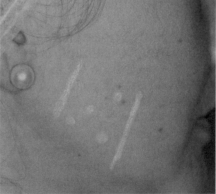

Fig. 16.1 Application points on the anterior temporalis and masseter muscles for bruxism and/or TMDs

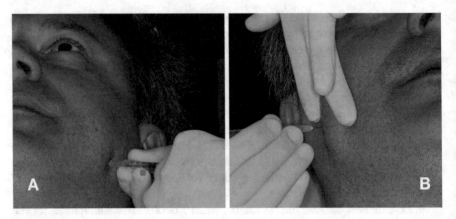

Fig. 16.2 BoNT/A injection into the masseter muscle

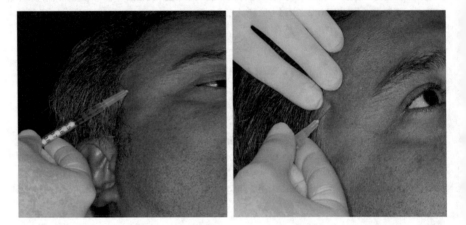

Fig. 16.3 BoNT/A injection into the anterior temporalis muscle

with nocturnal microarousals and is considered a sleep-related behavior, and awake bruxism (AB). The prevalence of bruxism in adult populations varies from 8% to 15% for SB and 22% to 30% for AB [29].

The continuous or repetitive contraction of masticatory muscles during bruxism is considered a risk factor for mechanical tooth wear, muscle and/or joint pain, joint blockage and noises, and prosthodontic/implant complications. Current therapies for bruxism are based on conservative strategies and focused on the management of the possible clinical consequences such as tooth wear, TMJ damage, and/or excessive muscle activity reduction [29, 30]. Oral appliances are an effective and widely used approach to control bruxism; unfortunately, there is insufficient scientific evidence supporting their long-term use [31, 32]. In the same manner, pharmacotherapy with muscle relaxants and centrally acting drugs is employed to decrease the masticatory force and frequency of the episodes, in order to reduce or prevent possible damage to oral structures [30].

Table 16.2 Evidence-based clinical guide for BoNT/A applications on dentistry-related conditions

Condition	Dose[a]	Delivery route	Application points	Expected outcomes
TMDs	30 U/masseter 10 U/anterior temporalis	Intramuscular	4–5 points within each muscle	Reduction of pain Improvement of psychological status
Bruxism	25–70 U/ masseter 10–30 U/ anterior temporalis	Intramuscular	4–5 points within each muscle	Reduction of pain (if present) Reduction of muscle force Improvement of sleep time Reduction of muscle size (when masseter hypertrophy is associate)
Trigeminal neuralgia	25 U	Intradermal Subcutaneous Submucosal	Distributed on painful site	Reduction of pain Reduction of the number of paroxysms Improvement of psychological status
Sialorrhea	30 U/parotid 20 U/subman	Intraglandular	1 point on each gland	Reduction of salivary flow

[a]Research suggests a dose conversion of 1:3 U from BoNT/A to abobotulinumtoxinA (Dysport, Ipsen®) [93]. However, since units are not interchangeable, it is recommended to follow manufacturer's dose guidelines

Preclinical Evidence and Mechanism of Action of BoNT/A for Bruxism

The therapeutic effectiveness of BoNT/A on bruxism is based on the decrease of muscle activity/force of the masticatory muscles (masseter, temporalis, pterygoid). It is well known that intramuscular injections of BoNT/A cause long-lasting and dose-dependent muscle paralysis; hence, it is valid to consider the toxin as a feasible approach to control bruxism [4, 33].

In vivo models resembling bruxism are not reported in the literature. In an attempt to assess the impact of BoNT/A on masticatory muscles and its possible adverse/side effects, unilateral injections of the toxin into the masseter of rabbits were performed [34]. The results showed a reduction of the electromyographic activity due to the paralysis of the treated muscles. Surprisingly, the chewing capacity of the animals was only slightly altered by BoNT/A, probably because of compensation by different masticatory muscles such as the medial pterygoid. An important observation was the reduction of muscle force and the presence of severely decreased bone quantity and quality in the underloaded locations. Although muscle force returned to basal values after 12 months, bone loss persisted until the end of the study.

All these data suggest that applications of BoNT/A can reduce masticatory muscle loading and decrease the severity of bruxism events. On the other hand, a possible long-term usage of the toxin and interference on masticatory muscle loading may compromise the mechanical properties of the TMJ and the mandibular bone [34–36]. However, there is still a lack of strong evidence supporting these possible side effects.

Evidence-Based Clinical Effectiveness

The existing knowledge regarding the use of BoNT/A in the control of bruxism is based mostly on a few randomized clinical trials [4, 37] and low-quality research [33]. Most studies have included only SB populations, since data regarding AB is available only from retrospective self-reports at single observation points [38], impeding the development of well-designed studies. A recently published systematic literature review on the applications of BoNT/A for SB [4] presented the toxin as a possible approach for controlling SB repercussions, minimizing symptoms and reducing the contraction of masticatory muscles. However, since the pathophysiology of bruxism is still uncertain [39], a direct action of this toxin on the cessation of bruxing activity is still unknown.

The therapeutic efficiency of BoNT/A for bruxism is based on decreasing contraction of the masticatory muscles [3, 40, 41], including masseter, anterior temporalis, and in some cases, lateral pterygoid. However, the analgesic properties of BoNTs are also important when the behavior is accompanied by pain.

Searching through the literature, we found a recently published high-quality randomized study assessing the efficacy of BoNT/A on SB. In this double-blind placebo-controlled trial [42], 23 patients diagnosed with SB by polysomnography were included. Applications of BoNT/A into the masseter (60 U) and temporalis (40 U) muscles reduced the number of bruxism events and tended to improve the total sleep time after 4 weeks. Additionally, a different study [43] also showed a decrease in the number of sleep events after bilateral masseteric injections of BoNT/A (80 U; Dysport, Ipsen®). This effect was maintained for up to 12 weeks; however, the small number of patients (6 bruxers and 6 healthy controls), the absence of a validated diagnostic criteria, and the treatment of just 1 masticatory muscle (masseter) suggest that these results should be interpreted cautiously.

Paralysis of masseter using BoNT/A was also suggested in cosmetics for the treatment of benign masseteric hypertrophy, a bilateral or unilateral condition attributed to a number of factors including masseteric hyperfunction and/or para-function (e.g., bruxism), and characterized by the enlargement of the masseter muscles [44, 45]. Despite the large number of trials describing the use of the toxin for this condition, the majority of them are not relevant or contain no robust evidence to support or refute the effectiveness and safety of BoNT/A [45]. For this reason, the development of high-quality clinical trials on this issue is encouraged.

Unloading the mandible using BoNT/A has also been proposed as a procedure to allow immediate placement of implants in bruxers [46]. There is a common fear

among practitioners that bruxism can overload dental implants, affecting osseointegration, compromising their mechanical integrity, and leading to implant failure
[47]. Nevertheless, bruxism is more likely to be a risk factor for mechanical dam-
ages of the implant-supported rehabilitations rather than a cause for biological complications such as osseointegration problems [47]. Despite all of this, literature
supporting this practice is very poor and more studies are still needed.

Summarizing the clinical evidence regarding the use of BoNT/A for bruxism, it
appears that more well-designed studies still need to be performed considering different bruxism populations, such as sleep and awake bruxers, dental implant hold-
ers, and bruxism-associated masseteric hypertrophy, in order to confirm the possible
benefits of this toxin.

Clinical Guide for the Application of BoNT/A for Bruxism

Until now, no standardized protocol for the control of bruxism using BoNT/A has
been established. Since bruxism affects masticatory muscles, the application of
BoNT/A in TMDs has been suggested and would be a suitable approach for the
treatment of this issue. Administration of BoNT/A into 4–5 injection points on the
masseter and temporalis could adequately spread this toxin within the treated muscles (Table 16.2 and Fig. 16.1).

In contrast to BoNT/A injections for TMDs, the neuromuscular effect of the
toxin is desired in patients with bruxism, and the employed doses may vary according to muscle size, patient age, gender, race, and/or even the severity of bruxism
activity. Therefore, a correct elaboration of anamnesis including the medical history
of the patient as well as a thorough clinical examination are critical steps to determine the protocol to be employed. Frequent doses range from 10 to 100 U in the
masseter and 0 to 30 U in the temporalis muscle [4, 41, 42]. The difference in the
doses used for various muscles is due to the differences in their volumes and the
positive correlation between the amount of toxin applied and the extension of the
elicited paresis [48] (Fig. 16.4).

One additional fact to consider is that currently there is no strong evidence supporting the effect of BoNT/A on the frequency of SB events. It is known that
repeated masticatory muscle activity during bruxism is caused by nocturnal microarousals which increase autonomic cardiac and motor neuronal networks [39],
leading to involuntary contractions of the masseter with or without grinding sounds
[49, 50]. BoNT/A acts by reducing muscle contraction but does not affect the
development of bruxism; therefore, the concomitant use of oral appliances is recommended to prevent the consequences of repeated masticatory muscle activity,
i.e., bruxism events.

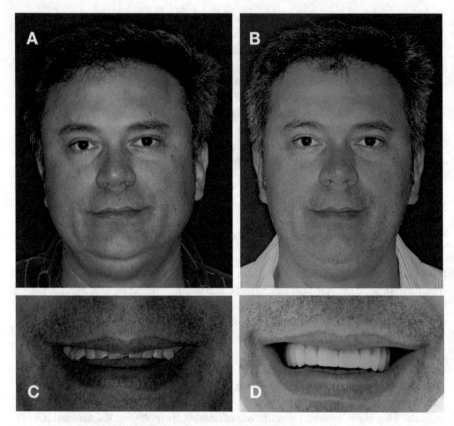

Fig. 16.4 (**a**) Before and (**b**) after BoNT/A injections for bruxism associated with masseter and temporalis hypertrophy. Note a bigger muscle volume on the left side. BoNT/A dosage of 30 and 40 U into right and left temporalis muscles. BoNT/A dosage of 50 and 70 U into right and left masseter muscles. (**c**) Tooth wear as a common clinical sign of bruxism. (**d**) Full mouth rehabilitation after controlling bruxism with BoNT/A

Botulinum Toxin Type A and Trigeminal Neuralgia

Trigeminal neuralgia (TN) is described as a typically unilateral condition characterized by paroxysmal, severe, sharp, and recurrent shock-like pain along the somatosensory distribution of the trigeminal nerve [5, 51, 52]. It is considered as one of the most distressing disorders of the orofacial region, increasing the risk of anxiety and depression among patients [5, 53–55]. The International Headache Society divides this condition into "classical TN," including all TN cases with unknown etiology other than vascular compression of the trigeminal nerve, and "secondary TN," induced by the compression of the trigeminal nerve by structural abnormalities or tumors [3, 52].

Commonly, only one division of the trigeminal nerve is affected by TN, with a higher prevalence of the maxillary branch (52%), followed by the mandibular branch (39%) [56]. Epidemiologic studies have shown the incidence of TN to be 4 to 5 per 100,000 individuals and 28.9 per 100,000 individuals per year in the United States and United Kingdom–Netherlands, respectively [5]. Additionally, a female/male ratio of 1.17:1 has been reported [56].

Treatment of TN is based on pharmacotherapy using anticonvulsant drugs, such as carbamazepine and oxcarbamazepine, as first-line agents. Unfortunately, approximately 25–50% of pharmacologically treated patients become refractory, requiring surgical procedures such as vascular decompression, partial sensory rhizotomy, and gamma knife radiosurgery [57]. However, effective surgical outcomes are not always permanent, and in addition to the possibility of developing neurologic deficits, reappearance of pain is relatively common among surgically treated patients [5].

Preclinical Evidence and Mechanism of Action

The majority of data from in vitro and in vivo studies support a positive effect of BoNT/A on TN [58–60]. In an experiment using stimulated cultures of trigeminal neurons, clinical effective doses of BoNT/A were able to decrease the amount of calcitonin gene-related peptide, a neurotransmitter commonly associated with the pathophysiology of migraine and other neuropathic pain conditions [61, 62].

Unfortunately, no animal model has been developed that can successfully duplicate the neuropathic pathophysiology of TN [63]; however, the model of infraorbital nerve constriction (IoNC), based on the loose ligation of the infraorbital nerve, is frequently used to investigate the action of BoNT/A on trigeminal neuropathic conditions, including TN [64, 65]. Filipovic et al. [66] studied the effects of BoNT/A on local allodynia and bilateral dural neurogenic inflammation induced by IoNC. Using a single injection of the toxin (3.5 U/kg) into the vibrissae pad of rats, dural extravasation and facial allodynia were reduced. Interestingly, the analgesic effect of BoNT/A was prevented by a colchicine injection (e.g., axonal blocker) into the trigeminal ganglia of the affected side, suggesting the necessity of axonal transport to reach trigeminal sensory neurons.

In a different study, long-lasting ipsilateral allodynia was developed in rats submitted to IoNC. An intradermal pretreatment injection of BoNT/A into the whisker pad of the animals decreased the exaggerated release of neurotransmitters from sensory neurons of the trigeminal root ganglia and, consequently, alleviated the pain-like behaviors [59].

As the pathogenesis of these models is entirely based on nerve damage, it is acceptable to affirm that the analgesic/antinociceptive mechanism of the toxin is the major contributor in the control of neuropathic pain conditions. In our opinion, these data suggest that BoNT/A may represent a valuable alternative as a centrally acting drug for trigeminal neuropathic conditions, including TN.

Evidence-Based Clinical Effectiveness

The clinical effectiveness of BoNT/A for TN is probably one of the most reviewed issues involving the analgesic activity of the toxin in the trigeminal region. The reason is based on the overlapping of TN as a condition related to more than one medical field (dentistry, neurology, surgery, etc.). However, when it affects the maxillary and/or the mandibular branch of trigeminal nerves, TN is commonly presented as a dental problem, with patients seeking help from dental practitioners [3, 56].

Two meta-analyses concluded that BoNT/A may be an effective and safe method for patients suffering from TN [5, 53]. According to the Therapeutics and Assessment Subcommittee of the American Academy of Neurology, the use of BoNT/A for TN can be already considered as a level A treatment (i.e., treatment efficacy supported by two or more high-quality studies), based on two high-quality randomized clinical trials [3, 6, 54, 67], described below:

One of these was a randomized, double-blind, placebo-controlled study [54] which showed that intradermal and/or submucosal administration of BoNT/A was more effective than placebo injections (saline solution) to control classical TN. Interestingly, BoNT/A not only decreased pain scores measured by the visual analogue scale, but also reduced the frequency of attacks as early as 2 weeks after treatment. The higher percentage of BoNT/A responders (15/22; 68.18%) compared to placebo (3/20; 15.00%) placed the toxin as a clinically effective treatment for TN.

The other study included 80 patients diagnosed with TN [67] and the therapeutic outcome of two different doses of intradermal/mucosal BoNT/A injections (25 U or 75 U) was assessed. The results revealed a significantly higher number of responders in the groups treated with BoNT/A, compared to placebo (saline solution). Responders were defined as patients demonstrating at least 50% pain reduction in comparison to baseline values. According to the Patient Global Impression of Change, a greater improvement was found in patients treated with BoNT/A compared to those receiving placebo injections.

Differences between various doses of BoNT/A and adverse reactions are discussed in the following sections.

Considering all the available data, the use of BoNT/A for TN can be considered an effective therapeutic modality, reducing pain and the frequency of attacks and improving anxiety, depression, and the patient's quality of life [3, 5, 6, 68].

Clinical Guide for the Application of BoNT/A for Trigeminal Neuralgia

It is important to mention that pain in TN is mostly promoted by Aβ-fibers, expressing allodynia triggered by gentle mechanical stimuli such as washing the face, touching gums with a toothbrush, or moving food inside the mouth [63]. Since Aβ-fibers innervate cutaneous mechanoreceptors responding to physical interactions

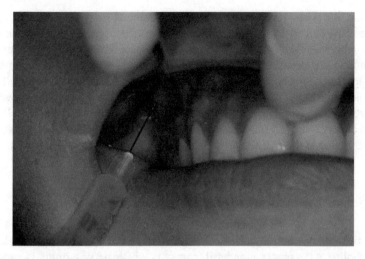

Fig. 16.5 Submucosal application of BoNT/A into an intraoral trigger point on the molar region of a patient diagnosed with classical TN

including pressure and vibration [56, 63], the intradermal or submucosal injection of the toxin in areas surrounding the trigger zones has proven to be the more effective approach to treat this neuropathic pain condition [5, 6, 54, 67] (Fig. 16.5).

A detailed clinical examination to recognize the affected trigeminal branch and delineate the painful area and trigger zone is required to define the best injection sites. There is still no consensus about the exact number of injections required to achieve a superior analgesic effect. Apparently, the spread of BoNT/A through the defined painful area will allow a better distribution of the toxin around the affected sensory region, generating a greater analgesic activity. Nevertheless, the number of injection points has not been defined and varies with each situation [53].

As mentioned in preceding sections, the analgesic activity of BoNT/A is not dose-dependent. Analgesic effects were similar between low and high doses (25 U vs 75 U) of this toxin in patients diagnosed with TN [67]. Both doses had a greater effect and a higher analgesic activity than a placebo injection (saline solution). It should be considered that higher doses of the toxin are associated with larger undesired neuromuscular effects (see Section "Adverse Effects/Reactions of BoNT/A Application on Dentistry-Related Conditions"); thus, great care must be taken even when intradermal or submucosal injections are employed (Table 16.2).

Botulinum Toxin Type A in Sialorrhea

Sialorrhea, drooling, or excessive salivary overflow is a socially disabling condition commonly associated with the loss of neuromuscular control due to different neurological disorders such as cerebral palsy, Parkinson's disease, and amyotrophic lateral sclerosis [69–71]. The prevalence of sialorrhea varies widely; however, it is estimated that about 10–37% of children with cerebral palsy are affected [72], and between 10% and 84% of people with Parkinson's disease and 20% of patients with amyotrophic lateral sclerosis or motor neuron disease develop this symptom [73].

Conservative treatments, including anticholinergic and antihistaminic pharmacotherapy, are frequently employed to reduce salivary overflow; however, they are associated with significant adverse effects (e.g., cognitive impairment, drowsiness, urinary retention, etc.) [74, 75]. Surgical procedures, such as salivary duct ligation, parotid denervation, and bilateral excision of sublingual glands, are less commonly considered due to the risk of irreversible deficits [69].

Preclinical Evidence and Mechanism of Action

The anticholinergic activity of BoNT/A is based on the inhibition of the release of acetylcholine at the presynaptic level (parasympathetic nerve terminals), producing chemical nerve blocking and, consequently, loss of neuronal functioning [76]. Despite the large number of clinical trials reporting the effectiveness of BoNT/A for sialorrhea, there is still a lack of experimental evidence on the effect of the neurotoxin on glandular tissues [77].

According to a recent review [77], different immunohistochemical experiments on rats and rabbits reached similar results regarding the effect of BoNT/A on salivary glands. The injection of this toxin into the parotid and/or submandibular glands of animals led to decreased immunoreaction of acetylcholinesterase, neuronal nitric oxide synthase, and SNAP25. This reduction was proportional to the length of exposure and the applied dose of the neurotoxin [78–83]. In addition, chemical "denervation" of the salivary glands caused diminished salivary flow and resulted in reduction of the size and weight of the treated glands [83].

Another preclinical experiment on rabbits injected with 5 U BoNT/A for 12 weeks demonstrated an increased salivary amylase concentration and decrease of submandibular salivary secretion, respectively. These changes were ascribed to acinar cell apoptosis, which occurred 1 week after BoNT/A administration causing (1) reduced salivary flow, (2) decreased expression of M3 muscarinic acetylcholine receptors involved in regulation of glandular fluids, and (3) a reduction of aquaporin 5 expression that has a significant role in the regulation of salivary fluid secretion [84].

Evidence-Based Clinical Effectiveness

The first attempt for the use of BoNT/A on sialorrhea was reported in 1997 [85], when patients diagnosed with amyotrophic lateral sclerosis and severe sialorrhea were successfully treated with intraglandular injections of the toxin. IncobotulinumtoxinA (Xeomin, Merz®) was recently approved by the US FDA in

2018 and by EU/EEA in 2019 for the treatment of chronic sialorrhea, becoming the first and only neurotoxin with this approved indication in the United States and EU [2]. This approval was based on the positive results from a phase III, randomized, double-blind, placebo-controlled, multicenter, 184-patient trial, designated as the "SIAXI" (Sialorrhea in Adults Xeomin Investigation) study [2].

The SIAXI study [2] included 184 patients diagnosed with Parkinson's disease (70.7%), atypical parkinsonism (8.7%), stroke (19.0%), and traumatic brain injury (2.7%). Patients were randomized into placebo (36 patients), or total doses of 75 U (74 patients) or 100 U (74 patients) incobotulinumtoxinA. Changes in unstimulated salivary flow and Global Impression of Change scale scores were evaluated after 4, 8, 12, and 16 weeks. Adverse effects were also recorded (see Section "Adverse Effects/Reactions of BoNT/A Application on Dentistry-Related Conditions"). The results showed that 100 U incobotulinumtoxinA caused a significant reduction of unstimulated salivary flow until the last observation on week 16 ($-0,10 \pm 0.033$ g/min; $p = 0.002$, mixed model repeated measurement analysis). In addition, a significant improvement of the Global Impression of Change score was registered for patients treated with 100 U of the toxin through the 16th week (0.52 ± 0.203; $p = 0.011$, mixed model repeated measurement analysis). Based on these results, incobotulinumtoxinA (100 U) was considered an effective and well-tolerated treatment for chronic sialorrhea in adults.

Applications of BoNT/B into the parotid and submandibular glands also resulted in a significant decrease in the volume of saliva compared to placebo injections in patients diagnosed with amyotrophic lateral sclerosis after 4 weeks of evaluation [86]. A global impression of improvement was also reported by 90% of the patients treated with BoNT/B, compared to 44% among participants assigned to the placebo group, positioning BoNT/B as an effective alternative for drooling as well.

Clinical Guide for the Application of BoNT/A for Sialorrhea

Despite the currently available research on the use of BoNT/A in drooling, standard specifications for the best application method of this toxin have not yet been issued. Information regarding the preferred administration technique (ultrasound guidance vs anatomic guidance), dosages at initial and following injections, and the type and number of salivary glands required for BoNT/A administration is still lacking. For these reasons, a Botulinum toxin International Consensus for the assessment, intervention, and aftercare of pediatric and adult drooling was established [87].

As a first step, a complete and detailed evaluation of the patient must be performed, including a clinical examination of the orofacial region, assessment of the psychosocial status, a dental examination, and the utilization of valid questionnaires such as the Drooling Impact Scale [88].

Regarding the best technique of administration, it seems like the use of ultrasound (for localization of the glands) or electromyography (to avoid intramuscular injection) can ensure the accuracy of the injection site and improve the safety of

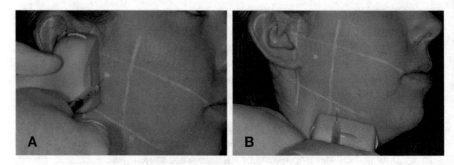

Fig. 16.6 (a) Injection into the parotid gland under sonographic guidance. (b) Injection into the submandibular gland under sonographic guidance

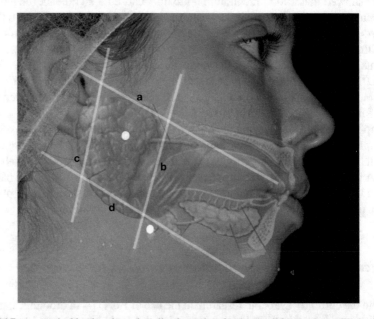

Fig. 16.7 Anatomical landmarks and application points for the parotid and submandibular glands. (a) The upper limit is represented by a line connecting the external acoustic meatus and the lateral corner of the mouth, (b) the front limit is represented by the masseter, (c) the back limit is established by the mandibular edge, and (d) the low limit is represented by the lower part of the mandible's body

BoNT/A applications on salivary glands, since patients treated without any guidance reported more frequent severe side effects (e.g., dysphagia, jaw dislocation, and chewing difficulties) [70, 71, 86]. Optimally, BoNT/A injections into salivary glands should be conducted under ultrasound guidance (Fig. 16.6), although experienced clinicians might rely on landmarks [87] (Table 16.2 and Fig. 16.7).

Protocols for injection of BoNT/A into salivary glands contemplate doses ranging from 40 U to 100 U for onabotulinumtoxinA (Botox, Allergan®) or 60 U to

300 U for abobotulinumtoxinA (Dysport, Ipsen®) [2, 89–92], considering a dosing conversion of 1:3 from onabotulinumtoxinA to abobotulinumtoxinA [93], in agreement with the International Consensus Statement [87]. A dose–effect relation must be considered for the anticholinergic action of BoNT/A, which means that higher doses will result in a greater reduction of saliva. Nonetheless, usually dosage recommendations are based on Western country populations and the safety profile could change depending on the ethnicity of patients; for example, Asian patients reported the need for lower doses of BoNT/A compared to European populations [94].

Another important point to consider is the number of treated salivary glands. Numerous studies have described procedures for single glands, injecting into either the parotid glands or the submandibular glands, whereas other investigations have described the treatment of both glands, simultaneously [95]. Nevertheless, the International Consensus Statement recommends the treatment of both salivary glands, parotid and submandibular, while the treatment of sublingual glands should be avoided due to their minor contribution to saliva production, relatively inaccessible anatomical location, and frequently associated side effects such as dysphagia [75, 95]. Considering the smaller size of the submandibular glands compared to the parotid, a smaller injection volume of BoNT/A seems to be a reasonable option and may be associated with a greater safety profile [96].

Botulinum Toxin Type A in Painful Traumatic Trigeminal Neuropathies

Painful traumatic trigeminal neuropathy (PTTN) is defined as any pain resulting from trigeminal nerve damage as a consequence of physical or surgical trauma such as dental extractions, dental implant therapy, endodontic treatments, and nerve injuries due to surgical procedures [97, 98]. A mean prevalence of 0.5–12% has been reported for PTTN among the general population and it is known to share similar pathophysiological characteristics with TN, such as burning and paroxysmal, constant, and/or severe pain attacks, which are mostly unilateral (90–95%) [97, 99].

PTTN has been poorly defined and has assumed different or overlapping designations over time, including atypical odontalgia, phantom tooth pain, persistent idiopathic facial pain, painful posttraumatic trigeminal neuropathy, idiopathic toothache, persistent dentoalveolar pain disorder, non-odontogenic tooth pain, and continuous neuropathic orofacial pain. For this reason, the therapeutic information regarding this problem is usually difficult to uncover, becoming a challenge for many practitioners [97].

The American Pain Society and the European Federation of Neurological Societies recommend the use of anticonvulsants, tricyclic antidepressants, inhibitors of serotonin and norepinephrine reuptake, and opioids to control this condition. Moreover, as a kind of neuropathic pain, the response rate to conventional analgesics such as acetaminophen or nonsteroidal anti-inflammatory drugs is usually minimal [98].

The number of studies on the use of BoNT/A for PTTN management is limited and mostly consists of case reports claiming the beneficial effect of this toxin on long-lasting dental pain [100]. One case showed that subcutaneously injected BoNT/A (10 U) improved the existing perception threshold and subjective pain symptoms caused by axonotmesis of the left inferior alveolar nerve with dysesthesia, after placement of dental implants [101]. Another report demonstrated a significant relief of pain in four patients with atypical refractory odontalgia after intraoral injections of BoNT/A (15 to 30 U). One patient was completely pain-free after BoNT/A administration, while the other three reported an intermittent mild pain. No side effects were noted [102]. In two cases of refractory PTTN, BoNT/A was shown to reduce pain frequency and intensity [103]. In the first case, 100 U of the toxin was diluted in lidocaine without vasoconstrictor and applied submucosally into six different intraoral points. A reduction of pain from 5 to 2 on a 0–10 scale was achieved 1–2 weeks following treatment. The patient related a significant improvement after treatment, but at the same time demonstrated transient side effects such as dryness of the injected area and facial asymmetry. In the second case, an individual with a 3-year history of refractory TN, reporting a pain intensity of 10 out of 10, was treated with extra- and intraoral injections of BoNT/A. Results showed a significant reduction of pain with facial asymmetry as a side effect (e.g., patient reported "dropping of her smile"). In this study, BoNT/A was considered as an efficient treatment for refractory PTTN, reducing pain intensity and frequency with minor side effects [103].

There is a lack of strong evidence demonstrating the effectiveness of BoNT/A for the treatment of PTTN. However, histopathologically, there are similarities between PTTN and TN, with the former being more varied and dependent on the degree of the nerve damage. The resemblance between these conditions suggests a possible benefit of the toxin for reducing the accompanying pain and the number of paroxysms experienced by neuropathic patients. Nevertheless, the development of additional clinical studies is encouraged to determine the actual benefit of BoNT/A in relieving PTTN.

Adverse Effects/Reactions of BoNT/A Application on Dentistry-Related Conditions

The reversible effects and the minute doses (in picogram range) used in the different therapeutic indications of BoNT/A make the toxin a generally safe treatment option [3, 104]. Fatal adverse effects due to orofacial treatments with BoNT/A are not reported; however, some minor and moderate side effects and/or adverse events have been described by clinicians and scientists (Table 16.3 and Fig. 16.8).

Minor side effects such as edema, itching, and pain at the injection sites are frequently reported and resolve spontaneously in most cases [104]. The use of topical anesthesia (e.g., EMLA cream) and antibacterial/anti-inflammatory creams on the application sites before/after BoNT/A injections can help reduce these symptoms [105].

Table 16.3 Main adverse effects/events reported after BoNT/A applications for dentistry-related conditions

| Condition | Possible adverse effects/events | | |
	Minor	Moderate	Severe
TMDs	Edema Itching Pain at injection side	Decrease on muscle size Muscle weakness Speech changes Reduced masticatory efficacy	Decrease of trabecular bone density and bone volume
Bruxism	Edema Itching Pain at injection side	Reduced masticatory efficacy Muscle weakness Speech changes	Decrease of trabecular bone density and bone volume
Neuropathic pain	Edema Itching Pain at injection side	Short-term facial asymmetry Undesired muscle paralysis	Not reported
Sialorrhea	Edema Itching Pain at injection side	Undesired muscle paralysis Dysphagia	Not reported

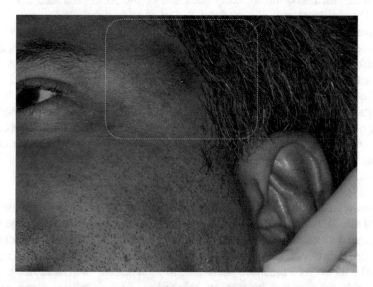

Fig. 16.8 Mild edema after BoNT/A injection into the temporalis muscle

Moreover, mild and transient adverse effects such as undesired muscle paralysis, muscle weakness, changes in speech, swallowing alterations, and chewing difficulties are also frequently reported after BoNT/A injections into the masticatory muscles (i.e., in cases of TMDs, bruxism, and/or masseteric hypertrophy) [36, 106, 107]. From a physiological point of view, the use of high doses and repeated injections of BoNT/A could lead to structural changes and atrophy of muscle fibers, producing a significant decrease in the size of the treated masticatory muscles, affecting mastication efficacy and oral functions of the patients [104]. However, it was demonstrated that injection of low doses of BoNT/A (30 U masseter/10 U temporalis) into masticatory muscles can reduce the pain associated with myogenic TMDs with significantly lower and reversible side effects compared to higher doses (50–75 U masseter/20–25 U temporalis) [24].

Muscle loading is also considered an important factor guiding facial bone growth. Consequently, inducing localized masticatory muscle atrophy could also alter the craniofacial growth and jaw development, as described by different studies conducted in animal and human populations [34, 104, 106, 107]. Bone changes associated with muscle atrophy due to BoNT/A injections in the masseter of rabbits have been described [34]. Furthermore, patients treated with BoNT/A for TMDs and masseter hypertrophy have been reported to show decreased trabecular bone density and bone volume in the mandibular angle area [106, 107]. Unfortunately, there is a lack of clinical trials evaluating the possible effects of repeated injections of high doses of BoNT/A on masticatory muscles, as most of the studies merely present side effects as secondary outcomes [107]. However, this evidence collectively suggests that if multiple injections of the toxins are considered, a careful follow-up for early detection of the aforementioned side effects should be contemplated.

Adverse reactions regarding the therapeutic use of BoNT/A for sialorrhea are not uncommon [87]. Dysphagia and chewing and swallowing difficulties due to the diffusion of the toxin into nearby muscular tissues, especially when applied in submandibular glands, are described as potential risks of the treatment [70, 86, 90]. However, the use of ultrasound to guide BoNT injections can help reduce the magnitude of these effects. Besides, the presence of dry mouth and thickening of saliva were also reported in drooling populations treated with BoNT/A, leading to problems during mastication of solid foods. For all these reasons, the recommendations of the International Consensus Statement for the use of BoNTs in sialorrhea should be carefully considered in order to reduce undesired effects of this toxin [87].

Finally, some general recommendations to avoid possible side effects include a careful attention to drug dilution and handling and storage of the toxin. The use of suggested doses, not exceeding recommended guidelines, reduces the potential of undesired side effects and adverse events. Moreover, the product should be reconstituted with the recommended saline solution; substances such as anesthetic solutions or water may not be used as substitutes. Also, handling errors such as injection of reconstituted products after the expiration date or the use of frozen products should be avoided as it may also help prevent unwanted effects of BoNT/A.

References

1. Hoque A, McAndrew M. Use of botulinum toxin in dentistry. N Y State Dent J. 2009;75:52–5.
2. Jost WH, et al. SIAXI: placebo-controlled, randomized, double-blind study of incobotulinumtoxinA for sialorrhea. Neurology. 2019;92:E1982–91.
3. Muñoz-Lora VRM, Cury AADB, Jabbari B, Lackovic Z. Botulinum Toxin Type A in Dental Medicine. 2019; https://doi.org/10.1177/0022034519875053.
4. De la Torre Canales G, Câmara-Souza MB, do Amaral CF, Garcia RCMR, Manfredini D. Is there enough evidence to use botulinum toxin injections for bruxism management? A systematic literature review. Clin Oral Investig. 2017; https://doi.org/10.1007/s00784-017-2092-4.
5. Morra ME, et al. Therapeutic efficacy and safety of botulinum toxin A therapy in trigeminal neuralgia: a systematic review and meta-analysis of randomized controlled trials. J Headache Pain. 2016;17:63.
6. Safarpour Y, Jabbari B. Botulinum toxin treatment of pain syndromes –an evidence based review. Toxicon. 2018;147:120–8.
7. Romero-Reyes M, Uyanik JM. Orofacial pain management: current perspectives. J Pain Res. 2014;7:99–115.
8. Gronseth G, French J. Invited article: practice parameters and technology assessments: what they are, what they are not, and why you should care. Neurology. 2008;71:1639–43.
9. French J, Gronseth G. Invited article : lost in a jungle of evidence we need a compass. Neurology. 2008;71:1634–8.
10. Manfredini D, Arveda N, Guarda-Nardini L, Segù M, Collesano V. Distribution of diagnoses in a population of patients with temporomandibular disorders. Oral Surg Oral Med Oral Pathol Oral Radiol. 2012;114:e35–41.
11. Muñoz- Lora VRM, De la Torre Canales G, Machado-Gonçalves L, Beraldo-Meloto C, Rizzatti-Barbosa CM. Prevalence of temporomandibular disorders in postmenopausal women and relationship with pain and HRT. Braz Oral Res. 2016;30:e100.
12. De La Torre Canales G, et al. Prevalence of psychosocial impairment in temporomandibular disorder patients: a systematic review. J Oral Rehabil. 2018;45:881–9.
13. Manfredini D, Ahlberg J, Winocur E, Guarda-Nardini L, Lobbezoo F. Correlation of RDC/TMD axis I diagnoses and axis II pain-related disability. A multicenter study. Clin Oral Investig. 2011;15:749–56.
14. Manfredini D, Borella L, Favero L, Ferronato G, Guarda-Nardini L. Chronic pain severity and depression/somatization levels in TMD patients. Int J Prosthodont. 2010;23:529–34.
15. Costa YM, Conti PCR, de Faria FAC, Bonjardim LR. Temporomandibular disorders and painful comorbidities: clinical association and underlying mechanisms. Oral Surg Oral Med Oral Pathol Oral Radiol. 2017;123:288–97.
16. De Laat A, Stappaerts K, Papy S. Counseling and physical therapy as treatment for myofascial pain of the masticatory system. J Orofac Pain. 2003;17:42–9.
17. Conti PCR, et al. Behavioural changes and occlusal splints are effective in the management of masticatory myofascial pain: a short-term evaluation. J Oral Rehabil. 2012;39:754–60.
18. Lackovic Z, Filipovic B, Matak I, Helyes Z. Activity of botulinum toxin type A in cranial dura: implications for treatment of migraine and other headaches. Br J Pharmacol. 2016;173:279–91.
19. Muñoz-Lora VRM, et al. Botulinum toxin type A reduces inflammatory hypernociception induced by arthritis in the temporomadibular joint of rats. Toxicon. 2017;129:52–7.
20. Matak I, Bölcskei K, Bach-rojecky L, Helyes Z. Mechanisms of botulinum toxin type A action on pain. Toxins (Basel). 2019;11:1–24.
21. Kurtoglu C, et al. Effect of botulinum toxin-A in myofascial pain patients with or without functional disc displacement. J Oral Maxillofac Surg. 2008;66:1644–51.
22. Patel AA, Lerner MZ, Blitzer A. IncobotulinumtoxinA injection for temporomandibular joint disorder: a randomized controlled pilot study. Ann Otol Rhinol Laryngol. 2017;126:328–33.

23. Ernberg M, Hedenberg-Magnusson B, List T, Svensson P. Efficacy of botulinum toxin type A for treatment of persistent myofascial TMD pain: a randomized, controlled, double-blind multicenter study. Pain. 2011;152:1988–96.
24. De la Torre Canales G, Alvarez-Pinzon N, Muñoz-Lora VRM, Vieira Peroni L, Farias Gomes A, Sánchez-Ayala A, Haiter-Neto F, Manfredini D, Rizzatti-Barbosa CM. Efficacy and Safety of Botulinum Toxin Type A on Persistent Myofascial Pain: A Randomized Clinical Trial. Toxins (Basel). 2020;12(6):395. https://doi.org/10.3390/toxins12060395.
25. Machado D, et al. Botulinum toxin type A for painful temporomandibular disorders: systematic review and meta-analysis. J Pain. 2019; https://doi.org/10.1016/j.jpain.2019.08.011.
26. Chen YW, Chiu YW, Chen CY, Chuang SK. Botulinum toxin therapy for temporomandibular joint disorders: a systematic review of randomized controlled trials. Int J Oral Maxillofac Surg. 2015;44:1018–26.
27. Hallett M. Explanation of timing of botulinum neurotoxin effects, onset and duration, and clinical ways of influencing them. Toxicon. 2015;107:64–7.
28. Lobbezoo F, et al. International consensus on the assessment of bruxism: report of a work in progress. J Oral Rehabil. 2018;45:837–44.
29. Manfredini D, Colonna A, Bracci A, Lobbezoo F. Bruxism: a summary of current knowledge on etiology, assessment, and management. Oral Surg. 2019:ors.12454. https://doi.org/10.1111/ors.12454.
30. Manfredini D, Ahlberg J, Winocur E, Lobbezoo F. Management of sleep bruxism in adults: a qualitative systematic literature review. J Oral Rehabil. 2015;42:862–74.
31. Jokubauskas L, Baltrušaitytė A, Pileičikienė G. Oral appliances for managing sleep bruxism in adults: a systematic review from 2007 to 2017. J Oral Rehabil. 2017; https://doi.org/10.1111/joor.12558.
32. Silva Gomes Ribeiro CV, Ribeiro-Sobrinho D, Muñoz Lora VRM, Morais Dornellas Bezerra L, Del Bel Cury AA. Association between mandibular advancement device therapy and reduction of excessive daytime sleepiness due to obstructive sleep apnea. J Oral Rehabil. 2019;46:i–i.
33. Redaelli A. Botulinum toxin A in bruxers. One year experience. Saudi Med J. 2011;32:156–8.
34. Rafferty KL, et al. Botulinum toxin in masticatory muscles: short- and long-term effects on muscle, bone, and craniofacial function in adult rabbits. Bone. 2012;50:651–62.
35. Matthys T, Ho Dang HA, Rafferty KL, Herring SW. Bone and cartilage changes in rabbit mandibular condyles after 1 injection of botulinum toxin. Am J Orthod Dentofac Orthop. 2015;148:999–1009.
36. Balanta-Melo J, Toro-Ibacache V, Kupczik K, Buvinic S. Mandibular bone loss after masticatory muscles intervention with botulinum toxin: an approach from basic research to clinical findings. Toxins (Basel). 2019;11:84.
37. Tinastepe N, Kucuk BB, Oral K. Botulinum toxin for the treatment of bruxism. Cranio. 2015;33:291–8.
38. Manfredini D, Winocur E, Guarda-Nardini L, Paesani D, Lobbezoo F. Epidemiology of bruxism in adults: a systematic review of the literature. J Orofac Pain. 2013;27:99–110.
39. Macaluso GM, et al. Sleep bruxism is a disorder related to periodic arousals during sleep. J Dent Res. 1998;77:565–73.
40. Srivastava S, Kharbanda S, Pal U, Shah V. Applications of botulinum toxin in dentistry: a comprehensive review. Natl J Maxillofac Surg. 2015;6:152.
41. Guarda-Nardini L, et al. Efficacy of botulinum toxin in treating myofascial pain in bruxers: a controlled placebo pilot study. Cranio. 2008;26:126–35.
42. Ondo WG, et al. Onabotulinum toxin-A injections for sleep bruxism. Neurology. 2018;90:e559–64.
43. Lee SJ, McCall WD, Kim YK, Chung SC, Chung JW. Effect of botulinum toxin injection on nocturnal bruxism: a randomized controlled trial. Am J Phys Med Rehabil. 2010;89:16–23.
44. Yeh YT, Peng JH, Peng HLP. Literature review of the adverse events associated with botulinum toxin injection for the masseter muscle hypertrophy. J Cosmet Dermatol. 2018;17:675–87.

45. Fedorowicz Z, van Zuuren EJ, Schoones J. Botulinum toxin for masseter hypertrophy. Cochrane Database Syst Rev. 2013;2013 CD007510 https://doi.org/10.1002/14651858. CD007510.pub3
46. Mijiritsky E, et al. Botulinum toxin type a as preoperative treatment for immediately loaded dental implants placed in fresh extraction sockets for full-arch restoration of patients with bruxism. J Craniofac Surg. 2016;27:668–70.
47. Manfredini D, Poggio CE, Lobbezoo F. Is bruxism a risk factor for dental implants? A systematic review of the literature. Clin Implant Dent Relat Res. 2014;16:460–9.
48. Dressler D, Adib Saheri F, Reis Barbosa E. Botulinum toxin: mechanisms of action. Arq Neuropsiquiatr. 2005;63:180–5.
49. Lavigne GJ, et al. Genesis of sleep bruxism: motor and autonomic-cardiac interactions. Arch Oral Biol. 2007;52:381–4.
50. Lavigne GJ, Kato T, Kolta A, Sessle BJ. Neurobiological mechanisms involved in sleep bruxism. Crit Rev Oral Biol Med. 2003;14:30–46.
51. Montano N, et al. Advances in diagnosis and treatment of trigeminal neuralgia. Ther Clin Risk Manag. 2015:11–289. https://doi.org/10.2147/TCRM.S37592.
52. Peker S, Sirin A. Primary trigeminal neuralgia and the role of pars oralis of the spinal trigeminal nucleus. Med Hypotheses. 2017;100:15–8.
53. Hu Y, et al. Therapeutic efficacy and safety of botulinum toxin type A in trigeminal neuralgia: a systematic review. J Headache Pain. 2013;14:72.
54. Wu CJ, et al. Botulinum toxin type A for the treatment of trigeminal neuralgia: results from a randomized, double-blind, placebo-controlled trial. Cephalalgia. 2012;32:443–50.
55. Wu TH, et al. Risk of psychiatric disorders following trigeminal neuralgia: a nationwide population-based retrospective cohort study. J Headache Pain. 2015;16:64.
56. Bowsher D. Trigeminal neuralgia: an anatomically oriented review. Clin Anat. 1997;10:409–15.
57. Cruccu G, Truini A. Refractory trigeminal neuralgia. CNS Drugs. 2013;27:91–6.
58. Durham PL, Cady R, Cady R. Regulation of calcitonin gene-related peptide secretion from trigeminal nerve cells by botulinum toxin type A: implications for migraine therapy. Headache J Head Face Pain. 2004;44:35–43.
59. Kitamura Y, et al. Botulinum toxin type a (150 kDa) decreases exaggerated neurotransmitter release from trigeminal ganglion neurons and relieves neuropathy behaviors induced by infraorbital nerve constriction. Neuroscience. 2009;159:1422–9.
60. Matak I, Bach-Rojecky L, Filipović B, Lacković Z. Behavioral and immunohistochemical evidence for central antinociceptive activity of botulinum toxin A. Neuroscience. 2011;186:201–7.
61. Williamson DJ, Hargreaves RJ. Neurogenic inflammation in the context of migraine. Microsc Res Tech. 2001;53:167–78.
62. Iyengar S, Ossipov MH, Johnson KW. The role of calcitonin gene-related peptide in peripheral and central pain mechanisms including migraine. Pain. 2017;158:543–59.
63. Dasilva AF, Dossantos MF. The role of sensory fiber demography in trigeminal and postherpetic neuralgias. J Dent Res. 2012;91:17–24.
64. Deseure K, Hans GH. Chronic constriction injury of the rat's infraorbital nerve (IoN-CCI) to study trigeminal neuropathic pain. J Vis Exp. 2015;2015:7–9.
65. Vos BP, Strassman AM, Maciewicz RJ. Behavioral evidence of trigeminal neuropathic pain following chronic constriction injury to the rat's infraorbital nerve. J Neurosci. 1994;14:2708–23.
66. Filipović B, Matak I, Bach-Rojecky L, Lacković Z. Central action of peripherally applied botulinum toxin type a on pain and dural protein extravasation in rat model of trigeminal neuropathy. PLoS One. 2012;7:1–8.
67. Zhang H, et al. Two doses of botulinum toxin type A for the treatment of trigeminal neuralgia: observation of therapeutic effect from a randomized, double-blind, placebo-controlled trial. J Headache Pain. 2014;15:1–6.

68. Shehata HS, El-Tamawy MS, Shalaby NM, Ramzy G. Botulinum toxin-type A: could it be an effective treatment option in intractable trigeminal neuralgia? J Headache Pain. 2013;14:92.
69. Dashtipour K, et al. RimabotulinumtoxinB in sialorrhea: systematic review of clinical trials. J Clin Mov Disord. 2017;4:9.
70. Petracca M, et al. Botulinum toxin A and B in sialorrhea: long-term data and literature overview. Toxicon. 2015;107:129–40.
71. Vashishta R, Nguyen SA, White DR, Gillespie MB. Botulinum toxin for the treatment of sialorrhea: a meta-analysis. Otolaryngol - Head Neck Surg (United States). 2013;148:191–6.
72. Lin YC, Shieh JY, Cheng ML, Yang PY. Botulinum toxin type a for control of drooling in Asian patients with cerebral palsy. Neurology. 2008;70:316–8.
73. Restivo D, et al. Botulinum toxin A for Sialorrhoea associated with neurological disorders: evaluation of the relationship between effect of treatment and the number of glands treated. Toxins (Basel). 2018;10:55.
74. Bavikatte G, Lin-Sit P, Hassoon A. Management of Drooling. Br J Med Pract. 2012;5:265–70.
75. Jost WH. The option of sonographic guidance in Botulinum toxin injection for drooling in Parkinson's disease. J Neural Transm. 2016;123:51–5.
76. Pirazzini M, Rossetto O, Eleopra R, Montecucco C. Botulinum neurotoxins: biology, pharmacology, and toxicology. Pharmacol Rev. 2017;69:200–35.
77. Oliveira JB, Evêncio-Neto J, Baratella-Evêncio L. Histological and immunohistochemical findings of the action of botulinum toxin in salivary gland: systematic review. Braz J Biol. 2016;77:251–9.
78. Ellies M, Laskawi R, Götz W, Arglebe C, Tormählen G. Immunohistochemical and morphometric investigations of the influence of botulinum toxin on the submandibular gland of the rat. Eur Arch Oto-Rhino-Laryngol. 1999;256:148–52.
79. Ellies M, Laskawi R, Schütz S, Quondamatteo F. Immunohistochemical evidence of nNOS and changes after intraglandular application of botulinum toxin A in cephalic salivary glands of adult rats. ORL J Otorhinolaryngol Relat Spec. 2003;65:140–3.
80. Ellies M, Laskawi R, Tormählen ‡ G, Götz W. The effect of local injection of botulinum toxin A on the parotid gland of the rat: an immunohistochemical and morphometric study. J Oral Maxillofac Surg. 2000;58:1251–6.
81. Ellies M, Schütz S, Quondamatteo F, Laskawi R. The effect of local injection of botulinum toxin A on the immunoreactivity of nNOS in the rat submandibular gland: an immunohistochemical study. Int J Pediatr Otorhinolaryngol. 2006;70:59–63.
82. Ellies M, Schütz S, Quondamatteo F, Laskawi R. Immunohistochemical investigations of the influence of botulinum toxin A on the immunoreactivity of nNOS in the parotid gland of the rat. J Oral Maxillofac Surg. 2006;64:397–401.
83. Xu H, et al. Pre- and post-synaptic effects of botulinum toxin a on submandibular glands. J Dent Res. 2015;94:1454–62.
84. Shan X-F, Xu H, Cai Z-G, Wu L-L, Yu G-Y. Botulinum toxin A inhibits salivary secretion of rabbit submandibular gland. Int J Oral Sci. 2013;5:217–23.
85. Bushara KO. Sialorrhea in amyotrophic lateral sclerosis: a hypothesis of a new treatment - botulinum toxin A injections of the parotid glands. Med Hypotheses. 1997;48:337–9.
86. Jackson CE, et al. Randomized double-blind study of botulinum toxin type B for sialorrhea in ALS patients. Muscle Nerve. 2009;39:137–43.
87. Reddihough D, Erasmus CE, Johnson H, McKellar GMW, Jongerius PH. Botulinum toxin assessment, intervention and aftercare for paediatric and adult drooling: international consensus statement. Eur J Neurol. 2010;17:109–21.
88. Reid SM, Johnson HM, Reddihough DS. The drooling impact scale: a measure of the impact of drooling in children with developmental disabilities. Dev Med Child Neurol. 2010;52:e23–8.
89. Intiso D. Therapeutic use of botulinum toxin in neurorehabilitation. J Toxicol. 2012;2012:802893.

90. Narayanaswami P, et al. Drooling in Parkinson's disease: a randomized controlled trial of incobotulinum toxin A and meta-analysis of botulinum toxins. Park Relat Disord. 2016;30:73–7.
91. Basciani M, et al. Botulinum toxin type B for sialorrhoea in children with cerebral palsy: a randomized trial comparing three doses. Dev Med Child Neurol. 2011;53:559–64.
92. Mazlan M, et al. A double-blind randomized controlled trial investigating the most efficacious dose of botulinum toxin-A for sialorrhea treatment in asian adults with neurological diseases. Toxins (Basel). 2015;7:3758–70.
93. Scaglione F. Conversion ratio between botox®, dysport®, and xeomin® in clinical practice. Toxins (Basel). 2016;8:65.
94. Bakheit AM, et al. The profile of patients and current practice of treatment of upper limb muscle spasticity with botulinum toxin type A: an international survey. Int J Rehabil Res. 2010;33:199–204.
95. Ondo W, Hunter C, Moore W. A double-blind placebo-controlled trial of botulinum toxin B for sialorrhea in Parkinson's disease. Neurology. 2004;62:37–40.
96. Evangelos A, et al. Volume matters: the influence of different botulinum toxin-A dilutions for sialorrhea in amyotrophic lateral sclerosis. Muscle Nerve. 2013;47:276–8.
97. Rafael B, Sorin T, Eli E. Peripheral painful traumatic trigeminal neuropathy: clinical features in 91 cases and proposal of novel diagnostic criteria. Oral Maxillofac Surg Clin North Am. 2016;28:371–80.
98. Finnerup NB, et al. Pharmacotherapy for neuropathic pain in adults: systematic review, meta-analysis and updated NeuPSIG recommendations. 2016;14:162–73.
99. Benoliel R, Kahn J, Eliav E. Peripheral painful traumatic trigeminal neuropathies. 2012:317–32. https://doi.org/10.1111/j.1601-0825.2011.01883.x.
100. Nathan N, et al. Topical review: potential use of botulinum toxin in the Management of Painful Posttraumatic Trigeminal Neuropathy. J Oral Facial Pain Headache. 2017;31:7–18.
101. Yoon SH, Merrill RL, Choi JH, Kim ST. Use of botulinum toxin type a injection for neuropathic pain after trigeminal nerve injury. Pain Med. 2010;11:630–2.
102. Cuadrado ML, García-Moreno H, Arias JA, Pareja JA. Botulinum neurotoxin type-A for the treatment of atypical odontalgia. Pain Med (United States). 2016;17:1717–21.
103. Herrero Babiloni A, Kapos FP, Nixdorf DR. Intraoral administration of botulinum toxin for trigeminal neuropathic pain. Oral Surg Oral Med Oral Pathol Oral Radiol. 2016;121:e148–53.
104. De la Torre G, et al. Botulinum toxin type A applications for masticatory myofascial pain and trigeminal neuralgia : what is the evidence regarding adverse effects ? Clin Oral Investig. 2019;23:3411–21.
105. Fung S, Phadke CP, Kam A, Ismail F, Boulias C. Effect of topical anesthetics on needle insertion pain during botulinum toxin type A injections for limb spasticity. Arch Phys Med Rehabil. 2012;93:1643–7.
106. Raphael KG, et al. Osteopenic consequences of botulinum toxin injections in the masticatory muscles: a pilot study. J Oral Rehabil. 2014;41:555–63.
107. Lee H-J, Kim S-J, Lee K-J, Yu H-S, Baik H-S. Repeated injections of botulinum toxin into the masseter muscle induce bony changes in human adults: a longitudinal study. Korean J Orthod. 2017;47:222–8.

Chapter 17
Botulinum Toxin Treatment in Veterinary Medicine: Clinical Implications

Helka Heikkilä

Abstract Botulinum toxin (BoNT) products are not licensed for veterinary use, but there are studies investigating its therapeutic potential in veterinary medicine, mainly in dogs and horses. Some efficacy has been reported for BoNT in the treatment of osteoarthritic and perioperative pain in dogs and in the treatment of lameness in horses in small controlled clinical trials. In addition, few case series have described the use of BoNT in the treatment of lower esophageal sphincter achalasia-like syndrome, urinary incontinence, and prostatic hypertrophy in dogs and in stringhalt in horses. Further thoroughly planned controlled clinical trials with objective outcome measures are needed to reveal the true relevance of BoNT in veterinary medicine.

Keywords Botulinum toxin injection · Canine pain therapy · Equine movement disorders · Intra-articular treatment

In contrast to human medicine, the therapeutic potential of botulinum toxin (BoNT) is not fully exploited in veterinary medicine, and BoNT products are not licensed for veterinary use. Conditions characterized by constant painful muscle overactivity, such as dystonias, are rarely seen or treated in animals, and the toxin has mainly been a concern among veterinary professionals due to unwanted events, where spoiled foliage has led to the death of many animals or whole packs [1–3].

However, BoNT has potential in pain therapy of veterinary patients, especially in companion animals. The direct antinociceptive effect of BoNT has been studied in the treatment of osteoarthritic and postoperative pain in dogs, and some evidence supports its use for pain therapy in this species. Additionally, the chemodenervation produced by BoNT might benefit laminitic equine patients in the future.

H. Heikkilä (✉)
Lahden eläinlääkäriasema, IVC Evidensia, Lahti, Finland
e-mail: helka.heikkila@evidensia.fi

© Springer Nature Switzerland AG 2020
B. Jabbari (ed.), *Botulinum Toxin Treatment in Surgery, Dentistry, and Veterinary Medicine*, https://doi.org/10.1007/978-3-030-50691-9_17

BoNT in the Treatment of Canine Osteoarthritis

Osteoarthritis (OA) is considered the leading cause of lameness and chronic pain in dogs. Estimates on its prevalence vary from 2.5% to 20% [4, 5]. In a recent UK study, OA was estimated to affect 200,000 dogs annually [5]. OA causes significant discomfort and pain and impairs the quality of life of the affected animals. As one of the most common reasons for euthanasia in dogs [6], OA also impacts lifespan, especially in working animals [7]. Multimodal treatment consisting of exercise modification, weight management, physiotherapy, nutraceuticals, and pain medication is recommended for OA treatment in dogs. In addition, some osteoarthritic canine patients are eligible for joint prosthesis. The requirement for oral analgesics in osteoarthritic dogs may be lessened by intra-articular (IA) treatment, which directly targets the painful joint.

IA-injected botulinum neurotoxin A (BoNT-A) has shown some efficacy in the treatment of osteoarthritic pain in dogs. Hadley et al. (2010) were the first to describe the effects of IA BoNT-A in dogs [8]. They conducted a pilot study lasting 12 weeks on five client-owned dogs with elbow or hip OA. All dogs received an IA injection of 25 U of onabotulinumtoxinA (Botox, Allergan Inc., USA) into the osteoarthritic joint. The response to treatment was assessed by measuring the ground reaction forces, i.e., weight-bearing, with a pressure platform. In addition, the owners graded their dog's locomotion and discomfort.

The ground reaction forces of the treated limbs improved in all dogs for a variable period of time, but remained inferior to those of the contralateral limbs, implying that the dogs remained somewhat lame. Two owners reported significant improvement, while moderate improvement, mild improvement, or no change was reported in the other three dogs at the end of the study. A mild increase in lameness in addition to redness and swelling over the injected joint was detected in two dogs. No other adverse events were detected during the study.

Although this was a small preliminary study without any control group, the improvement detected in the ground reaction forces was encouraging. There are no direct ways to measure pain in animals, and therefore, canine pain evaluation is based on the lack of normal behavior or on the presence of pain-associated behavior such as lameness. Measuring weight-bearing is an objective, quantitative, and unbiased method to evaluate lameness in dogs [9, 10].

The efficacy of IA BoNT-A injections in the treatment of chronic osteoarthritic pain was further investigated by Heikkilä et al. in 2014 in a placebo-controlled, randomized, double-blinded clinical study on 35 client-owned osteoarthritic dogs with chronic lameness due to OA in the stifle, elbow, or hip joint [11]. The dogs were randomized to receive either an IA injection of 30 U of onabotulinumtoxinA or placebo (saline) into the painful osteoarthritic joint. The primary outcome variables were ground reaction forces measured with a force plate and the Helsinki

Chronic Pain Index (HCPI), a questionnaire for dog owners validated for the evaluation of chronic canine orthopedic pain [12]. The subjective pain score evaluated by a veterinarian and the need for rescue analgesia were used as secondary outcome variables. The study lasted 12 weeks.

In BoNT-A-treated dogs, a significant improvement was detected in the ground reaction forces at the end of the study (week 12), while no change was observed in the dogs treated with placebo (Fig. 17.1). There was also a significant improvement from baseline in the HCPI of the dogs treated with BoNT-A, but not in the dogs

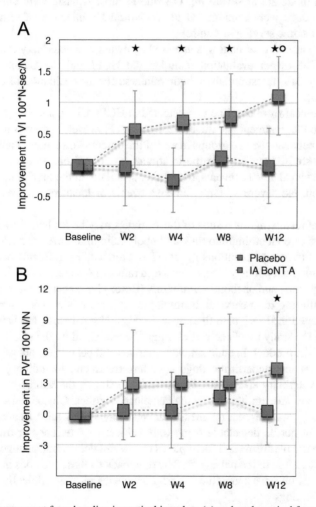

Fig. 17.1 Improvement from baseline in vertical impulses (**a**) and peak vertical forces (**b**) (mean and 95% CI) after intra-articular botulinum toxin A (*n* = 16) or intra-articular placebo (*n* = 15) in osteoarthritic dogs. Baseline, before the injections; IA BoNT A intra-articular botulinum toxin A; placebo, 0.9% saline, PVF peak vertical force, VI vertical impulse, W week. °*P* ≤ 0.005 between groups; ★*P* ≤ 0.05 within group. (Reprinted from the Heikkilä et al. [11], Elsevier (2014), with permission from Elsevier)

treated with placebo. The duration of the treatment effect could not be evaluated, since the effect was the largest at the end of the study.

No severe adverse events were detected. One dog developed a superficial skin infection over the injected hip joint 1 week after BoNT-A injection, and another one developed a mild disc protrusion during the study.

A more recent study by Nicacio et al. in 2019 investigated the efficacy of another botulinum toxin A preparation, IA abobotulinumtoxinA (Dysport, Ipsen Pharmaceuticals, Ireland), in the treatment of hip OA in 16 client-owned dogs [13]. Dogs with moderate or severe hip OA due to hip dysplasia were enrolled in the study. The dogs were randomized to receive an IA injection of either 25 U of BoNT-A or saline serving as control.

The response to treatment was assessed by owner and veterinary evaluations for 90 days. The owner evaluation included the HCPI and the Canine Brief Pain Inventory (CBPI) questionnaires, both validated for the evaluation of chronic pain in dogs [14].

Improvement from baseline was detected in HCPI, CBPI, and veterinary evaluation in both the treatment and the control groups. However, there was no significant difference between the two groups in any of the outcome measures at any time point during the study. Four dogs in the treatment group and one in the control group experienced local adverse events, not further specified, in the first 24 hours after the IA injection. No severe systemic adverse events or local muscle weakness were detected.

The conflict among the results of these studies may be explained by the fact that the dosages of onabotulinumtoxinA and abobotulinumtoxinA are not interchangeable. The different preparations of BoNT-A produced by different manufacturers differ in biological potency [15]. Conversion ratios of 4:1 and 3:1 for abobotulinumtoxinA (Dysport) and onabotulinumtoxinA (Botox) have been suggested for human patients suffering from cervical dystonia [15, 16], but this conversion ratio has not been evaluated in BoNT pain therapy or in dogs. Nevertheless, the lack of clinical efficacy in the study by Nicacio et al. might be explained by the smaller biological potency of the product. In addition, veterinarians and pet owners are prone to detect improvement in osteoarthritic dogs after any treatment, including placebo [17]; therefore, veterinary and owner assessments, including the validated owner questionnaires, are susceptible to a caregiver placebo effect. Objective outcome measures such as weight-bearing measurements may reveal mild treatment effects, which might not be detectable using only subjective veterinary or owner evaluations. Pressure platforms and force plates can detect very subtle changes in weight-bearing not visible to the naked eye. The drawback of these methods is that there is no consensus on what magnitude of improvement indicates clinically meaningful pain relief in dogs.

Despite several studies on IA BoNT in human patients [18], there is not much information on the possible adverse effects of the toxin inside the joint. Therefore,

Heikkilä and colleagues aimed to investigate whether the toxin affects the canine cartilage and whether it spreads from the joint after the IA injection [19]. They conducted a longitudinal, placebo-controlled, randomized clinical trial in six healthy laboratory Beagle dogs. The dogs were randomized to receive an IA injection of 30 U of onabotulinumtoxinA into the right or left stifle joint. An equivalent volume of saline serving as placebo was injected into the contralateral joint. The dogs were evaluated for clinical and cytological adverse effects and for spread of the toxin for 12 weeks. After 12 weeks the dogs were euthanized, the injected joints and the adjacent muscles and nerves were evaluated histologically, and autopsy was performed.

No clinical, cytological, or histological adverse effects were reported during the study. The electrophysiological recordings showed low compound muscle action potentials in two dogs in the BoNT-A-injected limb, suggesting that the toxin had spread from the joint. However, the clinical impact of such spread seemed to be low because the abnormalities detected in the electrophysiological recordings were not associated with any clinically meaningful neurological deficit. Autopsy and histopathological examinations of the joint and adjacent muscles and nerves did not reveal changes associated with IA BoNT-A.

BoNT as Adjuvant Surgical Pain Treatment in Dogs

Many dogs not intended for breeding are neutered. In addition, dogs undergo surgery for orthopedic and traumatic conditions and for neoplasia. Surgery in veterinary medicine has become less traumatic and invasive, and many procedures can be performed laparoscopically. On the other hand, especially in veterinary oncology, more extensive and complex surgeries are being performed. Meanwhile, perioperative pain management has greatly developed in recent years. The understanding of pain in animals and its consequences on the patients has deepened, and the monitoring of anesthesia has improved considerably, due to the availability of better equipment characterized by a broader spectrum. This has led to the use of a wider range of analgesic agents and methods. Current perioperative pain management can be a complex combination of constant-rate infusions and sedative, inductive, and inhalation agents, in addition to local analgesia and nerve blocks and non-steroidal antiinflammatory drugs.

It is not surprising, in this context, that also BoNT injections have been studied in the treatment of perioperative pain in dogs. Vilhegas et al. (2015) conducted a placebo-controlled, randomized, blinded study on the efficacy of BoNT-A injections in the treatment of perioperative pain [20]. Sixteen client-owned, middle-aged to old bitches of various breeds and sizes with malignant mammary gland tumors requiring bilateral chain mastectomy were enrolled in the study. The dogs were randomized to receive either a total dose of 7 U/kg of abobotulinumtoxinA divided into each mammary gland or injections of sterile saline as control. The injections were performed in the middle of each mammary gland 24 hours before surgery. Postoperative pain was evaluated by the modified Glasgow Composite Measure Pain Scale (modified-GCMPS) and the visual analogue scale (VAS) up to 72 hours after surgery. The modified-GCMPS is a validated questionnaire for veterinary professionals to evaluate postoperative pain in dogs based on pain-associated behavior [21]. Rescue analgesia was administered depending on the modified-GCMPS and VAS scores.

BoNT-A injections appeared effective in reducing postoperative pain, as the modified-GCMPS and VAS scores were significantly lower in the BoNT-A group compared with the control group. In addition, the need for rescue analgesia differed between the groups: In the BoNT-A group, two out of eight dogs needed rescue analgesia (two doses of rescue analgesia in total), compared with seven out of eight dogs in the control group (17 doses in total). The histopathological tumor classification, the number and size of the nodules, and the degree of inflammation did not differ between the groups. No adverse events were noted during the study, which ended at the time of suture removal, 10–14 days after the surgery.

This study presents a promising addition to multimodal perioperative pain therapy in dogs undergoing bilateral chain mastectomy, or possibly other invasive surgeries. In this study, the dogs were premedicated with BoNT-A injections into the center of the mammary gland 24 hours before surgery, although in a similar study on human breast cancer patients the toxin was injected intramuscularly during surgery [22]. Layeeque et al. proposed that the pain-relieving efficacy of BoNT-A injections in their study was mediated by the inhibition of pectoralis muscle spasms. In the study by Vilhegas et al., the mechanism of action was suggested to be the inhibition of neuropeptide release from afferent nociceptive nerve endings. Because the mammary glands were removed in the surgery, the toxin probably exerted its effects in the central nervous system rather than in the periphery. BoNT molecules have been shown to undergo retrograde transport via the axon from the peripheral nerve ending into the cell soma and to bridge synapses while preserving their activity [23, 24].

Bringing the dog to the clinic for premedication before surgery might be inconvenient for some dog owners. However, premedication with BoNT-A could be considered as an adjuvant pain therapy, especially for dogs in which nonsteroidal anti-inflammatory drugs are contraindicated.

Application of BoNT as Paralytic Agents in Dogs

Paralytic agents are seldom used in veterinary patients. Conditions leading to painful muscle overactivity are rare, and severely disabled animals are euthanized to spare them further suffering. There are no controlled studies on the paralytic effects of BoNT in animals, but a few case series and case reports have been published. In addition, two case series have exploited the toxin's anticholinergic effects in the treatment of lower urinary tract disease and ptyalism in dogs.

A recent retrospective case series described the use of BoNT-A in the treatment of lower esophageal sphincter achalasia-like syndrome (LES-AS) in 14 client-owned dogs [25]. The main clinical sign was regurgitation, and almost all the dogs had megaesophagus. A condition resembling human lower esophageal achalasia was diagnosed. All dogs were treated with mechanical dilatation of the lower esophageal sphincter following injections of BoNT-A. A total of 32 U of onabotulinum-toxinA was injected in the lower esophageal sphincter area. The dogs were presented for follow-up at a median of 21 days after treatment. The body weight of the dogs had markedly increased, the frequency of regurgitation reported by the owner was significantly reduced, and all owners reported subjective clinical improvement. Megaesophagus was not resolved and there were no changes in esophageal motility, but gastric filling had improved, explaining the clinical improvement. However, the median duration of the effect was only 40 days. Six dogs were further surgically treated. Two complications were reported after BoNT-A injections. One dog developed aspiration pneumonia and another developed gastroduodenal-esophageal intussusception and hiatal hernia requiring surgical treatment.

BoNT-A injections combined with mechanical dilatation thus appeared to be effective in the treatment of dogs suffering from LES-AS, but the short duration of the effect, which would require repeated procedures, was considered disappointing. The authors suggested that the response to BoNT treatment could be used to select the LES-AS patients which would benefit from surgery and that repeated BoNT injections could be used to allow the animals to grow before the definitive surgical treatment. It is not known how much of the improvement was due to the BoNT-A injections rather than to mechanical dilatation.

Three case reports describe the use of BoNT as a paralytic agent in dogs. Rogatko et al. (2016) reported a case in which repeated BoNT-A injections were successfully used for the treatment of neuromyotonia and myokymia in a dog [26]. The case was a five-year-old Maltese dog suffering from persistent muscle contractions and involuntary continuous muscle activity in the right thigh after receiving radiation therapy. The condition was refractory to conventional treatment. The affected muscles were injected with a total dose of 24 U of onabotulinumtoxinA, resulting in the resolution of the clinical signs in 10 days. The injections were successfully repeated at 3- to 4-month intervals for more than a year without adverse effects.

Another case report describes the use of BoNT injections to treat severe myoclonus in a 13-month-old mixed-breed midsized dog suffering from canine distemper encephalomyelitis [27]. It had developed tetraparesis and severe, debilitating myoclonus 8 months after the owner had found it in poor condition. After several other treatment methods had failed, a total amount of 100 U of onabotulinumtoxinA was injected into the most affected muscles. The procedure was repeated with 140 U of BoNT-A 18 days afterwards, after which the clinical signs subsided for several months: The dog was reported to be ambulatory and able to run long distances 180 days after the injections. The dog had an episode of hyperthermia and weakness of the thoracic limbs 15 days after the second injection, which were thought to be adverse events caused by the toxin. However, the weakness rapidly resolved within 2 days.

Rinaldi et al. (2014) described a case in which onabotulinumtoxinA injection was used to treat delayed gastric emptying in an Australian Shepherd which had developed functional gastric outflow obstruction after several surgeries due to bile leakage and peritonitis [28]. A total amount of 400 U of onabotulinumtoxinA (91 U/kg) was injected into the pylorus in a laparoscopically assisted procedure. Both the dog's condition and its gastric emptying were improved after the injections, but euthanasia due to pancreatitis was performed 11 days afterwards. Pancreatitis was most likely a consequence of the primary condition of the dog, but diffusion of the toxin into the pancreas could not be excluded. Despite the final undesirable outcome, the authors argued that BoNT-A injection as a potential therapeutic modality for pyloric spasm warrants further investigation.

Treatment of blepharospasm was one of the first indications for BoNT injections in medicine [29]. Despite this, only one case report describes the use of BoNT injections to treat this condition in a dog [30]. A total amount of 200 U of abobotulinumtoxinA was injected into the orbicularis oculi muscle of both eyes of a 3-year-old Great Dane suffering from bilateral essential blepharospasm refractory to conventional treatment. Improvement in the condition was evident within 3 days, and the spasms were reported to have completely disappeared 6 days after treatment. In the following 3 years, the dog received repeated injections at 3- to 4-month intervals.

In addition to dogs, one case report is available in which BoNT injections were used to treat congenital right hind limb arthrogryposis in a cat (2007) [31]. An 11-week-old cat was presented to a veterinarian for congenital right tarsal deformity and non-weight-bearing lameness. The cat received 20 U of onabotulinumtoxinA into the spastic right gastrocnemius muscle. Despite this treatment, the cat did not start to bear weight on the limb, and the condition was then successfully treated with surgery. This was the first report to describe the use of BoNTs in cats.

BoNT Injections in Lower Urinary Tract Disorders in Dogs

BoNT injections are considered effective in the treatment of lower urinary tract disorders such as neurogenic detrusor overactivity and non-neurogenic overactive bladder in human patients [32, 33]. The effects of intramuscularly injected BoNT in the bladder are thought to be produced by inhibition of the nociceptive and parasympathetic pathways, because its receptor and intracellular target proteins are not expressed in urothelial or bladder muscular cells [34].

The use of BoNT injections in dogs with lower urinary tract disease has been described. Lew et al. published a prospective case series in which BoNT injection was used to treat urinary incontinence in 11 client-owned bitches in 2010 [35]. The dogs suffered from clinical urinary incontinence with no detectable underlying reasons. The dogs represented various breeds and were aged 2–8 years. Nine of the dogs were neutered. The dogs were treated with 50–100 U of onabotulinumtoxinA, depending on the size of the animal. The toxin was injected submucosally into the bladder wall in a cystoscopic procedure. The evaluation of the treatment effect was left to the dog owners. One dog did not respond to treatment, while urinary incontinence decreased in all the other dogs, for a variable time period, in their owners' assessment. The duration of the treatment effect ranged from 1 to 13 months, the average being 5 months. Although controlled studies with objective outcome measures should be conducted, BoNT injections might provide an alternative treatment for dogs suffering from urinary incontinence refractory to conventional treatment.

A case series describing the effect of intraprostatic BoNT injections in the treatment of benign prostatic hyperplasia in dogs [36] is also available. Eight client-owned, intact, midsized, and middle-aged male dogs were included in the study. All dogs had clinical signs of benign prostatic hyperplasia such a hematuria, urethral bleeding, or constipation, and their prostate was enlarged. A total 250 U of onabotulinumtoxinA was injected into the prostate of the dogs, equally divided between the two lobes. The treatment effect was evaluated up to 16 weeks after treatment. In addition, semen was collected before and after the procedure.

Urethral bleeding resolved in all dogs and hematuria in all but one. The duration of the effect was not reached in the 16-week study. Two dogs that suffered from constipation before the injection did not show clinical improvement regarding this clinical sign. The prostatic diameter or volume did not change significantly from the baseline values. Interestingly, the treatment had no effect on the libido of the dogs, nor on the quality of their semen. Two dogs were allowed to mate successfully after the injection. No abnormalities were detected in the following pregnancy, gestation duration, or litter size.

Benign prostatic hyperplasia is a very common condition among older intact male dogs, affecting 80% of those over 5 years of age [37]. It is best treated by castration, although androgen suppression therapy is also commonly used if castration is declined by the dog owner or if anesthesia is contraindicated. This case series suggests that BoNT injection might be considered an alternative treatment for breeding male dogs suffering from benign prostatic hyperplasia. However, in a recent meta-analysis in human patients, BoNT injection showed no benefit over placebo in the treatment of benign prostatic hyperplasia in men, and the clinical efficacy of BoNT injections detected in previous studies has been attributed to a marked placebo effect [38].

One paper presents a dog in which severe ptyalism was successfully treated with BoNT-A injections into both mandibular salivary glands [39]. The dog was an

11-year-old Collie with ptyalism due to difficulty in swallowing because of esophageal adenocarcinoma. Ptyalism was reported to be decreased after the injections for the 12 weeks until the animal was euthanized. However, assessing the treatment effect of the toxin is difficult, because in addition to BoNT injection, an esophageal stent was placed at the same time to improve swallowing and relieve the mass effect produced by the carcinoma in the esophageal lumen.

BoNT injections have also been studied in dogs for application to human therapy of several disorders, including the induction of ptosis [40] and cricothyroid muscle paralysis [41], the reduction of prostatic contractility [42] and parasympathetic activation of the heart [43], the inhibition of biliary leakage [44], and the reduction of salivary gland [45] and nasal secretions [46].

BoNTs in Equine Veterinary Medicine

A few publications describe the use of BoNT in equine medicine. From the veterinary point of view, equids and companion animals differ in the aim of the treatment. In addition to reducing the amount of suffering of the individual animal, the aim of treatment in equids is often to fully recover the previous level of performance. Not reaching this aim might lead to economic loss for the owner and euthanasia of the animal. Perhaps the most promising studies investigate BoNT as adjuvant to laminitis pain therapy in horses, and one controlled study exploits the direct antinociceptive effects of BoNT in the treatment of horse lameness.

Laminitis is a common debilitating condition in equids, affecting approximately 1.5–24% of the equine population [47] and resulting in economic loss in the horse industry and discomfort and pain, lameness, loss of performance, and euthanasia of the affected animals. For long, laminitis was considered a dreaded consequence of severe systemic inflammation or, more rarely, of mechanical overload on the affected limb [48]. However, endocrinopathies such as pituitary pars media dysfunction and hyperinsulinemia associated with equine metabolic syndrome have recently been shown to be the leading causes of laminitis in equids [49]. Laminitis is characterized by the disruption of the lamellar tissue between the distal phalanx and the epidermis of the keratinized hoof wall. In a healthy animal, this lamellar region attaches the distal phalanx to the hoof capsule, resisting the pull of the deep digital flexor tendon attached to the caudal aspect of the distal phalanx. The disruption of this tissue results in pain, separation of the distal phalanx from the hoof wall, and displacement of the distal phalanx inside the hoof capsule [50, 51].

Equine laminitis remains a therapeutic challenge for veterinarians. The aim of the treatment is to treat the underlying causative factor, provide analgesia, and prevent further lamellar damage and displacement of the distal phalanx. Treatment depends on the underlying etiology and includes diagnosis and treatment of the underlying cause, pain and anti-inflammatory medication, exercise restriction, digital hypothermia, therapeutic orthotics and shoeing, and dietary modification [52].

Deep digital flexor tendon tenotomy has been reported to provide pain relief and improve prognosis in horses with chronic laminitis refractory to medical treatment [53]. The purpose of this procedure is to reduce the pull of the deep digital flexor tendon on the distal phalanx and prevent its displacement. With a similar aim, Carter and Reinfoe (2009) published a case series of seven laminitic horses in which the deep digital flexor muscle was chemically denervated with BoNT injections [50]. The horses were client-owned, suffering from acute or chronic laminitis, and of various ages and breeds. They received injections of 100–200 U of onabotulinumtoxinA into the deep digital flexor muscle of either one or both front limbs. The horses' response to treatment was followed for a period ranging from 6 weeks to 3 years. The injections resulted in improvement in the condition of six of the seven horses, most becoming pasture-sound and one becoming pain-free during riding in all gaits. One horse was euthanized 6 weeks after the injections because of persistent pain. No adverse events were reported.

The effects of BoNT-A on the deep digital flexor muscle were further investigated by both Wijnberg and Hardeman in 2013 [54, 55]. They showed with quantitative needle electromyography that BoNT-A injections reduce the activity of the deep digital flexor muscle in healthy horses, without systemic toxicity. In addition, Hardeman et al. reported that such chemodenervation does not cause lameness or change the weight distribution in the hoof of healthy horses, as iatrogenic gait abnormalities would prevent the use of this novel treatment in laminitis. There is some evidence of increased muscle force in the deep digital flexor muscle of laminitic ponies and horses [56]. Thus, reducing this force with BoNT injections might provide a safe, noninvasive, and reversible adjuvant treatment of laminitis. However, the clinical efficacy of this treatment remains to be investigated in a controlled prospective study in laminitic equine patients.

Wijnberg has also studied the efficacy of BoNT injections in two Dutch warmblood dressage horses suffering from stringhalt in 2009 [57]. Stringhalt is an uncommon horse gait abnormality characterized by the spasmodic hyperflexion of one or both tarsi while walking [58]. Systemic anticonvulsants have been proposed as a medical treatment, and surgical treatment consisting of lateral digital extensor tendon myotenectomy has resulted in improvement [59, 60]. Wijnberg and colleagues injected a total amount of 700 U of onabotulinumtoxinA into the hind limbs of the two horses in four separate occasions in 28 days. Hyperflexion and adduction were reduced in the affected hind limbs for approximately 12 weeks, but the gait abnormality was not totally abolished.

In addition to these results, the effect of a different BoNT serotype, botulinum neurotoxin B (BoNT-B), has been studied on anal pressure in healthy adult horses [61]. Reducing the anal tone is thought to be beneficial in the repair of perianal lacerations in mares after parturition. Seven horses received injections of rimabotulinumtoxinB (Myobloc, Solstice Neurosciences, USA) to their external anal sphincter and five received saline injections as control. One horse received 2500 U, while the others received 500–1500 U of BoNT-B. Anal pressure was monitored with a custom-made probe for up to 168 days after the injection. The treatment resulted in a 38–89% reduction in anal pressure, depending on the amount injected.

The greatest reduction was measured in the horse receiving 2500 U (4.4 U/kg), 15 days after treatment, after which anal pressure gradually increased to normal levels in 151 days. However, the same horse developed clinical signs of generalized botulism 10 days after the injection, including generalized weakness, low head carriage, diarrhea, and dysphagia, which resolved 24 days after the injection. The other horses did not experience clinical adverse effects.

Although BoNT injections reduced the anal pressure in healthy horses in this study, no studies have investigated how much BoNT injections benefit mares suffering from perineal lacerations. This study emphasizes the fact that generalized botulism may be a concern when using BoNT injections in horses, which are among the species most sensitive to botulism [62].

Two controlled studies investigated the direct pain-relieving effect of BoNT injection in horses. Gutierrez-Nibeyro and colleagues (2013) published a study on BoNT-B injections in the treatment of lameness due to degenerative injury of the podotrochlear apparatus in 2014 [63]. The podotrochlear apparatus consists of the navicular bone and the associated soft tissue structures in the hoof region. Injury to these structures can result in acute or chronic front limb pain. Oral and intra-articular anti-inflammatory drugs, controlled exercise, corrective shoeing, and extracorporeal shockwave therapy have been used for the treatment of chronic lameness due degenerative injury to the podotrochlear apparatus [64, 65]. Still, the majority fail to recover their previous level of performance [65]. Interestingly, the pain in the soft tissue structures of the podotrochlear apparatus is mediated by nerve fibers containing substance P, calcitonin gene-related peptide, and neurokinin-A [66], all neuropeptides inhibited by BoNT. In the study by Gutierrez-Nibeyro et al. (2013), seven client-owned Quarter Horses suffering from chronic, bilateral, degenerative injury to the podotrochlear apparatus received an injection of BoNT-B into the navicular bursa. The limb with more severe lameness was treated, while the ipsilateral limb was not injected and served as control. RimabotulinumtoxinB at 3.8–4.5 U/kg was injected into the navicular bursa. The response to treatment was evaluated by veterinarians assessing lameness from video recordings in random order over 14 days. Lameness severity significantly decreased from baseline in the treated limbs. However, despite this improvement, the horses remained lame. The authors speculated that this might have resulted from a too small dosage of BoNT-B or the fact that the pain did not arise exclusively from the navicular bursa. The control limbs were not injected, and therefore, it is not certain whether the reduction in lameness was produced by BoNT or by the injection itself.

In addition, the antinociceptive efficacy of IA BoNT-A has been studied in acute synovitis in four healthy experimental horses with somewhat surprising results [67]. Two horses received 50 U of onabotulinumtoxinA into the middle carpal joint of both limbs, while two horses serving as controls received injections of saline. Acute synovitis was induced with interleukin-1 β (IL-1β) injection into one of the injected joints of each horse 14 days afterwards, while the other injected joint served as control and received an injection of saline. The antinociceptive efficacy of BoNT-A was evaluated by veterinary evaluation and by a computer-assisted kinematic analysis of lameness after the IL-1β injection. The horses were euthanized 15 days after the start of the study and the injected joints were histopathologically evaluated.

Both the control horses developed prominent front limb lameness after the IL-1β injection. Interestingly, only one of the BoNT-A-treated horses developed lameness, while the other remained sound. Suppurative inflammation was detected in the histopathological examination of the synovia in all IL-1β-injected joints. No abnormal findings were noted in the joints injected with BoNT-A but not IL-1β. No adverse events were detected during the study.

The results of this study were surprising, as one horse responded to BoNT-A very well, while the other did not respond, although both had developed synovitis after the IL-1β injection. The discrepancy in the treatment response was not further explained in this study due to the small sample size.

Conclusion

Only a few controlled studies and some case series have assessed the benefit of BoNT injections in veterinary medicine, and these are summarized in Tables 17.1 and 17.2. As so often in this discipline, the number of animals in these studies is small, and many include only subjective outcome measures. The veterinary clinician might be tempted to extrapolate study results from human medicine. However, different species differ in sensitivity to different BoNT serotypes [68]. Even in the same species and with a single BoNT serotype, different biological potency has been reported between different BoNT preparations provided by different manufacturers [15]. Therefore, further thoroughly planned controlled clinical trials with objective outcome measures are needed to reveal the true relevance of BoNT in veterinary medicine.

Table 17.1 Controlled clinical trials on BoNT in veterinary patients

Category	Animals	Treatment	Control	Outcome measures	Study period	Results
Treatment of OA pain in dogs [13]	16 client-owned dogs with hip OA BoNT-A group: Age 6.3 Y (3.9 Y) Mean (SD) Weight 25.1 kg (12.7 kg) Control group: Age 4.6 Y (2.3 Y) Weight 24 kg (7.8 kg)	IA injection of 25 U of BoNT-A (Dysport) N = 8	IA injection of saline N = 8	HCPI, CBPI, veterinary evaluation	12 W	No difference between groups in improvement in HCPI or CBPI No adverse events

(continued)

Table 17.1 (continued)

Category	Animals	Treatment	Control	Outcome measures	Study period	Results
Postoperative pain treatment in dogs [20]	16 client-owned dogs with mammary gland tumors BoNT-A group Age 8.75 Y (3 Y) Mean (SD) Weight 13 kg (8 kg) Control group: Age 16 Y (12 Y) Weight 9.5 kg (2 kg)	Injection of 7 U/kg of BoNT-A (Botox) into mammary glands $N = 8$	Injection of saline into mammary glands $N = 8$	Modified GCMPS, VAS, rescue analgesia	10–14 D	Significantly less pain in BoNT-A group compared to control group No adverse events
Treatment of OA pain in dogs [11]	35 client-owned dogs with chronic stifle, hip, or elbow OA Age 6.3 Y (3.2 Y) Mean (SD) Weight 33.1 kg (8.8 kg) Various breeds	IA injection of 30 U of BoNT-A (Botox) $N = 16$	IA injection of saline $N = 15$	Ground reaction forces, HCPI, veterinary evaluation, rescue analgesics used	12 W	Significant improvement in BoNT-A group compared to control group and baseline. Local skin infection over injection site 1/35 dogs, disc protrusion 1/35 dogs
Treatment of chronic pain in horses [63]	7 client-owned horses with bilateral degenerative injury to podotrochlear apparatus Age 11 Y (5–14 Y) median (range) Weight 553 kg (490–590 kg)	Injection of 3.8–4.5 U/kg of BoNT-B (Myobloc) into the navicular bursa $N = 7$	Injection of saline into the navicular bursa, contralateral limb $N = 7$	Veterinary evaluation of lameness from video recordings	14 D	Significantly less lameness in BoNT-A treated limbs compared to saline-treated limbs No adverse events

BoNT-A botulinum toxin A, *CBPI* Canine Brief Pain Inventory, *D* day, *HCPI* the Helsinki Chronic Pain Index, *IA* intra-articular, *modified-GCMS* modified Glasgow Composite Measure Pain Scale, *OA* osteoarthritis, *VAS* visual analogue scale, *W* week, *Y* year

Table 17.2 Case series on BoNT in veterinary patients

Category	Study method	Animals	Treatment	Outcome measures	Study period	Results
Treatment of ME and LES-AS in dogs [25]	Retrospective	14 client-owned dogs with ME and LES-AS Age 2 Y (0.9–5.8 Y) median (IQR) Various breeds	Injection of 32 U of BoNT-A (Botox) into the esophageal sphincter and mechanical dilatation	Clinical severity evaluated by owner, BW, BCS, regurgitation frequency, VFSS parameters	3.5 M (2–4.8 M) median (IQR)	Clinical severity, BW, and BCS improved, regurgitation decreased in all dogs, gastric filling improved in 12/14 dogs No improvement in ME. Duration of effect 40 D (17–53 D) median (IQR) Aspiration pneumonia in 1/14 dogs, intussusception and hiatal hernia in 1/14 dogs
Treatment of prostatic hypertrophy in dogs [36]	Prospective	8 client-owned intact male dogs with benign prostatic hypertrophy Age 5.8 Y (2.1 Y) mean (SD) Weight 18.4 kg (8.2 kg)	Injection of 250 U of BoNT-A (Botox) into the prostate	Clinical signs evaluated by owner, prostatic size and volume evaluated by radiography, ultrasonography, and retrograde urethrocystography, semen analysis, serum DHT and testosterone concentration	16 W	Clinical signs resolved or decreased in all dogs No significant change in prostatic size or volume Semen quality was preserved No change in DHT or testosterone concentration No adverse events

(continued)

Table 17.2 (continued)

Category	Study method	Animals	Treatment	Outcome measures	Study period	Results
Treatment of urinary incontinence in dogs [35]	Prospective	11 client-owned bitches with urinary incontinence Age range 2–8 Y 9/11 neutered Various breeds	Injection of 50–100 U of BoNT-A (Botox) into the bladder wall	Clinical signs evaluated by owner, hematology, serum biochemistry, urine analysis	1–13 M	Urinary incontinence resolved for a variable time period in 10/11 dogs Mean duration of treatment effect 5 M No adverse events
Treatment of chronic OA pain in dogs [8]	Prospective	5 client-owned dogs with elbow or hip OA Age 11 Y (5–15 Y) median (range) Weight 27.1 kg (1.7–43.0 kg)	IA injection of 25 U of BoNT-A (Botox)	Ground reaction forces, clinical signs evaluated by owner	12 W	Variable improvement in ground reaction forces in all dogs Improvement in owner evaluation in 4/5 dogs Mild redness and pain over injection site in 2 dogs
Treatment of laminitis in horses [50]	Not specified	7 client-owned horses with laminitis Age 12 Y (8–23 Y) Median (range) Various breeds	Injection of 100–200 U of BoNT-A (Botox) into the deep digital flexor muscle in one or both front limbs	Obel grading by veterinarian	6 W–3 Y	Pain decreased and Obel grading improved in 6/7 horses 1/7 horses euthanized No adverse events

| Treatment of stringhalt in horses [57] | Prospective | 2 dressage horses with neurogenic, idiopathic stringhalt in one hindlimb. Age 6 Y and 3 Y. Weight 565 kg and 637 kg | Injection of total amount of 700 U of BoNT-A (Botox) into hindlimb muscles in 4 occasions within 28 D | Veterinary evaluation. Automated kinematic gait analysis system. Semiquantitative sEMG analysis | 12 W | Stringhalt signs decreased in both horses. Reduction in sEMG signals. Duration of effect 12 W |

BCS body condition score, *BoNT-A* botulinum neurotoxin A, *BW* body weight, *D* day, *IA* intra-articular, *LES-AS* lower esophageal achalasia-like syndrome, *ME* megaesophagus, *M* month, *OA* osteoarthritis, *sEMG* surface electromyography, *VFSS* videofluoroscopic swallow study, *W* week, *Y* year

References

1. Lindström M, Nevas M, Kurki J, Sauna-Aho R, Latvala-Kiesilä A, Pölönen I, et al. Type C botulism due to toxic feed affecting 52,000 farmed foxes and minks in Finland. J Clin Microbiol. 2004;42(10):4718.
2. Johnson AL, McAdams SC, Whitlock RH. Type A botulism in horses in the United States: a review of the past ten years (1998–2008). J Vet Diagn Investig. 2010;22(2):165–73.
3. Payne JH, Hogg RA, Otter A, et al. Emergence of suspected type D botulism in ruminants in England and Wales (2001 to 2009), associated with exposure to broiler litter. Vet Rec. 2011;168(24):640.
4. Johnston SA. Osteoarthritis: joint anatomy, physiology, and pathobiology. Vet Clin North Am Small Anim Pract. 1997;27(4):699–723.
5. Anderson KL, O'Neill DG, Brodbelt DC, Church DB, Meeson RL, Sargan D, et al. Prevalence, duration and risk factors for appendicular osteoarthritis in a UK dog population under primary veterinary care. Sci Rep. 2018;8(1):5641–12.
6. Bonnett BN, Egenvall A, Hedhammar A, Olson P. Mortality in over 350,000 insured Swedish dogs from 1995–2000: I. Breed-, gender-, age- and cause-specific rates. Acta Vet Scand. 2005;46(3):105.
7. Moore GE, Burkman KD, Carter MN, Peterson MR. Causes of death or reasons for euthanasia in military working dogs: 927 cases (1993–1996). J Am Vet Med Assoc. 2001;219(2):209–14.
8. Hadley HS, Wheeler JL, Petersen SW. Effects of intra-articular botulinum toxin type A (Botox®) in dogs with chronic osteoarthritis. Vet Comp Orthop Traumatol. 2010;9:254–8.
9. Voss K, Imhof J, Kaestner S, Montavon PM. Force plate gait analysis at the walk and trot in dogs with low-grade hindlimb lameness. Vet Comp Orthop Traumatol. 2007;20(4):299–304.
10. Volstad N, Nemke B, Muir P. Variance associated with the use of relative velocity for force platform gait analysis in a heterogeneous population of clinically normal dogs. Vet J. 2016;207:80–4.
11. Heikkilä HM, Hielm-Björkman AK, Morelius M, Larsen S, Honkavaara J, Innes JF, et al. Intra-articular botulinum toxin A for the treatment of osteoarthritic joint pain in dogs: a randomized, double-blinded, placebo-controlled clinical trial. Vet J. 2014;200(1):162–9.
12. Hielm-Björkman AK, Kuusela E, Liman A, Markkola A, Saarto E, Huttunen P, et al. Evaluation of methods for assessment of pain associated with chronic osteoarthritis in dogs. J Am Vet Med Assoc. 2003;222(11):1552–8.
13. Nicácio GM, Luna SPL, Cavaleti P, Cassu RN. Intra-articular botulinum toxin A (BoNT/A) for pain management in dogs with osteoarthritis secondary to hip dysplasia: A randomized controlled clinical trial. J Vet Med Sci. 2019;81(3):411–7.
14. Brown DC, Boston RC, Coyne JC, Farrar JT. Development and psychometric testing of an instrument designed to measure chronic pain in dogs with osteoarthritis. Am J Vet Res. 2007;68(6):631–7.
15. Sampaio C, Ferreira JJ, Simões F, Rosas MJ, Magalhães M, Correia AP, et al. DYSBOT: a single-blind, randomized parallel study to determine whether any differences can be detected in the efficacy and tolerability of two formulations of botulinum toxin type A--Dysport and Botox--assuming a ratio of 4:1. Mov Disord. 1997;12(6):1013–8.
16. Odergren T, Hjaltason H, Kaakkola S, Solders G, Hanko J, Fehling C, et al. A double blind, randomised, parallel group study to investigate the dose equivalence of Dysport and Botox in the treatment of cervical dystonia. J Neurol Neurosurg Psychiatry. 1998;64(1):6–12.
17. Conzemius MG, Evans RB. Caregiver placebo effect for dogs with lameness from osteoarthritis. J Am Vet Med Assoc. 2012;241(10):1314–9.
18. Safarpour Y, Jabbari B. Botulinum toxin treatment of pain syndromes -an evidence based review. Toxicon. 2018;147:120–8.
19. Heikkilä HM, Jokinen TS, Syrjä P, Junnila J, Hielm-Björkman A, Laitinen-Vapaavuori O. Assessing adverse effects of intra-articular botulinum toxin A in healthy Beagle

dogs: a placebo-controlled, blinded, randomized trial. Premkumar LS, editor. PloS One. 2018;13(1):e0191043.
20. Vilhegas S, Cassu RN, Barbero RC, Crociolli GC, Rocha TLA, Gomes DR. Botulinum toxin type A as an adjunct in postoperative pain management in dogs undergoing radical mastectomy. Vet Rec. 2015;177(15):391.
21. Murrell JC, Psatha EP, Scott EM, Reid J, Hellebrekers LJ. Application of a modified form of the Glasgow pain scale in a veterinary teaching centre in the Netherlands. Vet Rec. 2008;162(13):403–8.
22. Layeeque R, Hochberg J, Siegel E, Kunkel K, Kepple J, Henry-Tillman RS, et al. Botulinum toxin infiltration for pain control after mastectomy and expander reconstruction. Ann Surg. 2004;240(4):608–13; discussion 613–4.
23. Antonucci F, Rossi C, Gianfranceschi L, Rossetto O, Caleo M. Long-distance retrograde effects of botulinum neurotoxin A. J Neurosci. 2008;28(14):3689–96.
24. Bach-Rojecky L, Lacković Z. Central origin of the antinociceptive action of botulinum toxin type A. Pharmacol Biochem Behav. 2009;94(2):234–8.
25. Grobman ME, Hutcheson KD, Lever TE, Mann FA, Reinero CR. Mechanical dilation, botulinum toxin A injection, and surgical myotomy with fundoplication for treatment of lower esophageal sphincter achalasia-like syndrome in dogs. J Vet Intern Med. 2019;33(3):1423–33.
26. Rogatko CP, Glass EN, Kent M, Hammond JJ, de Lahunta A. Use of botulinum toxin type A for the treatment of radiation therapy-induced myokymia and neuromyotonia in a dog. J Am Vet Med Assoc. 2016;248(5):532–7.
27. Schubert T, Clemmons R, Miles S, Draper W. The use of botulinum toxin for the treatment of generalized myoclonus in a dog. J Am Anim Hosp Assoc. 2013;49(2):122–7.
28. Rinaldi ML, Fransson BA, Barry SL. Botulinum toxin A as a treatment for delayed gastric emptying in a dog. Can Vet J. 2014;55(7):673–7.
29. Kessler KR, Benecke R. Botulinum toxin: from poison to remedy. Neurotoxicology. 1997;18(3):761–70.
30. Meyer-Lindenberg A, Wohlfarth KM, Switzer EN. The use of botulinum toxin A for treatment of possible essential blepharospasm in a dog. Aust Vet J. 2003;81(10):612–4.
31. Bright SR, Girling SL, O'Neill T, Innes JF. Partial tarsal arthrodesis and botulinum toxin A injection for correction of tarsal arthrogryposis in a cat. J Small Anim Pract. 2007;48(1):39–42.
32. Arruda RM, Takano CC, Girão MJBC, Haddad JM, Aleixo GF, Castro RA. Treatment of non-neurogenic overactive bladder with OnabotulinumtoxinA: systematic review and meta-analysis of prospective, randomized, placebo-controlled clinical trials. RBGO Gynecol Obstet. 2018;40(4):225–31.
33. Cooley LF, Kielb S. A review of botulinum toxin A for the treatment of neurogenic bladder. PM&R. 2019;11(2):192–200.
34. Coelho A, Dinis P, Pinto R, Gorgal T, Silva C, Silva A, et al. Distribution of the high-affinity binding site and intracellular target of botulinum toxin type A in the human bladder. Eur Urol. 2010;57(5):884–90.
35. Lew S, Majewski M, Radziszewski P, Kuleta Z. Therapeutic efficacy of botulinum toxin in the treatment of urinary incontinence in female dogs. Acta Vet Hung. 2010;58(2):157–65.
36. Mostachio GQ, Apparício M, Motheo TF, Alves AE, Vicente WRR. Intra-prostatic injection of botulinum toxin type A in treatment of dogs with spontaneous benign prostatic hyperplasia. Anim Reprod Sci. 2012;133(3–4):224–8.
37. Johnston SD, Kamolpatana K, Root-Kustritz MV, Johnston GR. Prostatic disorders in the dog. Anim Reprod Sci. 2000;60–61:405–15.
38. Shim SR, Cho YJ, Shin I-S, Kim JH. Efficacy and safety of botulinum toxin injection for benign prostatic hyperplasia: a systematic review and meta-analysis. Int Urol Nephrol. 2016;48(1):19–30.
39. Hansen KS, Weisse C, Berent AC, Dunn M, Caceres AV, Todd KL, et al. Use of a self-expanding metallic stent to palliate esophageal neoplastic obstruction in a dog. J Am Vet Med Assoc. 2012;240(10):1202–7.

40. Bittencourt MKW, de Vasconcellos JPC, Bittencourt MD, Malagó R, Bacellar M. J Ocul Pharmacol Ther. 2013;29(4):431–6.
41. Cohen SR, Thompson JW, Camilon FS Jr. Botulinum toxin for relief of bilateral abductor paralysis of the larynx: histologic study in an animal model. Ann Otol Rhinol Laryngol. 1989;98(3):213–6.
42. Lin ATL, Yang AH, Chen KK. Effects of botulinum toxin A on the contractile function of dog prostate. Eur Urol. 2007;52(2):582–9.
43. Tsuboi M, Furukawa Y, Kurogouchi F, Nakajima K, Hirose M, Chiba S. Botulinum neurotoxin A blocks cholinergic ganglionic neurotransmission in the dog heart. Jpn J Pharmacol. 2002;89(3):249–54.
44. Brodsky JA, Marks JM, Malm JA, Bower A, Ponsky JL. Sphincter of Oddi injection with botulinum toxin is as effective as endobiliary stent in resolving cystic duct leaks in a canine model. Gastrointest Endosc. 2002;56(6):849–51.
45. Shaari CM, Wu BL, Biller HF, Chuang SK, Sanders I. Botulinum toxin decreases salivation from canine submandibular glands. Otolaryngol Head Neck Surg. 1998;118(4):452–7.
46. Shaari CM, Sanders I, Wu BL, Biller HF. Rhinorrhea is decreased in dogs after nasal application of botulinum toxin. Otolaryngol Head Neck Surg. 1995;112(4):566–71.
47. Wylie CE, Collins SN, Verheyen KLP, Newton JR. Frequency of equine laminitis: a systematic review with quality appraisal of published evidence. Vet J. 2011;189(3):248–56.
48. Baxter GM, Morrison S. Complications of unilateral weight bearing. Vet Clin N Am Equine Pract. 2008;24(3):621–42, ix.
49. Patterson-Kane JC, Karikoski NP, McGowan CM. Paradigm shifts in understanding equine laminitis. Vet J. 2018;231:33–40.
50. Carter DW, Renfroe BJ. A novel approach to the treatment and prevention of laminitis: botulinum toxin type A for the treatment of laminitis. J Equine Vet. 2009;29(7):595–600.
51. van Eps AW, Burns TA. Are there shared mechanisms in the pathophysiology of different clinical forms of laminitis and what are the implications for prevention and treatment? Vet Clin N Am Equine Pract. 2019;35(2):379–98.
52. Bamford NJ. Clinical insights: treatment of laminitis. Equine Vet J. 2019;51(2):145–6.
53. Eastman TG, Honnas CM, American BHJOT, 1999. Deep digital flexor tenotomy as a treatment for chronic laminitis in horses: 35 cases (1988–1997). J Equine Vet Sci. 2010;30(2):111.
54. Hardeman LC, van der Meij BR, Oosterlinck M, Veraa S, van der Kolk JH, Wijnberg ID, et al. Effect of Clostridium botulinum toxin type A injections into the deep digital flexor muscle on the range of motion of the metacarpus and carpus, and the force distribution underneath the hooves, of sound horses at the walk. Vet J. 2013;198:e152–6.
55. Wijnberg ID, Hardeman LC, van der Meij BR, Veraa S, Back W, van der Kolk JH. The effect of Clostridium botulinum toxin type A injections on motor unit activity of the deep digital flexor muscle in healthy sound Royal Dutch sport horses. Vet J. 2013;198:e147–51.
56. Hardeman LC, van der Meij BR, Back W, van der Kolk JH, Wijnberg ID. The use of electromyography interference pattern analysis to determine muscle force of the deep digital flexor muscle in healthy and laminitic horses. Vet Q. 2015;36(1):10–5.
57. Wijnberg ID, Schrama SEA, Elgersma AE, Maree JTM, De Cocq P, Back W. Quantification of surface EMG signals to monitor the effect of a Botox treatment in six healthy ponies and two horses with stringhalt: preliminary study. Equine Vet J. 2009;41(3):313–8.
58. Draper ACE, Trumble TN, Firshman AM, Baird JD, Reed S, Mayhew IG, et al. Posture and movement characteristics of forward and backward walking in horses with shivering and acquired bilateral stringhalt. Equine Vet J. 2015;47(2):175–81.
59. Huntington PJ, Seneque Slocombe RF, Jeffcot LB, McLean A, Luff ARI. Use of phenytoin to treat horses with Australian stringhalt. Aust Vet J. 1991;68(7):221–4.
60. Torre F. Clinical diagnosis and results of surgical treatment of 13 cases of acquired bilateral stringhalt (1991–2003). Equine Vet J. 2005;37(2):181–3.
61. Adam-Castrillo D, White NA II, Donaldson LL, Furr MO. Effects of injection of botulinum toxin type B into the external anal sphincter on anal pressure of horses. Am J Vet Sci. 2005;65(1):26–30.

62. Galey FD. Botulism in the horse. Vet Clin N Am Equine Pract. 2001;17(3):579–88.
63. Gutierrez-Nibeyro SD, Santos MP, White NA II, Brown JA, Adams MN, McKnight AL, et al. Effects of intrabursal administration of botulinum toxin type B on lameness in horses with degenerative injury to the podotrochlear apparatus. Equine Vet J. 2014;75(3):282–9.
64. Schoonover MJ, Jann HW, Blaik MA. Quantitative comparison of three commonly used treatments for navicular syndrome in horses. Am J Vet Res. 2005;66(7):1247–51.
65. Nibeyro SDG, White Na II, Wepy NM. Outcome of medical treatment for horses with foot pain: 56 cases. Equine Vet J. 2010;42(8):680–5.
66. Bowker RM, Linder K, Sonea IM, Holland RE. Sensory innervation of the navicular bone and bursa in the foal. Equine Vet J. 1995;27(1):60–5.
67. DePuy T, Howard R, Keegan K, Wilson D, Kramer J, Cook JL, et al. Effects of intra-articular botulinum toxin type A in an equine model of acute synovitis: a pilot study. Am J Phys Med Rehabil. 2007;86(10):777–83.
68. Peng L, Adler M, Demogines A, Borrell A, Liu H, Tao L, et al. Widespread sequence variations in VAMP1 across vertebrates suggest a potential selective pressure from botulinum neurotoxins. PLoS Pathog. 2014;10(7):e1004177.

Chapter 18
Future Perspectives of Botulinum Toxin Application in Dentistry

Shahroo Etemad-Moghadam

Abstract In recent years, the therapeutic application of botulinum neurotoxin (BoNT) has expanded to encompass a variety of issues beyond its well-known usage for hyperkinetic movement disorders, autonomic hyperactivity, and facial rejuvenation. Dentistry is one of the fields that has benefited greatly from botulinum toxin therapy, as evidenced by multiple clinical trials which provided evidence for usefulness of this mode of therapy in common issues encountered in the field of dentistry (described in Chap. 16). In this chapter, the future potentials for BoNT therapy in the field of dentistry and its use in oral and maxillofacial region with its rich network of nerves and muscles are described. In addition, this chapter focuses on preclinical and preliminary studies on the effect of intramuscular injections of BoNT on craniofacial growth and proposes the possibility of using this toxin to influence the dentofacial complex during growth. Existing data or suggestions on the use of BoNT in implant dentistry, tongue thrust, temporomandibular joint dislocation, bone/plate fractures, herpes simplex virus, angular cheilitis, and burning mouth syndrome are also presented.

Keywords Botulinum neurotoxin · Dentistry · Orthodontics · Gummy smile · Bone fracture

Introduction

The head and neck constitute a complex arrangement of structures composed of a variety of tissues, including muscles and nerves, which work in harmony to provide the normal functions inherent to this area. As meticulously discussed in Chap. 16, there are multiple well-documented uses of botulinum toxin (BoNT) in this region for which considerable studies, some with high levels of evidence, have been performed and are being used as reference by oral surgeons and dentists. However,

S. Etemad-Moghadam (✉)
Dental Research Center, Dentistry Research Institute, Tehran University of Medical Sciences, Tehran, Iran

© Springer Nature Switzerland AG 2020   359
B. Jabbari (ed.), *Botulinum Toxin Treatment in Surgery, Dentistry, and Veterinary Medicine*, https://doi.org/10.1007/978-3-030-50691-9_18

there are several other applications for this toxin which still lack a high level of scientific evidence and would benefit from further research based on randomized controlled trials, when possible. In this chapter, we present potential applications of BoNT for the treatment of less investigated issues in the orofacial complex and explore other ways to take advantage of this safe and accessible substance in different areas and specialties of dentistry. Whether BoNT will gain widespread acceptance for use in these areas would depend on future research to confirm or reject its application. The cases presented herein are intended to familiarize practitioners with additional approaches to applying BoNT in clinical situations, where there is a need to avoid invasive procedures or to supplement an existing treatment.

Orthodontics

Orthodontics is the art and science of providing the patient with an esthetically pleasing oral and facial appearance through correction of the teeth and jaws. It is sometimes paired with orthognathic surgery to treat dentofacial problems. Certain circumstances such as age, negative attitude towards orthodontic appliances, hesitance to undergo orthognathic surgery, and a number of medical conditions limit the use of orthodontic therapy [1], and therefore, patients need to be presented with alternatives that offer acceptable results. Additionally, a number of factors including muscular activity can compromise the outcome of orthognathic surgery leading to its instability and relapse [2]; the potential impact of these factors needs to be reduced as much as possible with simple techniques. Finally, if feasible, access to uncomplicated methods to manipulate growth and development of the dentofacial complex in a desirable direction could help avoid going through subsequent more intricate treatments.

Within this context, BoNT injection can be a valuable tool in orthodontic treatments and it may be used in different aspects of this specialty. A selection of applications ranging from treatment of existing issues to prevention of relapse and the possibility of manipulating growth is presented below:

Treating Existing Issues

Gummy Smile or Excessive Gingival Display

Definition Maxillary gingival display of more than 3 mm upon smiling is known as "gummy smile" and is regarded as unattractive by most people. Various etiologic factors have been identified for this condition, one of which is hyperactivity of the muscles responsible for lip elevation. Accordingly, different treatment methods ranging from orthodontic therapy to surgical procedures have been used to improve the esthetic appearance of these patients [3–5]. In many cases, patients and/or clinicians decide on nonaggressive methods that cause the least posttreatment morbidity, regardless of the specific etiologic factor. Therefore, BoNT injections would be a perfect choice, even in cases other than those caused by muscular hyperactivity that could be camouflaged with labial modification.

Treatment of Cases with Muscular Etiology   Excessive gingival display due to lip muscle hyperfunction includes individuals who demonstrate normal maxillary dimensions on cephalometric analysis, but display 2 mm of the upper incisors while their lips are at rest [3]. Gummy smilers have been shown to possess more powerful lip-elevating muscles compared to individuals with normal lip lines [3, 6]. To eliminate this problem, numerous surgical methods have been employed through the years [4] including muscle detachment from the underlying bone to lower the lip [7], partial amputation of the levator labii superioris muscle (with or without the addition of a spacer) [8, 9], subperiosteal cutting of the labial elevators through the exterior aspect of the nasal septum [10], and surgical remodeling of the gingiva and alveolar bone [11]. In addition to being complex, time-consuming and expensive surgical procedures carry the risk of complications such as formation and contraction of scar tissues [3, 12]. BoNT has been used to treat gummy smile for nearly a decade; however, a uniform and standardized application method is still lacking.

Muscles Involved in Gummy Smile Appearance   In order to achieve optimal treatment results with BoNT injections, the muscles responsible for lip activity and their best access points should be identified. Different studies have proposed different muscles as targets for injection, with the levator labii superioris alaeque nasi being the most commonly proposed target [13].

Mazzuco and Hexsel [12] analyzed muscle function and localized each of the muscle groups responsible for moving a specific part of the lip and used it to classify gummy smile into anterior, posterior, mixed, and asymmetric subtypes. They reported levator labii superioris alaeque nasi, levator labii superioris, zygomaticus minor, zygomaticus major, and risorius to be the major muscles associated with gingival exposure, providing a guide for patient-based injections (Fig. 18.1) [12].

Number of Injections   Different studies have reported between 1 and 3 injections per side, some with the additional use of electromyography [3, 4, 12, 13]. In order to minimize the number of injections, the Yonsei point was introduced as a single spot situated at the intersection of the levator labii superioris alaeque nasi, levator labii superioris, and zygomaticus minor muscles. This point could be easily located in both males and females, at the crossing of a horizontal line drawn 1 cm lateral from the ala and a vertical line drawn 3 cm above the lip line, when the lips are at rest (Fig. 18.2) [3]. Initially, the Yonsei point was established based on information gathered from Asian subjects [3], but further studies in other populations reported significant improvement of gummy smiles following single injections into this point [13–15].

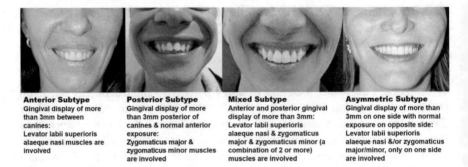

Anterior Subtype
Gingival display of more
than 3mm between
canines:
Levator labii superioris
alaeque nasi muscles are
involved

Posterior Subtype
Gingival display of more
than 3mm posterior of
canines & normal anterior
exposure:
Zygomaticus major &
zygomaticus minor muscles
are involved

Mixed Subtype
Anterior and posterior gingival
display of more than 3mm:
Levator labii superioris
alaeque nasi & zygomaticus
major & zygomaticus minor (a
combination of 2 or more)
muscles are involved

Asymmetric Subtype
Gingival display of more than
3mm on one side with normal
exposure on opposite side:
Levator labii superioris
alaeque nasi &/or zygomaticus
major/minor, only on one side
are involved

Fig. 18.1 Subtypes of gummy smile and the major muscles involved in each type. (Adapted from Ref. [12] and reproduced with permission from Publisher: Elsevier)

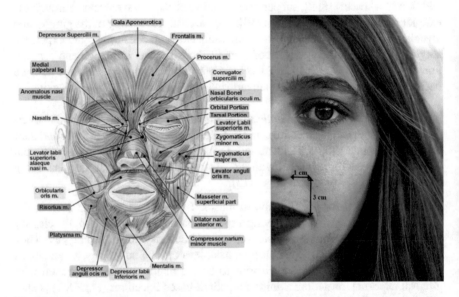

Fig. 18.2 The Yonsei point at the convergence of three muscles involved in lip function including levator labii superioris alaeque nasi, levator labii superioris, and zygomaticus minor muscles. (The schematic image (left) is reprinted from Kwon KH, Shin KS, Yeon SH, Kwon DG. Application of botulinum toxin in maxillofacial field: part I. Bruxism and square jaw. Maxillofac Plast Reconstr Surg. 2019 Oct 1;41(1):38 which has been made available under http://creativecommons.org/licenses/by/4.0/, the right image is obtained and modified from https://unsplash.com/ "internet's source of freely usable images")

Evidence for Effectiveness of BoNT A considerable number of reports, with the number of patients ranging from 1 to 52 [3, 4, 12–20], have indicated BoNT to be an effective method for the treatment of gummy smile. Nevertheless, there is a lack of randomized controlled trials on this subject. A total of 3 clinical trials specific to gummy smile and BoNT are listed in the Clinical Trials Registry (https://clinicaltrials.gov/). However, their status is "not yet recruiting" (NCT03717987), "withdrawn" (NCT03284047), and "unknown" (NCT03186547).

Three systematic reviews have evaluated BoNT in the treatment of gummy smile [21] and assessed its ideal dose [15] and duration of effectiveness [22]. According to their results, when administered by an experienced clinician, BoNT is a safe, reversible, and effective method to treat excessive gingival exposure, either as a separate treatment or as accompanying other techniques.

The levator labii superioris alaeque nasi was reported to be the most important muscle when using this protocol [21]. BoNT dosage generally depends on its formulation, potency, or the practitioner's experience and preference. A total dose of 5 IU onabotulinum toxin per side was reported to be effective, with subsequent follow-up administrations, as necessary. The Yonsei point was considered a convenient target for injection in all types of gummy smile [15]. There is a gradual reduction of the paralyzing effect of this toxin, which continues up to week 12 and, even then, may not completely return to baseline levels. Gummy smile patients remain free of excessive gingival exposure for at least 8 weeks, postinjection [22].

All three systematic reviews highlighted a lack of randomized controlled trials and high-quality studies for the use of BoNT in the treatment of gummy smile [15, 21, 22].

Considerations and Adverse Effects   Certain facts should be contemplated when selecting BoNT for the treatment of gummy smile:

- Gingival display is more pronounced in females compared to males and it becomes less conspicuous with age due to an increase in upper lip length following loss of soft tissue volume and support [23, 24]. Therefore, spontaneous correction is expected up to a certain level, particularly when dealing with male patients [23].
- Most adverse effects of BoNT are temporary and treatable in follow-up sessions; nonetheless, they should be considered when deciding to use it in clinical practice. Unwanted consequences of injection for the treatment of gummy smile reported in the literature include but may not be limited to asymmetric smile, difficulty in smiling, "sad smile" [12], pain and twitching at injection site, headache, vertigo [15, 21], "joker smile," protrusion of the lower lip, drooling [25], and in one case appearance of a horizontal depressed line when smiling [26].

Before administering BoNT, we have to make sure that the toxin is injected only into the muscle and does not enter the bloodstream; for this purpose, aspiration is suggested before completing the injection [23, 24].

Concluding Remarks   In conclusion, there is a need for further research and well-designed trials that can lead to the establishment of a set of universally accepted guidelines for the proper use of BoNT in the treatment of gummy smile. Researchers are currently working on this important task [27] and one of the pioneers in this field has suggested an injection protocol based on the amount of gingival display (Table 18.1) [28].

Preventing Issues Following Orthognathic Surgery

Treatment Relapse

One of the most common options for the treatment of dentoskeletal discrepancies is the combination of orthodontics and orthognathic surgery. A major consideration after achievement of the desired dentofacial appearance is to maintain the stability of hard and soft tissues, or in other words to prevent relapse. Treatment relapse is dependent upon a number of factors, one of which is the activity of facial muscles [2].

Following orthognathic surgery, the original relationship of the jaws is altered, and as a consequence, the muscular system tries to adapt by making modifications in the size and/or function of the involved musculature [29]. Masticatory muscles tend to return to their original state, which is due to the activation of stretch receptors. Therefore, BoNT would be a good option to consider when trying to sustain postoperative stability and prevent muscular tension [30]. This is especially true when comparing simple injections to the use of more invasive methods such as myotomy [31]. Additionally, considering that the majority of relapse following orthognathic surgery occurs within the first 6 months, the transient nature of BoNT would not be a problem in these cases [32].

Supporting Studies
- Patients with skeletal class II malocclusions have mandibular deficiency. When this condition is accompanied by anterior open bite, their treatment can involve counterclockwise rotation of the mandible and a high rate of posttreatment relapse is expected. A 21-year-old woman with this type of facial deformity was treated with presurgical orthodontic therapy, orthognathic surgery, and double genioplasty. This was immediately followed by injection of a total dose of 20 U BoNT (Meditoxin, Type A) into 4 points of the anterior belly of the digastric muscle (Fig. 18.3). A 15-month follow-up of this patient showed complete retention and no relapse [32].

The same injection has been suggested to treat open-bite patients who do not respond to comprehensive rubber traction [33].

Table 18.1 Injection guide based on the amount of gingival exposure as proposed by Polo. Adapted from reference 28, with permission from Publisher: Oxford University Press

Gingival exposure (mm)	Injection sites Number (location)	Dosage per side (U/site)	Total units (U)
4–5	1 (overlapping area of LLSAN/LLS)	2	4
5–7	1 (overlapping area of LLSAN/LLS)	2.5	5
7–8.5	2 (overlapping area of LLSAN/LLS; overlapping area of LLS/Zmi)	2	8
>8.5	2 (overlapping area of LLSAN/LLS; overlapping area of LLS/Zmi)	2.5	10

LLSAN levator labii superioris alaeque nasi, *LLS* levator labii superioris, *Zmi* zygomaticus minor

- Deep bite occurs when maxillary incisors cover more than the normal percentage of the mandibular incisors, and in some cases, the lower anterior teeth come into contact with the palatal surface of their opposing antagonists or the palatal mucosa. Along with retroclination of the maxillary incisors, deep bite is a major finding in class II division II individuals. Relapse has been reported in one-third of patients treated for this malocclusion. Twenty units of BoNT (Botox®, Allergan) was administered bilaterally into the mylohyoid muscles of 8 deep-bite class II division II adult patients treated with orthognathic surgery and compared to 24 controls with the same malocclusion and treatment method, except for the injections. According to the results, none of the BoNT-treated patients exhibited relapse, while more than half the controls showed signs of relapse after a maximum of 1-year follow-up. The backward pull of the mylohyoid muscles in response to advancement of the mandible during surgery was considered to be a responsible factor for relapse, which was relieved by BoNT injection in this study, hence, the decreased occurrence of relapse [34].

Concluding Remarks The mechanisms and likelihood of posttreatment relapse vary among different types of surgical procedures. Also, depending on the type and direction of surgery, muscles would be affected differently (traction versus pressure), resulting in distinct impacts on the bone and different amounts and forms of relapse [31, 32, 34, 35]. Therefore, targeting the specific muscles known to be affected by the particular type of surgery and reducing its negative impact on the supporting bone, would be extremely helpful in clinical practice. Consequently,

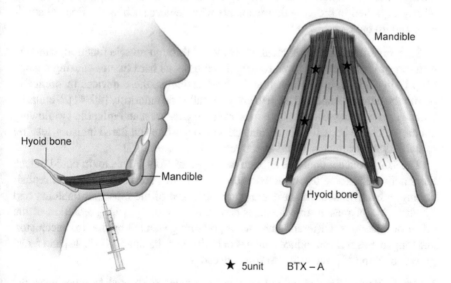

★ 5unit   BTX – A

Fig. 18.3 Injection of BoNT (Meditoxin Type A) into four points (stars) of the anterior belly of the digastric muscle. Five units were administered into each point. (Original figure is reprinted from Ref. [32] with minor changes to the legend, which has been made available under http://creativecommons.org/licenses/by/4.0/)

where ethically permissible, there is a need for well-designed, controlled clinical trials developed separately for the different surgical protocols and malocclusions in order to gain access to an acceptable approach to help reduce relapse.

Sculpturing Facial Bones During Growth

Premise As long as an individual is still growing, the position and growth direction of the teeth and jaws could be altered by noninvasive measures. However, after skeletal maturation, the clinician usually resorts to more aggressive procedures, such as surgery [36]. If skeletal development could be controlled through manipulation of soft tissues during growth, future orthognathic surgery might be avoided or less complicated.

Definition Growth and development of facial structures is an extremely complex process, as evidenced by the multiple theories intended to provide an explanation of the mechanisms responsible for its occurrence and progression [37]. One of the most important hypotheses was the functional matrix theory by Moss (1968), which strongly supported the role of extrinsic and epigenetic factors in cephalic development. While recognizing the contribution of genetics, emphasis was placed on external stimuli which induced a response in the supporting bone, ultimately leading to the promotion of bone growth [37, 38]. One of the major external stimuli in the dentofacial complex is that elicited by the masticatory muscles, which have been widely exploited in orthodontic treatments with devices such as the Frankel appliance and lip bumper.

Such myofunctional appliances are activated through muscle function, which in turn transmit (or prevent) force to dental and osseous hard tissues causing change [39]. Using shields in the buccal and labial vestibules, these devices theoretically permit the targeted bone and teeth to grow laterally and anteriorly [40, 41]. Similarly, tongue cribs are suggested to help overcome tongue thrust and infantile swallowing habits, which are occasionally associated with open-bite and flared incisors, leading to stability of treatments aimed at correcting these issues [42].

The same concept could be applied to the use of BoNT. This toxin could reduce the function and force of overactive muscles to allow hard-tissue growth or repositioning, where needed. An in-depth comprehension of the muscular anatomy and the direction of muscle movement is essential for more precise prediction of the effect of injections. Different amounts of pressure generated by the lip, buccinator, and tongue muscles can induce changes in both dental inclination [43, 44] and facial growth pattern [45], according to some investigators.

Initial Evidence Several animal studies have been conducted to investigate the effect of BoNT injection on facial bones during growth, which have shown the capability of BoNT to impact these structures [46–54] (Table 18.2). BoNT injection into the masseter of adult humans has resulted in modification of the alveolar bone, digastric fossa [55], condyle [55, 56], and mandibular angle [57] in some studies, but not others [58].

Application in Children The effect of BoNT on bones may be even more conspicuous in growing children who have not reached full development. In the head and neck regions, this toxin has been used for treating sialorrhea in 4- to 18-year-old individuals [59, 60], as off-label treatment in pediatric otolaryngology/laryngology patients older than 2 years [61], strabismus [62], conservative management of displaced condylar fracture in a 3-year-old child [63], and chronic migraine in adolescents [64].

We found one study in a growing child (an 8-year-old girl) who was injected with a total dose of 10 U BoNT into two points of her masseter muscle following orthodontic therapy to correct a masticatory movement disorder, facial asymmetry, and unilateral masseter hypertrophy. After this combined treatment, ramus height notably increased on the opposite (non-injected) side, correcting the transverse deviation of the upper jaw. It was concluded that mandibular growth could be modified by reduction of masseteric hypertrophy [65].

Concluding Remarks Clearly, there is a lack of strong evidence regarding the effect of muscle injections of BoNT on the growth and development of facial hard tissues, especially in children and adolescents. Considering that this age group, especially those with skeletal and dental malocclusions, may benefit most from this safe and simple approach, prospective studies and randomized controlled trials are necessary, when possible. The importance of BoNT treatment becomes more evident when considering the difficulties encountered in current routine treatments such as lack of compliance of young patients to use myofunctional devices [66], inability to manage the growth potential of soft tissues, unexpected complications in the rotation of the mandible, and relapse of more invasive methods such as distraction osteogenesis [47]. However, as mentioned in Chap. 16, the effect of muscle force on bone quantity/quality and mechanical properties of the temporomandibular joint should be given focused attention, when considering the use of BoNT. There is a long way to go before information from various studies can be incorporated into clinical treatments for this age group, especially considering that they are ethically regarded as a vulnerable population for use as subjects in clinical trials.

Treatment of Parafunctional Habits

Definition Habits are described as actions that are performed repeatedly and automatically. Parafunctional habits are behaviors that are enacted by a body organ in a manner beyond the original purpose/function of that organ. In the oral cavity, it includes actions other than mastication, swallowing, and talking which could appear in a wide array of behaviors such as bruxism, clenching, lip- or nail-biting, digit/object sucking, or chewing and tongue thrust. Muscular hyperactivity is a common

Table 18.2 Studies using muscular BoNT injections to evaluate craniofacial skeletal changes in growing rats

Authors	No. (groups)	Age	Study period	BoNT	Dose	Injection site	Assessment methods	Significant effects	Conclusions
Kim et al. 2008 [50]	80 (4)	4w	4w	BTXA®, Lanzhou Institute of Biological Products, Lanzhou, China	2.5 U, 0.05 ml	Bilateral Mst.	Histology, TUNEL, measurements on computer images from photographs of dry Mand.	Smaller lengths of the mandibular body, condyle, and coronoid process in addition to diminished heights of the anterior mandibular region, condyle, and coronoid process	Mandibular growth is affected by BoNT through its apoptotic impact on the condylar cartilage The influence of BoNT on growth should be considered before prescription to developing children
Tsai et al. 2009 [52]	11 (2)	30d	45d	BoNT/A, Botox, Allergan, Irvine, Calif.	1 U, 0.04 ml: (0.02 ml in each point)	2 points of the superficial and deep layers of the Mst.	Measurements on dry skulls by an electronic digital caliper	Reduced muscle weight after injection Some craniofacial and mandibular, but not maxillary measurements decrease when comparing between sides and groups	Mst. atrophy due to BoNT can change osseous growth and development, confirming the functional matrix theory indicating regulation of bone development by soft tissues

Authors	No. (groups)	Age	Study period	BoNT	Dose	Injection site	Assessment methods	Significant effects	Conclusions
Babuccu et al. 2009 [46]	49 (4)	15d	4 m	Botulinum toxin A; Botox, Allergan Pharmaceuticals, Ireland	0.4 IU, 0.05 ml	Unilateral Mst. or Temp.	Histology, direct cephalometric measurements	Atrophy in both injected muscles Decrease in all craniofacial/ mandibular dimensions after Temp. injection Decrease in most measurements after Mst. injection	Muscle paralysis due to BoNT, negatively impacts bone structures, during growth Further considerations should be given to the use of BoNT in pediatrics to control craniofacial deformities
Tsai et al. 2011 [49]	60 (4)	30d	45d	Botox®, Allergan Pharmaceuticals, Dublin, Ireland	1 U, 2.5 ml	Bilateral Mst. ± Temp.	DEXA, graphic software to analyze digital photographs of decalcified bone under an optical microscope	Lower muscle volume, cortical thickness, and BMD (skull and Mand., adjacent to muscle insertion areas) after injection	Reduced masticatory function has an impact on bone structure during growth
Park et al. 2015 [51]	60 (3)	4w	4w	Botox®, Allergan Inc., Irvine, CA,USA	3 U, 0.05 ml	Unilateral or bilateral Mst.	Measurements on computer images from photographs of dry Mand.	Smaller mandibular measurements in the BoNT-injected side compared to the saline side[a]	Unilateral BoNT injection induces unilateral changes in craniofacial development, regardless of the fact that the Mand. functions as a single unit

(continued)

Table 18.2 (continued)

Authors	No. (groups)	Age	Study period	BoNT	Dose	Injection site	Assessment methods	Significant effects	Conclusions
Seok et al. 2018 [53]	11 (2)	13d	47d	BoNT-A, Botulax® 50, HUGEL, Chuncheon, Korea)	0.5 U, 0.5 ml	Unilateral Mass	Measurements on micro-CT images	Reduction in some aspects of ramus height and mandibular plane angle and decreased bigonial mandibular width Mandibular midline deviation to BoNT side	Mst. BoNT administration decreases the development of the lower jaw
Ahn et al. 2019 [47]	10 (2)	13d	47d	Botulax® 50, BoNT type A, HUGEL, Chuncheon, Korea	0.5 U, 0.5 ml	Anterior belly of the DM	Micro-CT analysis	Decrease in the zygomatic arch and mandibular bicondylar width Increase in maxillary posterior arch width	Maxillofacial transverse bony width was affected by BoNT during growth possibly because of functional change of masticatory muscles in reaction to the decreased function of the DM

Authors	No. (groups)	Age	Study period	BoNT	Dose	Injection site	Assessment methods	Significant effects	Conclusions
Tsai et al. 2019 [48]	48 (4)	4w	42d	25 U/mL, Allergan Pharmaceuticals, Ireland	1 U, 0.04 ml	Bilateral Mst. ± Temp.	Electronic caliper, fluorescing line marking for calculation of bone apposition rate by fluorescence microscopy, micro-CT for sutural bone mineral density measurement	Weight reduction in injected muscles Diminished maxillary arch size only after injections into both muscles Decreased suture density dependent upon the muscle and muscle-suture position Reduced sutural apposition rate, most prevalent in paralysis of both muscles	Maxillofacial suture bone growth in developing rats can be influenced by masticatory muscle action

(continued)

Table 18.2 (continued)

Authors	No. (groups)	Age	Study period	BoNT	Dose	Injection site	Assessment methods	Significant effects	Conclusions
Choi et al. 2019 [54]	11 (2)	6w	12w	BoNT type A, Botulax®, Hugel, Inc., Korea	2 IU (2.5 IU per 0.1 ml): 0.91 IU in Mst., 0.73 IU in Temp., and 0.36 IU in Med.Ptr	Unilateral Mst. + Temp. + Med.Ptr followed by boosters, 6w later	3D analysis of micro-CT images, histochemical analysis (H&E and Masson trichrome)	Reduction in size + lateral tilting of Mand. causing asymmetry Supraeruption of U/ & L molars and downward canting of occlusal plane on BoNT side Decreased density of alveolar bone, smaller PDL space, and disorganized periodontal collagen fibers	The dentoalveolar complex responds to diminished occlusal forces by causing increased occlusal canting and pronounced skeletal asymmetry Diminished occlusal forces can be the result of BoNT injection, inducing depletion of masticatory functional loading

Mst. masseter, *Temp.* temporalis, *TUNEL* terminal deoxynucleotidyl transferase-mediated dUTP nick-end labeling, *DEXA* dual-energy X-ray absorptiometry, *BMD* bone mineral density, *DM* digastric muscle, *Med.Ptr.* medial pterygoid, *U/* & *L* upper and lower, *PDL* periodontal ligament, *w* week, *d* day

[a]Mandibular body, condylar, and coronoid process lengths and anterior region, condylar, and coronoid process heights

finding among these habits. Additionally, they can be destructive to the gnathic and dentoalveolar complex and/or any type of restoration placed within this system including fillings, crowns, bridges, and implants [67, 68]. Therefore, the use of BoNT to reduce the excessive force of these behaviors in order to minimize their negative effects could be an acceptable choice.

Here, we discuss the available literature on the use of BoNT in eliminating the effects of parafunctional habits on implants, and also, we hypothesize the impact that treating these habits could have on preventing dentoskeletal problems.

BoNT in Implant Dentistry

Definition Bruxism, clenching, and tongue thrust are the main parafunctional habits noted to be associated with implant failure [68]. Study results on the effect of bruxism on different aspects of implants are conflicting, with some regarding it as an important cause of biological and mechanical failure [68, 69] and others maintaining that its role is mainly mechanical, only resulting in issues such as screw loosening and porcelain/implant fractures as opposed to problems such as impaired osseointegration [70] (discussed in Chap. 16).

Clinical Evidence In a study by Mijiritsky et al. [71], the efficacy of preoperative administration of BoNT-A was evaluated in 13 bruxism patients receiving immediately loaded implants set in fresh extraction sockets for full-arch restorations and compared with 13 controls with the same characteristics. Injections of BoNT (Dysport) were delivered 3 weeks before surgery in the test group. For the temporal muscles on each side, a total dose of 70 U was injected into 4 points in an area located on the zygomatic arch and temporal region. For each masseter, a total dose of 90 U was administered into 3–4 points in proximity to the mandibular angle. Follow-up (18–51 months) revealed no implant failure in the test group. Of the 103 implants placed in this group, only 4 implants in one patient showed 1- to 2-mm bone loss. In contrast, among the 102 implants placed in the control subjects, 2 implants were lost in 1 individual and 3 implants in another patient demonstrated 2-mm bone loss.

Another recent study on bruxism patients receiving delayed loaded implants for full-arch restoration of the upper jaw showed less prosthetic complications in 5 patients injected with BoNT (masseter and temporal muscles) compared to the same number of controls without BoNT treatment at the end of a 2-year follow-up [72].

There are also case reports using Botox (Allergan) [73], 200 U Dysport [74], and 400 U Dysport [75] to inject masseter muscles before or during implant treatment in patients with bruxism and hypertrophic masseters with successful results.

Concluding Remarks It is noteworthy that despite promising findings reported in the literature, randomized controlled studies on this subject are still lacking. The need for trials on the efficacy of BoNT in implant dentistry has been noted since 2007 [76]. Randomized controlled trials for the possible use of BoNT during the "stability dip phase of integration" or periodic injections in patients with bruxism receiving full-arch immediately loaded implant-supported prosthetic rehabilitations are underway [77].

Theoretic Prevention of Dentoskeletal Issues

Tongue Thrust Parafunctional tongue thrust is defined as either an abnormal pressure of the tongue against the teeth in the course of swallowing or its passive anterior positioning during rest. The former is also known as an "atypical swallow" and its relation to malocclusion is controversial, while the latter has been more commonly associated with problems such as open bite, proclination of incisors, and lisping [78]. In any case, reduction of tongue pressure during orthodontic therapy and retaining it after treatment could help preserve the stability of the corrected dentoalveolar relation [79]. Some clinical studies have suggested that after orthodontic treatments, the tongue adapts to the new position of the teeth. The reduced tongue pressure following tongue crib utilization was shown to remain in a diminished state, even after removal of the tongue crib [80]. Therefore, considering that appliances such as tongue crib could be displeasing for the patient, BoNT may be a potential substitute and its transient nature would not be a problem due to the adaptive behavior of the tongue.

Tongue Injections Complications involving swallowing, speech, and chewing have been reported following administration of BoNT into the lingual muscles. To overcome these issues, injection into the extrinsic muscles of the tongue has been suggested while avoiding intrinsic muscles [81]. On the other hand, for an unrelated problem (dystonia) [82], lingual muscle injections by BoNT were reported to be safe when the clinician had a thorough knowledge of muscle anatomy.

Concluding Remarks BoNT could be considered as a treatment or an adjunct to other procedures that help resolve the symptoms caused by tongue thrust. Well-designed studies and randomized controlled trials, when possible, can help elucidate the effectiveness and safety of BoNT for the treatment of those tongue thrusts that lead to clinical problems.

Oral and Maxillofacial Surgery

As discussed in Chap. 16, popular uses of BoNT by oral surgeons include treatment of temporomandibular disorders, sialorrhea, orofacial pain [83, 84], and promotion of facial wound/scar healing [85–87]. Other areas where application of this toxin could be considered as a therapeutic option but requires further investigation are listed below:

Temporomandibular Joint Dislocation

Definition and Existing Treatment Options   Temporomandibular joint dislocation occurs when the condyle moves anteriorly to a location in front of the articular eminence during jaw movement and causes a lock in an open position. Subsequently, the masticatory muscles react by going into spasm and prevent the condyle from relocating to its normal position. When there are recurrent episodes of dislocation, a number of treatment modalities based on the responsible etiologic factor are used. These include occlusal adjustment and parafunctional habit therapy, autologous blood injection, surgical intervention and administration of BoNT as an adjunct to – or independent of – intermaxillary fixation and surgery [88–90].

Clinical Application of BoNT   Despite the fact that BoNT treatment for temporomandibular dislocation is off-label, its application has been suggested to be included as a new indication [91]. BoNT injection with or without the use of electromyography to treat temporomandibular dislocation has mostly been presented as case reports and case series of patients with or without other underlying diseases [92–100]. The largest number of patients (32) was studied by Yoshida et al. [92], who also reported the longest follow-up among these studies (75 months). In general, favorable outcomes, with minimal and usually transient side effects, have been reported for BoNT treatment of dislocations [91–93, 95–100].

A study compared intraoral pterygoid injection of 35 U Botox® (Allergan) with intermaxillary fixation in 20 patients and followed them for 6 months. The BoNT group, in contrast to the intermaxillary fixation patients, showed significant improvement in pain levels based on the visual analogue scale [101].

According to a recent review by Renapurkar and Laskin [102], as well as other investigations [88, 90, 91], level 1 evidence studies for the treatment of temporomandibular dislocation have not been published and most investigations have provided level 4 evidence.

Dosage   Single-muscle injections of Botox® (Allergan) [92, 93, 96, 101], Dysport [93, 95], and BoNT-A (Lanzhou) [99] were used with doses ranging from 20 U to 50 U, 50 M U (mouse unit) to 150 MU, and 25 U to 50 U, respectively. According to Daelen et al. [95], "In terms of quoted MU, the toxin preparation Botox is apparently 3-5 times more potent than Dysport."

Muscle(s)   The lateral (external) pterygoid was accessed either intraorally [92, 96, 101] or extraorally [93–95, 99, 100] for unilateral or bilateral injections, depending on the patient and study. The superficial masseter and lateral pterygoid were both injected extraorally in one patient, with the masseter receiving injections at 4 points on the mandibular angle [95]. In another case, injections were administered in the lateral pterygoid and the anterior bellies of both digastric muscles [94].

Access Intraorally, the pterygoid was located at the mucobuccal fold of the distal root of the upper second molar. For injection, a posterior-superior angle of 30° to the occlusal plane and 20° medially was used to insert the needle to a depth of 20–30 mm [92]. In another study [96], the needle insertion point was located halfway on the anterior ramus border and was entered superiorly and medially while the patient was requested to open the mouth.

For extraoral injection, the insertion point was located 1 cm anterior to the condyle, directly under the anterior zygomatic process while the mouth was open with a distance of 1.5 cm between the incisors. The needle was entered transversely pointing towards the contralateral temporomandibular joint [95]. In another investigation, two injections were administered: one was 1 cm inferior to the central zygomatic arch and the other, 0.5–1 cm in back of the first injection site, immediately anterior to the mandibular condyle. The mouth was closed and the insertion was made at 90° angle to a depth of 3–4 cm [99].

A comparison between intra- and extraoral injections for the treatment of anterior disc displacement with reduction was made; there was no significant difference in joint click, pain reduction, and joint tenderness between the techniques. However, the patients were more comfortable with the intraoral approach and it took a shorter amount of time [103].

Duration of Effect The temporary effect of BoNT has been a concern for some clinicians; however, a number of patients receiving a single injection have been reported to be symptom-free after 6–7 months [92, 94, 99, 100]. Others have used prophylactic injections before reappearance of symptoms [95, 96] or additional injections, when necessary [92–96]. A 2- to 4-month wait period has been suggested between injections [95]. It has been postulated that, at first, patients might need repeated administrations of BoNT, but after a minimum of 4 injections, a decrease or cessation of relapse may be expected, at least during the following 6 months. The reason for this experience was proposed to be related to the pterygoid not fully recovering its initial level of hyperactivity, or in other terms, the pterygoid may have sustained "involution" [93]. Another explanation was that in addition to permanent muscle weakening, perhaps there is a formation of fibrotic tissue around the temporomandibular joint following limitation of movement [96].

It should be noted that the effect of BoNT injection is not immediate and it may require 4–5 days [104], 3–10 days [96], or 2–14 days [92] to demonstrate effectiveness, which has led to reoccurrence of dislocation early after administration in some patients [99]. This is why some authors have recommended close observation [92], limiting movement of the jaws or mandibular fixation for the first few days after injection [99].

Concluding Remarks Due to ethical and logistical issues, inclusion of a control group may not be feasible and large numbers of double-blind randomized controlled trials may not become available in the near future [92, 93, 102]. Regardless, the need for level 1 evidence has been highlighted in the literature. Until such information becomes available, treatment doses and intervals should be selected according to existing evidence, preferably starting from the lowest dose and highest intervals possible and adjusting them as required [92, 93, 96].

The number of injections has been reported to increase in dislocations due to neurological dysfunction compared to those with habitual dislocations and no hyperactivity [92].

Trauma and Bone/Plate Fractures

Bone Fracture

Premise The attachment of muscle and bone promotes movement and loading and, in the orofacial complex, controls maxillofacial growth and dental occlusion. The masticatory and facial muscles work in concert to support these functions. Therefore, any disruption in the balance of this system, as in the case of fractures, could lead to undesirable outcomes, with various complications depending on factors such as the severity of the dissociation, direction of the fracture line, and age of the patient, among others [30, 55, 105]. BoNT could be used to relax the components that have been forced to exert unwanted pressure as a consequence of the injury.

Example Following an angle fracture of the mandible, the body and ramus are no longer connected and, therefore, each segment is controlled by its attached muscles. Generally speaking, the jaw-closing muscles are mostly attached to the ramus, while the ones connected to the body assist in jaw opening [33]. When the fracture has an unfavorable horizontal pattern (Fig. 18.4), ramal and body muscles pull in different directions and can complicate surgical procedures and their outcomes [105]. Relaxing the undesirable pulls of muscles by BoNT injection can be an effective approach to be used as an adjunct to surgery. The strength of muscles inhibiting reduction of fractures could be decreased with BoNT and used as a promising method in conservative treatment procedures. Confirming the "unfavorable" pattern as opposed to the "favorable" pattern of fracture is important when considering treatment (Fig. 18.4).

Preliminary Evidence Two animal studies on femoral bone presented opposing results regarding the effectiveness of BoNT in fracture reduction management. One reported reduced callus diameter and improved histological and biomechanical healing parameters [106], while the other demonstrated an absence of callus and woven bone formation and reduced biomechanical characteristics [107]. The shape and mechanism of the fractures differed between these investigations: the standard closed fracture used in the former study protected the vasculature and periosteum which might have contributed to the superior results by increasing the blood supply.

BoNT Application in Studies

Angle Fractures

Treatment of angle fractures through open reduction leads to attachment loss between the ramus and masseter, tilting the balance in favor of muscles connected to the mandibular body, promoting postsurgical open bite.

A 21-year-old man with a prior history of 2 surgeries and rubber traction for bilateral angle fracture presented with malocclusion and wound dehiscence. His third surgery did not resolve the open bite and it persisted, even after 1 week of rubber traction. A total dose of 20 units BoNT-A (Meditoxin) was injected into 4 points of the anterior belly of the digastric muscles (5 units each) on the 10th day after surgery, leading to complete resolution of the open bite, 3 days postinjection. Elastic traction was removed after observation of stable occlusion and a 6-month follow-up did not show recurrence of the open bite and additional injections were not considered necessary [33].

Symphysis Fracture

An incomplete fracture of the symphysis associated with a displaced condylar fracture of a 3-year-old boy was treated with intermaxillary fixation and an asymmetrical occlusal splint. This resulted in failure, demonstrated by 90° angulation between the condyle and ramus, due to caudal traction of the mandible by the masseter and temporalis muscles and medial traction of the condyle by the medial pterygoid. Therefore, a total dose of 20 IU BoNT was extraorally injected into 6 points along the temporalis, 15 IU extraorally into 5 linear points on the masseter, and 6 IU transorally into 2 points of the medial pterygoid, with an additional transoral injection of 6 IU into the masseter muscle. BoNT administration led to full recovery and fusion of the condyle with no adverse side effects [63].

Condylar Fracture

Bilateral condylar fractures lead to anterior open bite due to premature molar contacts caused by the horizontal traction of the lateral pterygoids and upward pull of the masseter causing the ramus to override the condyle. Ten patients with unilateral subcondylar or condylar neck fractures with no considerable angulation or dislocation were treated by closed reduction through injection of 100 units of BoNT (Botox, Allergan) into the muscles of the injured side, after which maxillomandibular fixation was performed with an asymmetric occlusal splint for 10 days, followed by application of intermaxillary guiding elastics for 2 months. A concentration of 20 IU/ml was used to deliver 30 IU into the masseter and anterior fibers of the temporalis muscles extraorally. Medial and lateral pterygoid muscles were accessed intraorally to receive a total of 40 IU toxin around the fractured bone fragments. Healings were uneventful and there was no complaint of complications such as malocclusion, deviation, or temporomandibular issues. Normal muscle functions were reestablished after 3–6 months [108].

Zygomatic Fractures

Displaced zygomatic fractures are usually treated by rigid fixation to prevent muscle traction, especially by the masseter which is regarded as a main reason for displacement of the zygoma after reduction. BoNT has been used presurgically, to decrease the number of fixation sites and surgical procedures. Five men with zygomatic fractures (with or without fractures of other bones) were extraorally injected with 100 IU BoNT (Botox, Allergan) into 5 points of the ipsilateral masseter, 12 to 24 hours before rigid fixation with mini- and/or microplates and screws. During a 5- to 12-month follow-up, no esthetic or functional complications were seen and muscle contractions returned after 3 to 6 months. It was concluded that masseter

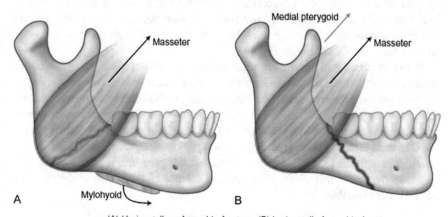

(A) Horizontally unfavorable fracture; (B) horizontally favorable fracture.

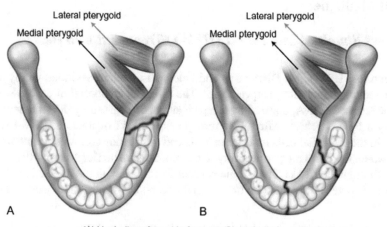

(A) Vertically unfavorable fracture; (B) vertically favorable fracture.

Fig. 18.4 Different directions of fracture lines relative to muscle insertion sites predict whether a fracture is favorable or unfavorable. (Reprinted from Ref. [105], with permission from publisher: Elsevier)

paralysis of individuals with zygomatic fractures could reduce the number of fixation sites and make the use of weaker plate systems possible. However, the study
lacked control patients for comparisons [109].

Plate Fracture

Plates are utilized for fixation of bone segments. In a study using bilateral sagittal
split ramus osteotomy for orthognathic surgery on 16 skeletal class III patients,
immobilization of rami was achieved through single four-hole extended titanium
miniplates. A total of 25 units BoNT-A was administered into 5 points of each masseter muscle of 8 patients immediately after surgery, while the rest received no
injections. After a maximum of 6 months of follow-up, the number of plate fractures
was significantly lower in the group who underwent BoNT treatment compared to
those without BoNT administration [31].

Titanium plates and screws are regarded as the gold standard for orthognathic
immobilization. However, several issues related to these materials have prompted
the need for their removal after treatment, leading to the introduction of bioresorbable fixation systems. Despite the favorable features of bioresorbable substances,
they have been reported to be weaker and possess inferior skeletal stability compared to their titanium counterparts in some types of orthognathic surgeries such as
mandibular setback [31, 35]. By reducing muscular pressure, it seems that BoNT
may help overcome this weak point, making the use of the bioresorbable fixation
systems more feasible.

Oral Medicine

Herpes Simplex Virus Type-1 (HSV-1) Treatment with BoNT

Definitions HSV-1 is a DNA virus and belongs to the herpesviridae family with
other members including herpes zoster. The virion is composed of a core with a
double-stranded DNA, covered by a capsid and encompassed by the tegument and
finally a lipid envelope. After entry through skin breaks or mucosa, HSV-1 repli-
cates in the epithelial cells and causes lysis and destruction followed by inflammation which increases the permeability of the blood-nerve barrier. Viral particles then
enter through the free endings of the neurons in contact with the infected epithelial
cells and travel through axons to neuronal cell bodies where they become latent
for life.

The oral region is innervated by the trigeminal nerve, and therefore, the trigeminal ganglion is the primary site for latency subsequent to oral infections. Reactivation
occurs following diminished immune response and exogenous stimuli which ultimately leads to increased replication. HSV-1 is then transported from the cell body,

through the axon to the nerve terminals, resulting in reinfection of the epithelial cells [110, 111].

The association between BoNT and herpesviridae (if any) is complex, and conflicting findings have been reported.

Positive Effect of BoNT on HSV-1 Reactivation It has been suggested that BoNT may have an inhibitory effect on the reactivation of HSV. A 33-year-old woman with simultaneously occurring impetigo and eczema herpeticum on the face and hands along with an extended history of atopic dermatitis and 5- to 6-year involvement with labial HSV recurrence was injected intradermally with BoNT after receiving treatment for her eczema and impetigo. Four points were selected on the skin of the upper lip and each were injected with 1 U onabotulinumtoxinA. New lesions erupted on another site away from the injection area after 4 weeks, followed by an outbreak of the eczema and a new HSV lesion on yet another site. A further treatment round was administered using 15 units of abobotulinumtoxinA (Dysport) resulting in prevention of outbreaks at the original areas, but 2 other recurrences took place within the next 3 months, again at a non-treated region. Ultimately, the authors reported complete resolution of the treated areas with repeated BoNT injections every 4 months for 19 months [112].

A double-blind, randomized, placebo-controlled, crossover study titled "Botulinum Toxin A for Herpes Labialis" has been registered at ClinicalTrials.gov (NCT01225341) with the aim of determining the effectiveness/safety of BoNT (onabotulinumtoxinA) for the prevention of herpes labialis. Injection of BoNT or bacteriostatic normal saline was considered to be administered into the orbicularis oris muscle at the site of re-eruption in 20 participants. Recurrence and duration of herpes labialis lesions, lesion size, and pain were to be assessed. Recruitment was completed but no results have been posted.

Negative Effect of BoNT on Herpesviridae Reactivation In contrast to the above-mentioned study, others have found a negative effect of BoNT on re-eruption of HSV or herpes zoster lesions. Narang et al. [113] reported HSV-1 stromal keratitis recurrence, 3 weeks after treating refractory epiphora with BoNT. The patient was a 59-year-old female, with a history of bilateral stromal keratitis, which had remained quiescent for the past 2 years. Stimulating factors such as psychogenic and surgical stress were considered as possible explanations for the HSV-1 recurrence; however, the authors suggested a possible association between viral reactivation and BoNT injection and recommended that clinicians exercise caution when considering BoNT for treatment in previously HSV-infected patients.

Similarly, another study also observed viral keratitis recurrence 1 week after BoNT administration for treatment of spastic entropion in a 55-year-old man who was infected with HSV-1, 6 years ago, and had not experienced recurrences for the past 1 year. The authors stated that despite involvement of other elements in the reactivation of HSV, the role of BoNT injection could not be entirely ruled out and suggested caution in patients receiving ocular BoNT with a history of herpes simplex viral keratitis [114].

A third study reported development of herpes zoster in the face of two (55- and 48-year-old) female patients approximately 1 week after BoNT injection into the glabella, forehead, and lateral periorbital regions for cosmetic purposes. The authors recommended considering re-eruption of herpes zoster if a patient reports prodromal symptoms or skin eruptions following BoNT therapy. However, they did not regard the incidents of these occurrences high enough to warrant prophylactic antiviral therapy for all patients before BoNT injection [115].

The exact effect (if any) of BoNT on infections caused by herpesviridae is unpredictable, unless supported by future well-designed studies.

Other Uses for BoNT in the Oral and Maxillofacial Region

Angular Cheilitis

Angular cheilitis or inflammation of the corner(s) of the mouth is clinically manifested as redness, cracks/fissures, crusting, and ulceration of the oral commissure(s). Various situations could lead to this condition, but the most common is infection. When deep creases develop at the corners of the mouth for any reason (age, malocclusion, shortening of vertical dimension, etc.), they collect saliva and skin maceration occurs, which is usually further complicated by colonizing of candida and infectious agents [116]. BoNT has been proposed either independently or in conjunction with other modalities such as dermal fillers, to physically eliminate the deep commissure lines leading to prevention of saliva collection and the ability to obtain a dry environment free from contamination [117, 118]. Its recommended use involves the injection of a total of 20 U BotoxCE with 5 U in 2 different points of the depressor muscles on both sides and results are expected within 2 weeks. The muscles suggested for injections included depressor anguli oris, mentalis and orbicularis oris [117]. A 60-year-old patient with a 2-year history of bilateral angular cheilitis refractory to pharmacotherapy has been reported to have been successfully treated with BoNT [119].

Burning Mouth Syndrome

Burning mouth syndrome presents as a burning sensation of the mouth accompanied by symptoms such as oral mucosal dryness, salivary gland functional issues, and taste problems. Its diagnosis is based on exclusion of other clinical and laboratory abnormalities [120]. Restivo et al. [121], relying on the focal analgesic effect of BoNT, bilaterally injected a total dose of 16 U incobotulinumtoxinA into the lip and anterior tongue (4 U each) of 4 patients (3 with diabetes) who had burning mouth syndrome involving the lower lip and anterior two-thirds of the tongue.

Simultaneously, 2 patients with similar pain scores and symptoms received the same volume of saline into the same injection sites. All 4 BoNT-treated patients were free of symptoms within 48 hours, which lasted up to 16–20 weeks, while in the 2 control patients, the burning sensation did not resolve. BoNT was suggested as an efficacious treatment for burning mouth syndrome, especially when other less invasive treatment options fail to provide comfort.

Summation

BoNT injections are generally safe, uncomplicated, reversible, and relatively inexpensive and comfortable for the patient. Standardization of injection sites, methods, numbers, and dosage of this toxin is required for many dentistry-related issues. There are still several conditions in the head and neck which could potentially benefit from BoNT therapy, but require accumulation of additional data for clinical application. A thorough and detailed knowledge of the facial muscles and their direction of movement is essential for all practitioners inclined to use BoNT injections in clinical practice.

References

1. Shah AA, Sandler J. Limiting factors in orthodontic treatment: 1. Factors related to patient, operator and orthodontic appliances. Dent Update. 2006;33(1):43–4, 46-8, 51-2.
2. Haas Junior OL, Guijarro-Martínez R, de Sousa Gil AP, da Silva Meirelles L, Scolari N, Muñoz-Pereira ME, Hernández-Alfaro F, de Oliveira RB. Hierarchy of surgical stability in orthognathic surgery: overview of systematic reviews. Int J Oral Maxillofac Surg. 2019;48(11):1415–33. https://doi.org/10.1016/j.ijom.2019.03.003.
3. Hwang WS, Hur MS, Hu KS, Song WC, Koh KS, Baik HS, Kim ST, Kim HJ, Lee KJ. Surface anatomy of the lip elevator muscles for the treatment of gummy smile using botulinum toxin. Angle Orthod. 2009;79(1):70–7. https://doi.org/10.2319/091407-437.1.
4. Polo M. Botulinum toxin type A in the treatment of excessive gingival display. Am J Orthod Dentofac Orthop. 2005;127(2):214–8.
5. Dilaver E, Uckan S. Effect of V-Y plasty on lip lengthening and treatment of gummy smile. Int J Oral Maxillofac Surg. 2018;47(2):184–7. https://doi.org/10.1016/j.ijom.2017.09.015.
6. Peck S, Peck L, Kataja M. The gingival smile line. Angle Orthod. 1992;62(2):91–100; discussion 101-2.
7. Litton C, Fournier P. Simple surgical correction of the gummy smile. Plast Reconstr Surg. 1979;63:372–3.
8. Miskinyar SA. A new method for correcting a gummy smile. Plast Reconstr Surg. 1983;72:397–400.
9. Ellenbogen R. Correspondence and brief communications. Plast Reconstr Surg. 1984;73:697–8.
10. Rees TD, LaTrenta GS. The long face syndrome and rhinoplasty. Persp Plast Surg. 1989;3:116.
11. Ezquerra F, Berrazueta MJ, Ruiz-Capillas A, Sainz-Arregui J. New approach to the gummy smile. Plast Reconstr Surg. 1999;104:1143–50.

12. Mazzuco R, Hexsel D. Gummy smile and botulinum toxin: a new approach based on the gingival exposure area. J Am Acad Dermatol. 2010;63(6):1042–51. https://doi.org/10.1016/j.jaad.2010.02.053.

13. Duruel O, Ataman-Duruel ET, Berker E, Tözüm TF. Treatment of various types of gummy smile with botulinum toxin-A. J Craniofac Surg. 2019;30(3):876–8. https://doi.org/10.1097/SCS.0000000000005298.

14. Al Wayli H. Versatility of botulinum toxin at the Yonsei point for the treatment of gummy smile. Int J Esthet Dent. 2019;14(1):86–95.

15. Duruel O, Ataman-Duruel ET, Tözüm TF, Berker E. Ideal dose and injection site for gummy smile treatment with botulinum toxin-A: a systematic review and introduction of a case study. Int J Periodontics Restorative Dent. 2019;39(4):e167–73. https://doi.org/10.11607/prd.3580.

16. Araujo JP, Cruz J, Oliveira JX, Canto AM. Botulinum toxin type-A as an alternative treatment for gummy smile: a case report. Dermatol Online J. 2018;24(7). pii: 13030/qt75f0h8kz

17. Sucupira E, Abramovitz A. A simplified method for smile enhancement: botulinum toxin injection for gummy smile. Plast Reconstr Surg. 2012;130(3):726–8. https://doi.org/10.1097/PRS.0b013e31825dc32f.

18. Polo M. Botulinum toxin type A (Botox) for the neuromuscular correction of excessive gingival display on smiling (gummy smile). Am J Orthod Dentofac Orthop. 2008;133(2):195–203. https://doi.org/10.1016/j.ajodo.2007.04.033.

19. Al-Fouzan AF, Mokeem LS, Al-Saqat RT, Alfalah MA, Alharbi MA, Al-Samary AE. Botulinum toxin for the treatment of gummy smile. J Contemp Dent Pract. 2017;18(6):474–8.

20. Suber JS, Dinh TP, Prince MD, Smith PD. OnabotulinumtoxinA for the treatment of a "gummy smile". Aesthet Surg J. 2014;34(3):432–7. https://doi.org/10.1177/1090820X14527603.

21. Nasr MW, Jabbour SF, Sidaoui JA, Haber RN, Kechichian EG. Botulinum toxin for the treatment of excessive gingival display: a systematic review. Aesthet Surg J. 2016;36(1):82–8. https://doi.org/10.1093/asj/sjv082.

22. Chagas TF, Almeida NV, Lisboa CO, Ferreira DMTP, Mattos CT, Mucha JN. Duration of effectiveness of Botulinum toxin type A in excessive gingival display: a systematic review and meta-analysis. Braz Oral Res. 2018;32:e30. https://doi.org/10.1590/1807-3107bor-2018.vol32.0030.

23. Seixas MR, Costa-Pinto RA, de Araújo TM. Checklist of aesthetic features to consider in diagnosing and treating excessive gingival display (gummy smile). Dent Press J Orthod. 2011;16(2):131–57. https://doi.org/10.1590/S2176-94512011000200016.

24. Few JW Jr. Commentary on: gummy smile treatment: proposal for a novel corrective technique and a review of the literature. Aesthet Surg J. 2018;38(12):1339–40. https://doi.org/10.1093/asj/sjy220.

25. Mostafa D. A successful management of sever gummy smile using gingivectomy and botulinum toxin injection: a case report. Int J Surg Case Rep. 2018;42:169–74. https://doi.org/10.1016/j.ijscr.2017.11.055.

26. Chen G, Oranges CM, Giordano S, Huang R, Wang W. Horizontal animation deformity as unusual complication of neurotoxin modulation of the gummy smile. Dermatol Online J. 2019;25(8). pii: 13030/qt49s9h9zh

27. Pedron IG. Comment on "Botulinum toxin type-A as an alternative treatment for gummy smile: a case report". Dermatol Online J. 2019;25(6). pii: 13030/qt1qk3183b

28. Polo M. Commentary on: botulinum toxin for the treatment of excessive gingival display: a systematic review. Aesthet Surg J. 2016;36(1):89–92. https://doi.org/10.1093/asj/sjv126.

29. Coclici A, Hedeşiu M, Bran S, Băciuţ M, Dinu C, Rotaru H, Roman R. Early and long-term changes in the muscles of the mandible following orthognathic surgery. Clin Oral Investig. 2019;23(9):3437–44. https://doi.org/10.1007/s00784-019-03019-3.

30. Seok H, Kim SG. Correction of malocclusion by botulinum neurotoxin injection into masticatory muscles. Toxins (Basel). 2018;10(1). pii: E27 https://doi.org/10.3390/toxins10010027.

31. Shin SH, Kang YJ, Kim SG. The effect of botulinum toxin-A injection into the masseter muscles on prevention of plate fracture and post-operative relapse in patients receiving orthognathic surgery. Maxillofac Plast Reconstr Surg. 2018;40(1):36. https://doi.org/10.1186/s40902-018-0174-0. eCollection 2018 Dec.

32. Kang YJ, Cha BK, Choi DS, Jang IS, Kim SG. Botulinum toxin-A injection into the anterior belly of the digastric muscle for the prevention of post-operative open bite in class II malocclusions: a case report and literature review. Maxillofac Plast Reconstr Surg. 2019;41(1):17. https://doi.org/10.1186/s40902-019-0201-9. eCollection 2019 Dec

33. Seok H, Park YT, Kim SG, Park YW. Correction of post-traumatic anterior open bite by injection of botulinum toxin type A into the anterior belly of the digastric muscle: case report. J Korean Assoc Oral Maxillofac Surg. 2013;39(4):188–92.

34. Mücke T, Löffel A, Kanatas A, Karnezi S, Rana M, Fichter A, Haarmann S, Wolff KD, Loeffelbein DJ. Botulinum toxin as a therapeutic agent to prevent relapse in deep bite patients. J Craniomaxillofac Surg. 2016;44(5):584–9. https://doi.org/10.1016/j.jcms.2016.01.021.

35. Luo M, Yang X, Wang Q, Li C, Yin Y, Han X2. Skeletal stability following bioresorbable versus titanium fixation in orthognathic surgery: a systematic review and meta-analysis. Int J Oral Maxillofac Surg. 2018;47(2):141–51. https://doi.org/10.1016/j.ijom.2017.09.013.

36. Reid RR. Facial skeletal growth and timing of surgical intervention. Clin Plast Surg. 2007;34(3):357–67.

37. Carlson DS. Theories of craniofacial growth in the postgenomic era. Semin Orthod. 2005;11(4):172–83.

38. Castaldo G, Cerritelli F. Craniofacial growth: evolving paradigms. Cranio. 2015;33(1):23–31. https://doi.org/10.1179/0886963414Z.00000000042.

39. Alam, M. 2011, A to Z orthodontics. Volume 11: functional orthodontic appliance (Kota Bharu: PPSP Publication).

40. McNamara JA Jr, Huge SA. The functional regulator (FR-3) of Fränkel. Am J Orthod. 1985;88(5):409–24.

41. Werner SP, Shivapuja PK, Harris EF. Skeletodental changes in the adolescent accruing from use of the lip bumper. Angle Orthod. 1994;64(1):13–20; discussion 21-2.

42. Huang GJ, Justus R, Kennedy DB, Kokich VG. Stability of anterior openbite treated with crib therapy. Angle Orthod. 1990;60(1):17–24; discussion 25-6.

43. Kurabeishi H, Tatsuo R, Makoto N, Kazunori F. Relationship between tongue pressure and maxillofacial morphology in Japanese children based on skeletal classification. J Oral Rehabil. 2018;45(9):684–91. https://doi.org/10.1111/joor.12680.

44. Hansen SE. The influence of genotype and perioral musculature on maxillary and mandibular development [dissertation]. Pittsburgh Univ; 2018.

45. Alabdullah M, Saltaji H, Abou-Hamed H, Youssef M. Association between facial growth pattern and facial muscle activity: a prospective cross-sectional study. Int Orthod. 2015;13(2):181–94. https://doi.org/10.1016/j.ortho.2015.03.011.

46. Babuccu B, Babuccu O, Yurdakan G, Ankarali H. The effect of the Botulinum toxin-A on craniofacial development: an experimental study. Ann Plast Surg. 2009;63(4):449–56. https://doi.org/10.1097/SAP.0b013e31818d4559.

47. Ahn J, Kim SG, Kim MK, Jang I, Seok H. Botulinum toxin A injection into the anterior belly of the digastric muscle increased the posterior width of the maxillary arch in developing rats. Maxillofac Plast Reconstr Surg. 2019;41(1):20. https://doi.org/10.1186/s40902-019-0203-7. eCollection 2019 Dec.

48. Tsai CY, Wang CW, Chang CW. Effects of masticatory muscle function affected by BTX on maxillofacial bone growth through the sutural modification. Orthod Craniofac Res. 2019;22(2):112–7. https://doi.org/10.1111/ocr.12290.

49. Tsai CY, Shyr YM, Chiu WC, Lee CM. Bone changes in the mandible following botulinum neurotoxin injections. Eur J Orthod. 2011;33(2):132–8. https://doi.org/10.1093/ejo/cjq029.

50. Kim JY, Kim ST, Cho SW, Jung HS, Park KT, Son HK. Growth effects of botulinum toxin type A injected into masseter muscle on a developing rat mandible. Oral Dis. 2008;14(7):626–32. https://doi.org/10.1111/j.1601-0825.2007.01435.x.

51. Park C, Park K, Kim J. Growth effects of botulinum toxin type A injected unilaterally into the masseter muscle of developing rats. J Zhejiang Univ Sci B. 2015;16(1):46–51. https://doi.org/10.1631/jzus.B1400192.

52. Tsai CY, Chiu WC, Liao YH, Tsai CM. Effects on craniofacial growth and development of unilateral botulinum neurotoxin injection into the masseter muscle. Am J Orthod Dentofac Orthop. 2009;135(2):142.e1–6; discussion 142-3. https://doi.org/10.1016/j.ajodo.2008.06.020.

53. Seok H, Kim SG, Kim MK, Jang I, Ahn J. Effect of the masseter muscle injection of botulinum toxin A on the mandibular bone growth of developmental rats. Maxillofac Plast Reconstr Surg. 2018;40(1):5. https://doi.org/10.1186/s40902-018-0146-4. eCollection 2018 Dec.

54. Choi JW, Kim HJ, Moon JW, Kang SH, Tak HJ, Lee SH. Compensatory dentoalveolar supraeruption and occlusal plane cant after botulinum-induced hypotrophy of masticatory closing muscles in juvenile rats. Arch Oral Biol. 2019;101:34–42. https://doi.org/10.1016/j.archoralbio.2019.03.003.

55. Kahn A, Kün-Darbois JD, Bertin H, Corre P, Chappard D. Mandibular bone effects of botulinum toxin injections in masticatory muscles in adult. Oral Surg Oral Med Oral Pathol Oral Radiol. 2019. pii: S2212-4403(19)30397-9; https://doi.org/10.1016/j.oooo.2019.03.007.

56. Raphael KG, Tadinada A, Bradshaw JM, Janal MN, Sirois DA, Chan KC, Lurie AG. Osteopenic consequences of botulinum toxin injections in the masticatory muscles: a pilot study. J Oral Rehabil. 2014;41(8):555–63. https://doi.org/10.1111/joor.12180.

57. Lee HJ, Kim SJ, Lee KJ, Yu HS, Baik HS. Repeated injections of botulinum toxin into the masseter muscle induce bony changes in human adults: a longitudinal study. Korean J Orthod. 2017;47(4):222–8. https://doi.org/10.4041/kjod.2017.47.4.222.

58. Chang CS, Bergeron L, Yu CC, Chen PK, Chen YR. Mandible changes evaluated by computed tomography following Botulinum Toxin A injections in square-faced patients. Aesthet Plast Surg. 2011;35(4):452–5. https://doi.org/10.1007/s00266-010-9624-5.

59. Savarese R, Diamond M, Elovic E, Millis SR. Intraparotid injection of botulinum toxin A as a treatment to control sialorrhea in children with cerebral palsy. Am J Phys Med Rehabil. 2004;83(4):304–11; quiz 312-4, 336.

60. Calim OF, Hassouna HNH, Yildirim YS, Dogan R, Ozturan O. Pediatric Sialorrhea: submandibular duct rerouting and intraparotid botulinum toxin A injection with literature review. Ann Otol Rhinol Laryngol. 2019;128(2):104–12. https://doi.org/10.1177/0003489418808305.

61. Shogan AN, Rogers DJ, Hartnick CJ, Kerschner JE. Use of botulinum toxin in pediatric otolaryngology and laryngology. Int J Pediatr Otorhinolaryngol. 2014;78(9):1423–5. https://doi.org/10.1016/j.ijporl.2014.06.026.

62. Rowe FJ, Noonan CP. Botulinum toxin for the treatment of strabismus. Cochrane Database Syst Rev. 2017;3:CD006499. https://doi.org/10.1002/14651858.CD006499.pub4.

63. Akbay E, Cevik C, Damlar I, Altan A. Treatment of displaced mandibular condylar fracture with botulinum toxin A. Auris Nasus Larynx. 2014;41(2):219–21. https://doi.org/10.1016/j.anl.2013.08.002.

64. Ali SS, Bragin I, Rende E, Mejico L, Werner KE. Further evidence that Onabotulinum toxin is a viable treatment option for pediatric chronic migraine patients. Cureus. 2019;11(3):e4343. https://doi.org/10.7759/cureus.4343.

65. Cho YM, Kim SG, Choi DS, Jang I, Cha BK. Botulinum toxin injection to treat masticatory movement disorder corrected mandibular asymmetry in a growing patient. J Craniofac Surg. 2019; https://doi.org/10.1097/SCS.0000000000005606.

66. Wishney M, Darendeliler MA, Dalci O. Myofunctional therapy and prefabricated functional appliances: an overview of the history and evidence. Aust Dent J. 2019;64(2):135–44. https://doi.org/10.1111/adj.12690.

67. Bucci R, Koutris M, Lobbezoo F, Michelotti A. Occlusal sensitivity in individuals with different frequencies of oral parafunction. J Prosthet Dent. 2019;122(2):119–22. https://doi.org/10.1016/j.prosdent.2018.10.006.

68. Resnik RR, Misch CE. Treatment planning complications. In: Misch's avoiding complications in oral implantology, vol. 1: Mosby; 2018. p. 54–147. https://doi.org/10.1016/B978-0-323-37580-1.00003-2.
69. Kwon KH, Shin KS, Yeon SH, Kwon DG. Application of botulinum toxin in maxillofacial field: part III. Ancillary treatment for maxillofacial surgery and summary. Maxillofac Plast Reconstr Surg. 2019;41(1):45. https://doi.org/10.1186/s40902-019-0226-0. eCollection 2019 Dec
70. Manfredini D, Poggio CE, Lobbezoo F. Is bruxism a risk factor for dental implants? A systematic review of the literature. Clin Implant Dent Relat Res. 2014;16(3):460–9. https://doi.org/10.1111/cid.12015.
71. Mijiritsky E, Mortellaro C, Rudberg O, Fahn M, Basegmez C, Levin L. Botulinum toxin type A as preoperative treatment for immediately loaded dental implants placed in fresh extraction sockets for full-arch restoration of patients with bruxism. J Craniofac Surg. 2016;27(3):668–70. https://doi.org/10.1097/SCS.0000000000002566.
72. Yilmaz C, Dogan A, Kizilaslan S, Gültekin A, Ersanli S. Botulinum toxin type a usage for preoperative treatment for dental implants placed in maxillary arches for full-arch restoration of patients with bruxism. Clin Oral Impl Res. 2017;28(S14):193. https://doi.org/10.1111/clr.192_13042.
73. Malcmacher L, Kosinski T. Bruxism, Botox, and dental implants. Dent Today. 2017;36(4):94. 96-7
74. Ihde S. Utilisation prophylactique de la toxine botulique en implantologie dentaire. Implantodontie. 2005;14(2):51–5.
75. Ihde S. Utilisation thérapeutique de la toxine botulique dans le traitement d'entretien en implantologie dentaire. Implantodontie. 2005;14(2):56–61.
76. Ihde SKA, Konstantinovic VS. The therapeutic use of botulinum toxin in cervical and maxillofacial conditions: an evidence-based review. Oral Surg Oral Med Oral Pathol Oral Radiol Endod. 2007;104:e1–e11.
77. Freund B, Bongard S, Zarb JP, Jones C. Full arch implant rehabilitation: parafunctional problems and solutions: https://www.oralhealthgroup.com/features/full-arch-implant-rehabilitation-parafunctional-problems-and-solutions/
78. Law CS, Habits O. In: Nowak AJ, Christensen JR, Mabry TR, Townsend JA, Wells MH, editors. Pediatric dentistry: infancy through adolescence. 6th ed. Philadelphia: Saunders; 2019. p. 386–393.e2.
79. Dean JA. Managing the developing occlusion. In: McDonald and Avery's dentistry for the child and adolescent. 10th ed. St. Louis: Elsevier Publication; 2016. p. 415–78.
80. Taslan S, Biren S, Ceylanoglu C. Tongue pressure changes before, during and after crib appliance therapy. Angle Orthod. 2010;80(3):533–9. https://doi.org/10.2319/070209-370.1.
81. Laskawi R. The use of botulinum toxin in head and face medicine: an interdisciplinary field. Head Face Med. 2008;4:5. https://doi.org/10.1186/1746-160X-4-5.
82. Yoshida K. Botulinum neurotoxin therapy for lingual dystonia using an individualized injection method based on clinical features. Toxins (Basel). 2019;11(1). pii: E51 https://doi.org/10.3390/toxins11010051.
83. Muñoz Lora VRM, Del Bel Cury AA, Jabbari B, Lacković Z. Botulinum toxin type A in dental medicine. J Dent Res. 2019;98(13):1450–7. https://doi.org/10.1177/0022034519875053.
84. Safarpour Y. Jabbari 2.Botulinum toxin treatment of pain syndromes -an evidence based review. Toxicon. 2018;147:120–8. https://doi.org/10.1016/j.toxicon.2018.01.017.
85. Gassner HG, Brissett AE, Otley CC, Boahene DK, Boggust AJ, Weaver AL, Sherris DA. Botulinum toxin to improve facial wound healing: a prospective, blinded, placebo-controlled study. Mayo Clin Proc. 2006;81(8):1023–8.
86. Kim SH, Lee SJ, Lee JW, Jeong HS, Suh IS. Clinical trial to evaluate the efficacy of botulinum toxin type a injection for reducing scars in patients with forehead laceration: a double-blinded, randomized controlled study. Medicine (Baltimore). 2019;98(34):e16952. https://doi.org/10.1097/MD.0000000000016952.

87. Wang Y, Wang J, Zhang J, Hu C, Zhu F. Effectiveness and safety of botulinum toxin type A injection for scar prevention: a systematic review and meta-analysis. Aesthet Plast Surg. 2019;43(5):1241–9. https://doi.org/10.1007/s00266-019-01358-w.

88. Abrahamsson H, Eriksson L, Abrahamsson P, Häggman-Henrikson B. Treatment of temporo-mandibular joint luxation: a systematic literature review. Clin Oral Investig. 2019; https://doi.org/10.1007/s00784-019-03126-1.

89. Szkutnik J, Wójcicki M, Berger M, Bakalczuk M, Litko M, Łobacz M, Rahnama-Hezavah M. Treatment of habitual luxation of temporomandibular joint – literature review. Eur J Med Technol. 2018;2(19):17–21.

90. Elledge ROC, Speculand B. Conservative management options for dislocation of the temporomandibular joint. In: Matthews N, editor. Dislocation of the temporomandibular joint. Cham: Springer; 2018.

91. Prechel U, Ottl P, Ahlers OM, Neff A. The treatment of temporomandibular joint dislocation. Dtsch Arztebl Int. 2018;115(5):59–64. https://doi.org/10.3238/arztebl.2018.0059.

92. Yoshida K. Botulinum neurotoxin injection for the treatment of recurrent temporomandibu-lar joint dislocation with and without neurogenic muscular hyperactivity. Toxins (Basel). 2018;10(5). pii: E174 https://doi.org/10.3390/toxins10050174.

93. Ziegler CM, Haag C, Mühling J. Treatment of recurrent temporomandibular joint dislocation with intramuscular botulinum toxin injection. Clin Oral Investig. 2003;7(1):52–5.

94. Vázquez Bouso O, Forteza González G, Mommsen J, Grau VG, Rodríguez Fernández J, Mateos Micas M. Neurogenic temporomandibular joint dislocation treated with botu-linum toxin: report of 4 cases. Oral Surg Oral Med Oral Pathol Oral Radiol Endod. 2010;109(3):e33–7. https://doi.org/10.1016/j.tripleo.2009.10.046.

95. Daelen B, Thorwirth V, Koch A. Treatment of recurrent dislocation of the temporomandibular joint with type a botulinum toxin. Int J Oral Maxillofac Surg. 1997;26(6):458–60.

96. Martínez-Pérez D, García Ruiz-Espiga P. Recurrent temporomandibular joint dislocation treated with botulinum toxin: report of 3 cases. J Oral Maxillofac Surg. 2004;62(2):244–6.

97. Stark TR, Perez CV, Okeson JP, Recurrent TMJ. Dislocation managed with botulinum toxin type A injections in a pediatric patient. Pediatr Dent. 2015;37(1):65–9.

98. Moore AP, Wood GD. Medical treatment of recurrent temporomandibular joint dislocation using botulinum toxin A. Br Dent J. 1997;183(11-12):415–7.

99. Fu KY, Chen HM, Sun ZP, Zhang ZK, Ma XC. Long-term efficacy of botulinum toxin type A for the treatment of habitual dislocation of the temporomandibular joint. Br J Oral Maxillofac Surg. 2010;48(4):281–4. https://doi.org/10.1016/j.bjoms.2009.07.014.

100. Oztel M, Bilski WM, Bilski A. Botulinum toxin used to treat recurrent dislocation of the temporomandibular joint in a patient with osteoporosis. Br J Oral Maxillofac Surg. 2017;55(1):e1–2. https://doi.org/10.1016/j.bjoms.2016.05.012.

101. Shehata B, Darwish S, Aly T, Younis G. Treatment of recurrent temporomandibular joint dislocation with botulinum toxin. Alex Dent J. 2015;40(2):200–7. https://doi.org/10.21608/adjalexu.2015.59152.

102. Renapurkar SK, Laskin DM. Injectable agents versus surgery for recurrent temporoman-dibular joint dislocation. Oral Maxillofac Surg Clin North Am. 2018;30(3):343–9. https://doi.org/10.1016/j.coms.2018.04.009.

103. Altaweel AA, Elsayed SA, Baiomy AABA, Abdelsadek SE, Hyder AA. Extraoral versus intraoral botulinum toxin type A injection for management of temporomandibular joint disc displacement with reduction. J Craniofac Surg. 2019;30(7):2149–53. https://doi.org/10.1097/SCS.0000000000005658.

104. Shorey CW, Campbell JH. Dislocation of the temporomandibular joint. Oral Surg Oral Med Oral Pathol Oral Radiol Endod. 2000;89(6):662–8.

105. Odono LT, Brady CM, Urata M. Mandible fractures. In: Facial trauma surgery; 2020. p. 168–85). Content Repository Only! https://doi.org/10.1016/B978-0-323-49755-8.00022-0.

106. Aydin A, Memisoglu K, Cengiz A, Atmaca H, Muezzinoglu B, Muezzinoglu US. Effects of botulinum toxin A on fracture healing in rats: an experimental study. J Orthop Sci. 2012;17(6):796–801. https://doi.org/10.1007/s00776-012-0269-x.

107. Hao Y, Ma Y, Wang X, Jin F, Ge S. Short-term muscle atrophy caused by botulinum toxin-A local injection impairs fracture healing in the rat femur. J Orthop Res. 2012;30(4):574–80. https://doi.org/10.1002/jor.21553.
108. Canter HI, Kayikcioglu A, Aksu M, Mavili ME. Botulinum toxin in closed treatment of mandibular condylar fracture. Ann Plast Surg. 2007;58(5):474–8.
109. Kayikçioğlu A, Erk Y, Mavili E, Vargel I, Ozgür F. Botulinum toxin in the treatment of zygomatic fractures. Plast Reconstr Surg. 2003;111(1):341–6.
110. Miranda-Saksena M, Boadle RA, Aggarwal A, Tijono B, Rixon FJ, Diefenbach RJ, Cunningham AL. Herpes simplex virus utilizes the large secretory vesicle pathway for anterograde transport of tegument and envelope proteins and for viral exocytosis from growth cones of human fetal axons. J Virol. 2009;83(7):3187–99. https://doi.org/10.1128/JVI.01579-08.
111. Petti S, Lodi G. The controversial natural history of oral herpes simplex virus type 1 infection. Oral Dis. 2019; https://doi.org/10.1111/odi.13234.
112. Gilbert E, Zhu J, Peng T, Ward NL. Decreased labial herpes simplex virus outbreaks following botulinum neurotoxin type A injection: a case report. J Drugs Dermatol. 2018;17(10):1127–9.
113. Narang P, Singh S, Mittal V. Bilateral herpes simplex keratitis reactivation after lacrimal gland botulinum toxin injection. Indian J Ophthalmol. 2018;66(5):697–9. https://doi.org/10.4103/ijo.IJO_904_17.
114. Ramappa M, Jiya PY, Chaurasia S, Naik M, Sharma S. Reactivation of herpes simplex viral keratitis following the botulinum toxin injection. Indian J Ophthalmol. 2018;66(2):306–8. https://doi.org/10.4103/ijo.IJO_714_17.
115. Graber EM, Dover JS, Arndt KA. Two cases of herpes zoster appearing after botulinum toxin type a injections. J Clin Aesthet Dermatol. 2011;4(10):49–51.
116. Federico JR, Basehore BM, Zito PM. Angular Chelitis. [Updated 2019 Aug 14]. In: StatPearls [Internet]. Treasure Island (FL): StatPearls Publishing; 2019. Jan-. Available from: https://www.ncbi.nlm.nih.gov/books/NBK536929/.
117. Katz H, Blumenfeld A, inventors; Allergan Inc, assignee. Botulinum toxin dental therapy for angular cheilosis. United States patent application US 11/029,546. 2006.
118. Bae GY, Na JI, Park KC, Cho SB. Nonsurgical correction of drooping mouth corners using monophasic hyaluronic acid and incobotulinumtoxinA. J Cosmet Dermatol. 2019; https://doi.org/10.1111/jocd.13010.
119. Kwon CI, Shin YB, Jo JW, Jeong HB, Moon YS, Jung EC, Kim CY, Yoon TJ. P272: A case of angular cheilitis treated with botulinum toxin. Program Book (Old Green Collection). 2018;70(1):413.
120. Bender SD. Burning Mouth Syndrome. Dent Clin N Am. 2018;62(4):585–96. https://doi.org/10.1016/j.cden.2018.05.006.
121. Restivo DA, Lauria G, Marchese-Ragona R, Vigneri R. Botulinum Toxin for Burning Mouth Syndrome. Ann Intern Med. 2017;166(10):762–3. https://doi.org/10.7326/L16-0451.

Index

Printed in the United States
by Baker & Taylor Publisher Services